Dealing With
FOOD ALLERGIES

A PRACTICAL GUIDE TO DETECTING CULPRIT FOODS AND EATING A HEALTHY, ENJOYABLE DIET

JANICE VICKERSTAFF JONEJA, PhD, RDN

Bull Publishing Company
Boulder, Colorado

Bull Publishing Company
P.O. Box 1377
Boulder, CO 80306
800-676-2855
www.bullpub.com

ISBN 0-923521-64-X

Manufactured in the United States of America

Library of Congress Cataloging-in-Publication Data

Joneja, Janice Vickerstaff.
Dealing with food allergies: a practical guide to detecting
culprit foods and eating a healthy, enjoyable diet /
by Janice Vickerstaff Joneja
p. cm.
Includes index.
ISBN 0-923521-64-X
1. Food allergy—Popular works. I. Title.
RC596.J665 2003
616.97′5—dc21
2002151489

PUBLISHER: James Bull
DESIGN AND COMPOSITION: Shadow Canyon Graphics
MANUSCRIPT EDITOR: Margaret Moore
PROJECT MANAGER: Erin Mulligan
COVER DESIGN: Lightbourne

— CONTENTS —

PART III
Determining the Culprit Foods and Food Components:

— PREFACE —

Twenty-five years ago I found myself in a strange dilemma. My training as a scientist and my thinking and emotional response as a mother landed me in a situation where I felt helpless in both roles. My infant son had been diagnosed with severe asthma. He had suffered with eczema almost from birth, first on his face, hands and legs, and later on just about every area of his skin. By the time he was five years old he was dependent on oral steroids for control of both conditions. Whenever we tried to reduce his intake of Prednisone below 10 mg per day, he would develop severe, and on more than one occasion, life-threatening asthma, which his pediatrician diagnosed as *status asthmaticus.* At the lower dosages of Prednisone, the eczema on his hands became extreme; frequently the eczematous patches became infected with common skin bacteria, and his fingers swelled to double their normal size. He would often go to kindergarten wearing little white cotton gloves to cover the oozing sores and to keep in place the steroid-containing ointment that I liberally applied to his hands.

When he was about two years old I began to notice reactions that I gradually realised were being triggered by specific foods. Orange juice would result in him running through the house, screaming. When I tried to hold him to stop the rampage, I felt his whole body quivering and shaking, and it was clear that he had no control over this reaction. Such behavior could be triggered predictably and consistently by his drinking a glass of orange juice, but occurred at no other time. By the age of about four, this response had thankfully stopped. However, whenever he drank orange, or any other citrus juice for many years, he would start scratching, particularly his hands. This seemed a clear indication that it most likely was an exacerbating factor for his eczema, which often starts with itching. Another food that would consistently cause similar scratching was chocolate. Halloween and birthday parties were occasions for bartering – all the chocolates, chocolate cake, and cookies were assessed, and exchanged for a toy or other desired treasure of equal value. It became a game that the whole family enjoyed.

Strangely, though, whenever I mentioned these "food allergies" to my son's doctors, the response was polite dismissal. It is likely that, because his father was also a physician, they were reluctant to openly label his mother "neurotic" and "over-protective" as so many parents of allergic children were in those days (the mid-1970s). Only one doctor, his respirologist, was frank enough to declare, "There's no such thing as food allergy!" Certainly at that time and sadly, occasionally today, the idea that asthma and eczema have an allergic etiology, especially the idea that *food* allergy might be involved, was, and is, categorically denied by too many medical practitioners. It was not until he was proven to be anaphylactic to peanuts that his medical advisors would entertain the idea that my son might *also* have food allergy, *in addition* to his other problems.

What made the whole situation so bizarre for me was the fact that my early training in immunology took place in the university department where the chairman was none other than Professor Philip Gell, one of the co-discoverers of the antibody responsible for allergy (IgE),. He was also one of the first scientists to develop the classification of the hypersensitivity reactions responsible for allergy, a system that is still recognized today. In essence I learned the immunology of allergy from the undoubted "master" of the subject, and followed this with research in medical microbiology and immunology, gaining a Ph.D. in the field, and later an appointment as Assistant Professor in Microbiology at the University of British Columbia. As a graduate student I actually taught a course in the immunology department (at that time called the Department of Experimental Physiology) where the science of allergy immunology had its inception–and yet when it came to helping my own son with his allergies–I was no more effective than any other parent.

As all parents will, I consulted every "expert" in an effort to help my son, but with increasing alarm and confusion, I realized that the field of allergy, especially food allergy, was fraught with controversy. There was a regrettable lack of scientific research, and even less credible clinical data. As a result, the field was open to every form of "alternative medical practice", ranging from the pseudo-scientific (and therefore almost plausible) to the frankly frightening. I consulted everyone, from those who use electroacupuncture (Vega tests), biokinesiology (testing muscle strength while the patient holds a vial containing the suspect food), urine analysis, hair analysis, iridologists, practitioners of radionics, practitioners who consult crystals – anyone who might help! This phase of my search for answers provided one valuable piece of information: when a field lacks scientific validation that is based on research conducted according to the tenets of traditional scientific method, it is vulnerable to infiltration by anyone offering hope–real or not. This old "snake oil" ruse was certainly the case with food allergy.

The real tragedy in this situation is the fact that, because the science is sparse, "traditional" medical practitioners tend to avoid the field, which is then taken over by "pseudo-scientists". The result is that the legitimate scientist and the ethical clinician do not wish to be associated with an area of practice lacking scientific and medical validation. Research in the area is not funded by granting agencies, and allergists with the temerity to enter the arena risk losing credibility and the respect of their peers.

My concern and confusion were increased to an alarming extent with the events that occurred in my son's thirteenth year. For several months he had been experiencing severe migraines. At their worst they happened three or four times a week with severe pain and vomiting. He would spend twenty-four hours in his darkened bedroom with each episode. Finally he was hospitalized, and every appropriate test was conducted. Special care was taken with these tests, since his own father was the only neurologist (and, incidentally, the only psychiatrist – he is, and was, a Fellow of the Royal College of Physicians and Surgeons of Canada in both specialties) in town at the time. No pathology was detected that could account for the migraines. His pediatrician prescribed a "parentectomy"; she had reached the conclusion that stress within the family home was responsible for our son's problems, and suggested that we should consider making arrangements for his living elsewhere. {As an aside, later he did attend boarding school, from Grade 9 to 12, where his allergies were in fact far worse than they had been at home!}. Fortunately for us, his parents who were in danger of living the rest of our lives in the shadow of the guilt engendered by the thought that we alone were responsible for the debilitating ill-health of our only son, a cause for the migraines was discovered. Once again it was related to food.

Based on his observation that he felt nauseated and ill after eating meat, our son decided to become a strict vegetarian. In accordance with his request, when he returned home from his two-week stay in the hospital, with symptoms unchanged in severity and frequency, I provided meals completely free from food derived from any animal source. The most amazing and gratifying result of this drastic change in diet was that he immediately and completely became free from migraines! For several years he remained a strict vegan in his food choices. He did not eat any meat, poultry, fish, egg, milk, or milk products. He found that ice cream, milk, cheese or other milk-based food caused immediate vomiting. In spite of his continuing anaphylactic reaction to peanuts (even the smallest quantity of peanut as a "hidden ingredient" in a food, accidentally eaten, resulted in immediate throat swelling and the onset of anaphylaxis, requiring prompt medical intervention) he was able to eat any other legume with impunity. This was fortunate, since his main sources of protein were dried peas, beans, lentils, and soy. I became an expert in bean-based gourmet cooking!

The only time that he has experienced a distressing recurrence of headaches since his thirteenth birthday is when he has eaten pork or beef. Years later, as a result of careful food challenges, we discovered that the primary cause of his migraines was pork, followed to a lesser extent by beef. Although he is not now vegetarian, as long as he avoids pork, beef, and foods containing these meats he remains free from those distressing migraine headaches. Interestingly, as a result of our careful food challenges, we discovered that he is also highly sensitive to sulfites—a situation that I now know to be quite common in steroid-dependent asthmatics. (The methods that we use for specific food challenges in the Allergy Nutrition Clinic are provided in great detail in the book).

The most important outcome of the experiences with my son's allergic conditions (and to some extent, my daughter's) was, for me, the realization that in spite of my specialized knowledge about the scientific bases of the clinical signs I was witnessing at first hand, I, and the medical specialists involved in their care, were unable to be of any real assistance in addressing the cause(s) of my children's allergic diseases. The recognition of the limited resources available to my children, to me, and to the untold numbers of people in similar situations has prompted me to pursue what has been my primary objective in the past fifteen years. Whereas previously I was a laboratory scientist, conducting research into the *mechanisms* responsible for microbial and immunological diseases, now I am focused on the clinical application of the knowledge gained from laboratory science for the benefit of people experiencing the results of such diseases. This type of "evidence-based" research is becoming increasingly important in medicine, and in no context is it more valid than in the pursuit of understanding and controlling the different ways in which our bodies interact with the food we eat —especially when the food that should nurture becomes a cause of distress.

In 1991 I was instrumental in the establishment of a unique service—the Allergy Nutrition Research Program at Vancouver Hospital and Health Sciences Centre in Vancouver, British Columbia. The program comprises three components:

◆ An outpatient clinic where patients can obtain help in the identification and management of their adverse reactions to foods. A physician's referral is required for all patients attending the Allergy Nutrition Clinic. To date more than 3,000 patients and their families have obtained assistance in the management of their food sensitivities in the clinic.

◆ An information resource, which provides information on current research in food allergy for health care professionals such as physicians, public health nurses and dietitians. The dissemination of this material includes seminars, lectures, workshops, radio and television interviews, the publication of books, manuals, audio and video resources, and articles in peer-reviewed medical and scientific journals.

◆ Research in adverse reactions to foods, both in the laboratory, and in the clinical setting.

This book is a response to numerous requests from patients, physicians, dietitians, and publishers, who have recognized a pressing need for a publication that explains the science of food allergy and food intolerance in terms that the non-medical, non-scientific person can understand. But more importantly, it is written to provide a way for food-sensitive people to live with their problem.

It is a resource that provides complete, practical methods of management of the diet so that the food sensitive person can eat healthily while avoiding the foods that make them sick. Before that can be achieved, of course, it is essential that the food components and food additives that are responsible for food intolerances are accurately identified, and this process is the essence of the book. No diagnostic test alone will reveal the identity of the specific foods that are causing a person's symptoms. Every allergist and medical practitioner in the field recognizes that identification of the culprit food requires careful elimination and challenge. This process will prove that eliminating the food avoids the symptoms, and, importantly, that eating the food will cause the symptoms to reappear.

It is not an easy journey through the maze of food sensitivity, and many factors in addition to the food itself will influence the expression of your symptoms. Nevertheless, there is a lot you can do to improve your health and increase your enjoyment of life, despite your sensitivity to food. With the strong foundation of science, and a clear vision of the essential nutritional value of food, your goal can be achieved in safety.

Come, follow me through the dense forest of misunderstanding and confusion. I have been there before you, and my greatest wish is that you will benefit from what I have learned. I hope this book will provide you and your family with the tools you need, and a path to reach a place where you can live in peace with your body, and where once again food will provide the nurture and comfort that it was always meant to do.

— PART I —

THE SCIENTIFIC BACKGROUND OF FOOD ALLERGY AND FOOD INTOLERANCE: WHAT IS REALLY GOING ON?

— INTRODUCTION —

LET'S TALK ABOUT FOOD

Food is central to every aspect of our life on every level: physical, psychological, and emotional. On the physical level no other relationship is as close; the food we eat becomes an integral part of our bodies. The building blocks for every cell in our body—bones, internal organs, brain, blood, skin, hair, and all the rest—come from the food we eat. Even more sobering is the thought that the sperm and eggs that will form our children and grandchildren will likewise be constructed from the molecules we get from our food. The energy for every bodily function is also supplied by the food we eat. Digestion, the circulation of our blood, the functioning of our brains, walking, working, loving, every internal physiological process, and every moment—these are all fueled by chemicals in our food.

Social life, so important to our psychological and emotional health, almost always revolves around food. Our celebrations—birthdays, weddings, holy days, holidays, and even death—invariably involve sharing the food appropriate to the occasion. Almost all religious ceremonies and festivals involve special food. Like the bread and wine of the Christian communion, the shared meal in the Gurdwara after the religious service in Sikh society, the special foods of Moslem Ramadan, the traditional foods of Jewish festivals, every religious and ethnic group has its own particular foods that are part of the cultural heritage of the people. From earliest childhood, food comes to represent family, community, nurturance, friendship, and belonging. When the experience has been pleasurable, food becomes a source of comfort and solace throughout life, like the family, culture, and religion with which it is associated. Sharing food is also

3

frequently associated with our careers and working life. Company dinners and picnics, "working lunches," and client meals are all strategies to improve relationships between co-workers with the aim of boosting productivity and increasing the success of the company and its employees. What better way to impress the boss than the carefully prepared and presented home-cooked meal? He or she feels pampered, cared for, satisfied, and (the point of the exercise!) extremely benevolent toward the provider of the meal. Food is central to the endeavor. But—imagine any of the above situations and remove food. The picture becomes very different.

Most of us are fortunate enough to be able to take our relationship with food for granted. We feel hungry—we eat. We attend a birthday party, wedding, holiday celebration—we expect, and receive, food. And we feel happy, cared for, part of the group, nourished physically and emotionally. But for those people who have an unhappy relationship with food, the same situations can be painful, stressful, and alienating. There are many reasons why food becomes a source of distress rather than pleasure. These extend from the inherited (inborn) errors of metabolism (for example, diseases such as phenylketonuria, galactosemia, and porphyria, with which readers having these disorders will be familiar) when consuming the wrong food can lead to irreparable damage, to eating disorders such as anorexia nervosa and bulimia where food is a cause of psychological and emotional misery. Perhaps the response to food that is most confusing, distressing (both physically and psychologically), and difficult to understand, and therefore manage, is when eating produces symptoms that do not fall into these extremes: the condition we know as "food allergy" or, more accurately, food sensitivity.

Food allergy and intolerance of foods and food additives can impose enormous pressures on sufferers and their families. When allergic people are in danger of a life-threatening anaphylactic reaction (a response that involves the whole body), they and their family and friends live in continual fear of exposure to the culprit food, and they maintain constant vigilance in seeking out and avoiding the "enemy food." This often leads to an obsessive preoccupation with food, which is viewed as a lethal threat. In extreme cases this may result in food phobia, nutritional deficiency, and extreme anxiety states. Even when the allergy is not life-threatening, nutritional, economic, and social stresses can compromise the quality of life of food-sensitive people and their families.

In situations where the reaction is not clinically visible (for example, the person does *not* break out in hives, develop nasal congestion, or have an asthma attack), observers tend to discredit the sufferer's complaints, causing frustration and psychological stress to the food-sensitive person. It then becomes necessary for the sufferer to obtain a definite diagnosis in order for him or her to establish credibility. In these situations, a person will often turn to practitioners of alternative medicine and rely on less than scientifically sound tests to validate his or her reactions to certain foods.

DETECTING AND AVOIDING THE CULPRIT FOODS

People often obtain information from diverse sources and follow sometimes nutritionally unsafe diets for a prolonged period of time in the belief that if they can avoid "the wrong foods" for long enough they will feel better. This does sometimes happen under rather unfortunate circumstances: If a very restricted diet is followed for any extended period of time, a semistarved state will lead to immune system suppression, and the symptoms of allergy, which are caused by a hypersensitive immune system, will disappear. But then so might the patient, whose immune system is also now less able to fight infections and other threats to the body's health. Of course, another important reason why symptoms do not disappear even on the most rigorously controlled diet is that they were not caused by foods in the first place.

The ultimate aim in managing and living with food sensitivity is the detection and elimination of the specific antagonistic foods, and the formulation of a nutritionally sound diet to ensure optimal health. This is often a tedious, time-consuming process and requires a tremendous amount of knowledge, skill, commitment, and dedication on the part of both the food-sensitive person and the clinician who is supervising his or her treatment.

However, when someone has been feeling chronically sick, and then suddenly feels well for the first time in many years, as so often happens, the reward more than justifies the time and effort that have gone into the endeavor. The detection of foods, food components, and food additives that are responsible for, or contribute to, a food sensitivity is often difficult because there really are no definitive laboratory tests to determine a person's food sensitivities. Many different immunological and physiological reactions contribute to the symptoms of adverse reactions to foods, so it would not be possible for a single test to detect them all. Frequently, we have little to guide us in the initial selection of food and formulation of a diet that will avoid symptoms, but at the same time be nourishing and provide complete balanced nutrition.

This book is designed to provide you with the information and tools that you (and your medical team) will require to detect your specific food sensitivities and to design a nutritionally adequate diet to ensure your good health. Although people often look for the ultimate "hypoallergenic diet," such a thing does not exist. What is hypoallergenic for one person could be life-threatening for another. Each person is an individual. Their inherited tendencies, previous medical history, lifestyle, and response to both food and nonfood factors (such as airborne and environmental allergens) will all contribute to the way in which their body reacts to the "foreign" foods and chemicals that enter it. This first part of the book will explain exactly what "food allergy" and "food intolerance" mean in terms of how the food-sensitive person's body responds and copes with food, and what actually causes a person to react in this way. The second part provides detailed instructions for the practical application of this information. It is designed for food-allergic persons, ideally with the support and direction of their physician and a qualified dietician, to detect their own "antagonistic foods" and to implement the dietary guidelines and lifestyle that will lead them to greatly improved health and well-being.

DISCLAIMER

The information provided here is as up-to-date, accurate, and as practical as possible in a field that is moving very quickly and is full of controversy. Any strategies suggested in this book should be discussed with and managed by a suitably qualified physician, and implementation should be supervised by a registered dietitian/nutritionist for maximum benefit.

The author and publisher disclaim any responsibility for any adverse consequences resulting from the use of drugs, diets, or procedures mentioned in this book.

Trade names of food products are used only as examples. The trade names given are not meant as a complete list of all available formulations or as recommendations of any particular product.

— CHAPTER 1 —

WHAT IS FOOD SENSITIVITY?

Our bodies are like complex factories that function day and night without pause in a never-ending cycle of renewal and decay. New cells and tissues are created, old worn-out matter is broken down, recycled or excreted, and our organs continue to function, day in and day out, without requiring any direction from us. We provide the building blocks and the source of energy for these processes through the food we eat, the liquids we drink, and the air we breathe. Everything runs smoothly in its appointed manner until a glitch in the system creates havoc, and we then have to deal with the consequences of this malfunction.

Food allergies and intolerances are just one example of "things going wrong," but because we cannot stop eating, we can't ignore the signs. We must come to terms with how our body is acting and take steps to adjust to the situation. In making changes, especially ones as far-reaching as how we eat, we need to understand exactly what we are trying to achieve so that we can make the correct modifications and then stay with them. So this book, which will guide you through the complexities of eating in the way that your particular system requires, even when food seems to cause nothing but problems, is going to start by answering that really important question: What is happening when my body rejects food?

We cannot avoid a discussion of science. In order to understand what happens when things go wrong, you need to know how your body functions normally. Section I will take you step by step through the processes of immunology, biochemistry, and physiology that are involved when your body reacts adversely to food. Don't be dismayed by the seemingly overwhelming science—each step leads logically to the next, and each is explained in a way that will help you understand. Any terms that seem obscure will be found in the Glossary (page 463)—use this as a dictionary until you become familiar with the terminology.

Perhaps the most important concept that you will learn in this section comes as a surprise to many people: *Food does not cause allergy or intolerance reactions!* Food in itself is harmless—it cannot cause disease. It is our body's *response* to the food, or more accurately, something in the food, that causes the symptoms we experience. Even when food is poisonous, it is so because our bodies lack the resources to detoxify the material (a biochemical process).

An allergy is caused by our immune system reacting to a foreign material (food) that is incapable of causing disease on its own. In the process of rejecting the "foreign material," the immune system releases chemicals that cause the symptoms we call allergy. In other words, a food *allergy* is a rejection of the food by our immune system that can sometimes be quite devastating in its severity. In contrast, *intolerance* of a food is often due to an error in the way our bodies process it, not an actual rejection of it. Food intolerance reactions are usually milder than allergies and do not involve the immune system.

Food allergy is perhaps one of the most confusing and misunderstood conditions in medical practice. Physicians, other health care professionals, and patients alike are often unsure about what symptoms are caused by food allergy, how it is diagnosed, and what is the best way to manage it. The greatest obstacle in understanding the problem is the misconception that "food allergy" is a distinct disease. In fact, "food allergy" refers to a response of our bodies that can result in many different symptoms, in diverse organ systems. Furthermore, a food that causes symptoms in one person is often quite harmless when eaten by another.

It is standard medical practice that when a person develops symptoms, his or her doctor orders specific tests in the process of making a diagnosis. When the doctor has made the diagnosis, he or she will then recommend a treatment, which in most cases will control the disease. In the case of food allergy, the only time the specific cause can be easily identified is in the occurrence of **anaphylaxis:** when a specific food triggers an immediate and sometimes life-threatening response. However, unlike a specific medical condition in which the same cause in different people causes the same disease, the food that causes anaphylaxis in one person rarely causes the same symptoms in others. *The symptoms are caused by the allergic person's unique response to the food,* **not** *by the food itself.* For example, an infectious bacterium such as *Salmonella* will cause the symptoms of severe food poisoning in just about everyone who eats the contaminated food. In contrast, a person who is highly allergic to peanuts can develop life-threatening anaphylactic shock after consuming the smallest quantity of food, whereas the majority of people can eat a whole bag of peanuts without any ill effects.

DEFINITIONS OF KEY TERMS

Allergy refers to a response of the immune system. It involves immunological processes similar to (but not exactly the same as) those that fight and reject an agent that can cause disease, such as a pathogenic (disease-causing) microorganism.

Hypersensitivity is the term scientists use to describe the immunological process that results in allergy. The terms *allergic reaction* and *hypersensitivity reaction* are often used interchangeably.

Food intolerance refers to a reaction that does *not* involve the immune system. It is caused by a problem in the way the body processes the food or food additive. The term *food intolerance* is not interchangeable with either *food allergy* or *hypersensitivity*.

Food sensitivity is a rather nonspecific term that refers to the fact that a person reacts adversely to a food or component of the food when it is not clear whether the reaction is due to allergy or intolerance. The term *food sensitivity* is therefore interchangeable with either *food allergy* or *food intolerance*, but it does not give any indication of the reason for a person's symptoms.

All of this will become clear as you read Chapters 3 and 4.

SOME OTHER USEFUL TERMS

Allergen is the term we use to refer to anything that can trigger the immune system to respond with an allergic reaction. It may be such things as pollen, animal dander, mold, insect venom, medication, or food.

Antigen is the term scientists use for anything that triggers the immune system to respond. This may be a disease-causing microorganism or an allergen. All allergens are antigens; not all antigens are allergens.

To complicate the situation further, most adverse reactions to foods are not caused by an allergic reaction, but by "food intolerances." Food intolerance reactions are quite different from food allergy both in the way the body responds to the food and in the management of the condition. The term we often use to describe the situation in which eating a food results in distressing symptoms is **food sensitivity**. This term covers both food allergy and food intolerances and is often used in place of both, or when it is unclear whether the condition is an allergic reaction or a food intolerance.

The term **food allergy** is reserved for a response of the immune system that is triggered when a food is eaten by a person who has been *sensitized* to it. **Sensitization** is the process whereby the immune system is alerted to something foreign entering the body, which it believes to be a threat to the body's health. Thereafter, whenever that same foreign material enters the body, the immune system responds by releasing its "weapons" to destroy the foreign invader. This is the usual way in which the immune system protects us from diseases such as viral and bacterial infections. All of the food we eat comes from foreign plants and animals, so it is not surprising that sometimes this foreign material is mistakenly identified as "alien" to the body. In fact, what is more surprising is that most of us can eat this foreign material without our immune systems responding at all! This process, called "tolerance," will be discussed in greater detail in later chapters. Figure 1-1 illustrates the ways in which our bodies can respond to food: tolerance or allergy.

HOW THE IMMUNE SYSTEM RESPONDS IN AN ALLERGIC REACTION

The key event in food allergy occurs when the immune system identifies a specific food as a foreign invader and orders the release of special chemicals to protect the body. These chemicals act on body tissue and result in a specific set of symptoms. In the 1960s, all reactions of the immune system that are not involved in protecting us from diseases caused by viruses, bacteria, and similar threats to the body were termed "hypersensitivity reactions" by the internationally renowned Professors Gell and Coombs. Such reactions include allergy. Therefore, another term for an allergic reaction is a *hypersensitivity reaction*, which is often used in medical texts in place of "allergy." (On a personal note, I was greatly privileged to learn my first immunology under the tutelage of Professor Gell, who was chairman of the university department where I was a student, and his distinguished colleagues.)

In contrast, any adverse reaction to a food or food additive that is *not* caused by a response of the immune system is called food intolerance. Because there are many ways in which food can cause symptoms in the body that are not due to an immunological (related to the immune system) response, the term covers a large number of different physiological mechanisms. For convenience, we shall refer to adverse reactions to food as *"food sensitivity"* when it is unclear whether the reaction is an allergy or an intolerance.

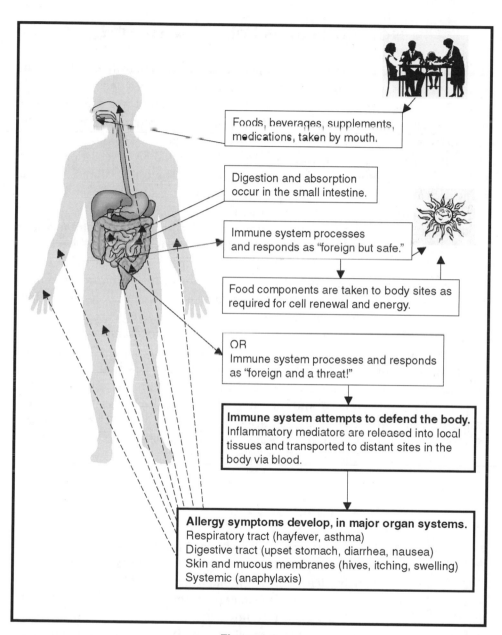

Foods, beverages, supplements, medications, taken by mouth.

Digestion and absorption occur in the small intestine.

Immune system processes and responds as "foreign but safe."

Food components are taken to body sites as required for cell renewal and energy.

OR
Immune system processes and responds as "foreign and a threat!"

Immune system attempts to defend the body. Inflammatory mediators are released into local tissues and transported to distant sites in the body via blood.

Allergy symptoms develop, in major organ systems.
Respiratory tract (hayfever, asthma)
Digestive tract (upset stomach, diarrhea, nausea)
Skin and mucous membranes (hives, itching, swelling)
Systemic (anaphylaxis)

Figure 1-1
The Ways Our Bodies Can Respond to Food:
"Tolerance" or "Allergy"

HOW COMMON IS FOOD SENSITIVITY?

It is difficult to determine how many people are actually sensitive to foods and suffer symptoms as a result of eating or drinking. The absence of any reliable laboratory tests that can prove a person is allergic or intolerant to a specific food or food additive makes estimating how frequently such reactions occur very difficult. Because there are so many different immunological and nonimmunological reactions involved in food sensitivity symptoms, it would be unrealistic to expect that a single laboratory test could identify them all. The only accurate way that clinicians can determine a person's reactivity to a food, beverage, or food additive is by eliminating the food from the diet, followed by challenge (reintroducing the food) under conditions in which neither the doctor nor the patient knows whether he or she is eating the test food or the placebo (sugar pill). This is known as the double-blind placebo-controlled food challenge (DBPCFC). Unfortunately, this process is too expensive and time-consuming to be a routine procedure. However, based on the statistics that are available, it is usually accepted that food allergy occurs in up to 8% of children under the age of five years, and that 2% of children in this age group have an allergic reaction to cow's milk proteins. Most children outgrow their food allergies by the age of five years, and allergy in adults is relatively uncommon. Most authorities estimate that less than 2% of adults have true food allergy; some consider the figure of less than 1% to be more accurate. However, intolerance (non-immune-system related reactions) of food components, naturally occurring chemicals, and food additives is a frequent experience, and some practitioners estimate the incidence of food intolerance to be as high as 50% of the adult population.

SYMPTOMS OF FOOD SENSITIVITY

Symptoms of food intolerance usually appear in three major organ systems: the digestive tract, the respiratory tract, and the skin. In the digestive tract, nausea, vomiting, cramping pain, diarrhea, abdominal distension (bloating), and excessive gas are common indicators of food allergy. In the respiratory tract, sneezing, nasal congestion (stuffy nose), runny nose, itching and watering of the eyes, itching in the throat, throat tightening, wheezing, shortness of breath, and chest tightening might be signs of allergy. Skin reactions include eczema, hives, facial swelling, and rashes, especially with itching. These symptoms might occur after eating the food, or when the skin and mucous membranes come into contact with *allergens*. An allergen is the term we use to indicate the component of the food or other material, such as pollen, animal dander, mold, or insect venom, that causes allergy. (Mucous membranes are the tissue systems in internal organs exposed to the outside, such as the mouth, digestive tract, respiratory tract and lungs, and the urogenital tract). The most common contact reactions occur on the hands and in the mouth after direct exposure to raw foods.

The most severe allergic reaction is anaphylaxis. In anaphylactic reactions to food, the response is systemic, meaning that the reaction is not confined to any single organ system. Multiple organ systems are involved, and symptoms develop rapidly throughout the body. In the most severe anaphylactic reactions, the symptoms can start within 1 to 2 minutes of eating the food. Thereafter, the reaction builds up over a period of 1 to 3 hours and it can result in anaphylactic shock and death from cardiorespiratory arrest. Fatal food anaphylaxis is fortunately very rare. Authorities have estimated that there are an average of 100 cases of fatal food anaphylaxis every year in the United States and that there are 10 cases per year in Canada. Nevertheless, even one case is too many, and we must be very alert to taking the most appropriate precautions in such situations.

FOODS THAT CAUSE FOOD SENSITIVITY REACTIONS

In theory, any food should be capable of causing an allergic reaction. All foods contain molecules capable of triggering the immune system—we call these molecules *antigens*. However, for many reasons that include both the structure of the antigens and peoples' immunological responses to them, the foods that cause the majority of allergic reactions tend to be few in number. We refer to antigens that trigger an allergic response as *allergens*.

Adverse reactions to foods and beverages can appear in many forms and can result in a confusing array of symptoms. Sometimes, the realization that a person's ill health is caused by his or her diet is reached only when all other causes have been ruled out, often after many (sometimes painful) diagnostic tests. At other times, the culprit food is instantly recognized, especially when the result is a frightening, severe anaphylactic reaction. Dr. T. J. David, a British pediatrician, summarizes the current medical attitudes towards the subject of adverse reactions to foods quite succinctly in his book *Food and Food Additive Intolerance in Childhood*:[1] "Some doctors have hoped that the current popular vogue for food intolerance, if ignored studiously enough, would go away. Others are inclined to see reactions to food around every corner."

---

[1] T. J. David, *Food and Food Additive Intolerance in Childhood*. Oxford, U.K.: Blackwell Scientific Publications, 1993.

— CHAPTER 2 —

SIGNS AND SYMPTOMS OF FOOD SENSITIVITY

An adverse reaction to a food can result in a variety of symptoms and may seem quite different in different people. Some people develop hives, others have an upset stomach, while others might have a migraine headache or even an asthma attack. Some practitioners have tried to put people into categories depending on their specific **target organ** (the site in the body where they usually "express" their reaction). Some people are "skin reactors" and break out in hives, develop swelling, especially of the face and mouth, and itch quite severely after eating an allergenic food. Others are "respiratory reactors," who tend to develop nasal stuffiness (rhinitis), irritated eyes, and even asthma. A third group are the "headache sufferers," who develop migraine headaches or other types of headaches in response to "alien foods." The fourth group, which seems on average to contain the largest number of people, are the "gut reactors," who develop stomach pains, bloating, diarrhea, gas, and sometimes nausea and vomiting after eating an allergenic food. It is probably not surprising that this grouping of people also reflects their responses to stress—it would seem that each person has their own "weak point" and it is here that they first experience an "attack" on the body. Of course, many people have symptoms in more than one of these systems, but there is usually one that is most vulnerable.

Because of each individual's unique response, it is not surprising that food allergy is experienced in a variety of ways. This often makes diagnosis of food allergy very difficult for the doctor. After all, most medical conditions have very specific symptoms, which makes their diagnosis quite straightforward when the appropriate tests are carried out. When we are dealing with food allergy, the most common initial approach is to rule out any other cause for the patient's symptoms before suspecting food as the culprit.

15

When we consider the variety of foods that make up our daily diet–even when we eat only pure foods–we realize that they are all derived from plants and animals that are completely foreign to our bodies. It is quite surprising that most of us consume all of these foods without any ill effects. Humans have adapted amazingly well to the vast range of foreign proteins and chemicals that we now consume in our daily diets. The internationally renowned allergists Professors Jonathan Brostoff and Stephen Challacombe, in the preface to their encyclopedic textbook on food allergy and intolerance,[1] point out that "the majority of us are tolerant from an immunological point of view of large quantities of foreign protein to which the body is exposed each day." However, when this tolerance is compromised, we become ill.

There is frequent controversy among medical practitioners about which symptoms are caused by food allergy, or intolerance of food or food additives, because of the lack of laboratory tests that can indisputably identify the precise food responsible for a person's allergy or intolerance symptoms. It is universally accepted that conditions such as hay fever, asthma, and allergic conjunctivitis are often caused by airborne allergens; that hives, mouth and facial swelling, and throat tightening and itching can result from food allergies; and that rashes can result from direct contact with allergens such as nickel, latex, and poison ivy. Anaphylactic reactions to injected allergens such as X-ray dyes, local anesthetics, and wasp and bee stings are well recognized. Anaphylactic reactions to foods, though rare, are always headline news.

In nonmedical books, journals, and magazines there are many reports of symptoms that are supposed to be due to food allergy. In fact, it is difficult to cite a symptom that has not been attributed to this cause. Many symptoms, which depend on anecdotal reports from the sufferer, are frequently not taken seriously by traditional medical practitioners. Often physicians suggest a psychological basis for symptoms that cannot be verified by laboratory tests. This is frustrating and causes resentment for both patient and doctor.

WHERE SYMPTOMS OCCUR IN THE BODY

Symptoms of food allergy and intolerance usually appear in three major organ systems: the digestive tract, the respiratory tract, and the skin. As we learn more about food sensitivity, however, it is increasingly apparent that adverse reactions can occur in any organ system. Table 2-1 summarizes the types of reactions presently accepted as possibly due to adverse reactions to allergens.

---

[1] J. Brostoff and S. J. Challacombe (eds.), *Food Allergy and Intolerance* (London and Philadelphia; Bailliere Tindall, 1987), Preface, p. xviii.

Table 2-1
EXAMPLES OF ALLERGIC CONDITIONS AND SYMPTOMS

RESPIRATORY TRACT
Allergic or perennial rhinitis (hay fever)
Rhinorrhea (runny nose)
Allergic conjunctivitis (itchy, watery, reddened eyes)
Serous otitis media (earache with fluid drainage)
Asthma
Laryngeal edema (throat tightening due to swelling of tissues)

SKIN AND MUCOUS MEMBRANES
Atopic dermatitis (eczema)
Urticaria (hives)
Angioedema (swelling of deeper tissues, especially the mouth and face)
Pruritus (itching of skin, eyes, ears, mouth)
Contact dermatitis
Oral allergy syndrome

DIGESTIVE TRACT

Diarrhea	Abdominal pain
Constipation	Indigestion
Nausea and vomiting	Belching
Abdominal bloating and distention	

NERVOUS SYSTEM
Migraine
Other headaches
Spots before the eyes
Listlessness
Hyperactivity
Lack of concentration
Tension-fatigue syndrome
Irritability
Chilliness
Dizziness

OTHER

Urinary frequency	Excessive sweating
Bed-wetting	Pallor
Hoarseness	Dark circles around the eyes
Muscle aches	
Low-grade fever	

The most severe allergic reaction is called an anaphylactic reaction, which involves every organ system in the body and, in most extreme cases, can lead to life-threatening anaphylactic shock and death.

ANAPHYLACTIC REACTIONS TO FOODS

An **anaphylactic reaction** is a severe rapid reaction involving most organ systems. In the most extreme cases, the reaction turns into **anaphylactic shock** with cardiovascular collapse, resulting in death. Due to the risks associated with such a reaction, *anyone at risk of severe food allergy should be aware of the signs suggesting the potential for anaphylaxis and should follow the dietary measures necessary for preventing it.*

SYMPTOMS OF AN ANAPHYLACTIC REACTION

◆ The first symptoms are usually in the mouth, with burning, itching, or irritation of the lips, inside the mouth, and throat.

◆ This may be followed by nausea, vomiting, abdominal pain, and diarrhea as the food enters the digestive system.

◆ As the food antigen enters the general circulation, the sensation of being unwell, feeling anxious, feeling warm, generalized itching, faintness, and sometimes nasal irritation and sneezing develop.

◆ Skin reactions include hives, itching, and reddening.

◆ Chest tightness, bronchospasm, rhinitis, voice hoarseness, and irritated eyes might occur, but may be absent in some cases.

◆ The pulse may be rapid, weak, irregular, and difficult to detect.

◆ In severe cases these symptoms are rapidly followed by loss of consciousness, and death may occur from suffocation (due to edema, or tightening, of the larynx, epiglottis, and pharynx) or often from shock and cardiac arrhythmia.

◆ Death due to anaphylactic shock may occur within minutes of ingesting the offending food.

◆ Not all of the above symptoms occur in each case of anaphylaxis, and they may appear in any order; the above descriptions refer to the response most commonly experienced.

Characteristics of Anaphylactic Reactions

The longer it takes for symptoms to appear after eating the food, the less severe the anaphylactic reaction is likely to be. Severe reactions occur within minutes and up to one hour of eating, but the onset of a reaction may be delayed up to two hours. In a very significant number of reported cases of anaphylactic reactions to foods, the patient was asthmatic. This indicates that *people with asthma are more likely to experience anaphylactic reactions to foods*. When a patient is receiving allergy shots, or is allergic to wasp and bee venom, the potential for an anaphylactic reaction increases.

FOODS RESPONSIBLE FOR ANAPHYLACTIC REACTIONS

Almost any food can cause an anaphylactic reaction, but the foods most commonly responsible include **peanuts, nuts, shellfish, fish, cow's milk, and eggs.** Anaphylactic reactions to **cow's milk, eggs, wheat, and chicken** most often occur in children under the age of three years. Table 2-2 lists the foods that have been reported in medical journals as the cause of anaphylactic reactions. This list gives *examples* only and does not include every food that is capable of inducing an anaphylactic reaction. *Anaphylactic reactions are entirely unique to each individual.*

EXERCISE-INDUCED ANAPHYLAXIS

In a surprisingly large number of cases, anaphylactic reactions to foods in adults have occurred while the person is participating in rigorous exercise. Exercise-induced anaphylaxis is now considered to be a specific disease entity and is different from the usual anaphylactic reaction (in which symptoms occur immediately after eating food). Exercise-induced anaphylaxis can occur up to two hours after eating or drinking and always involves physical exertion. Foods that are known to have been associated with exercise-induced anaphylaxis include **celery, shellfish (shrimp, oysters), squid, peaches, and wheat.** However, there is evidence that exercise-induced anaphylaxis may not in fact be caused by an allergic reaction to a specific food. Instead, the changes in the body chemistry from the stress of exertion when the digestive process is taking place at the same time may trigger the reaction after a heavy meal.

Precautions for Persons Who Experience Anaphylactic Reactions to Foods

The most important measure to prevent anaphylaxis is to avoid contact with the food or beverage that causes it. People who have experienced an anaphylactic reaction are usually prescribed an Anakit™ or Epipen™ by their doctor for use

Table 2-2
SPECIFIC FOODS THAT HAVE BEEN REPORTED TO CAUSE FATAL AND NONFATAL ANAPHYLACTIC REACTIONS
(NOT A COMPLETE LIST)

Nuts
Peanut
Pecan
Pistachio
Cashew
Brazil

Shellfish
Crab
Shrimp
Lobster
Limpet

Grains
Wheat
Rice

Vegetables
Potato
Celery
Pea
Pinto bean
Soy
Chickpea
Corn

Milk products
Cow's milk (usually in children under 5 years)
Milk products such as cheese and ice cream

Poultry
Chicken

Beverages
Chamomile tea
Wine

Seeds
Millet
Sunflower
Sesame
Flax
Psyllium

Fish
Cod
Halibut

Fruits
Orange
Tangerine
Mango
Banana
Kiwi fruit

Egg
Hen

when they are accidentally exposed to the allergen. The kit contains injectable adrenaline (epinephrine) and an oral antihistamine. Their doctor will advise them to take the antihistamine, inject the adrenaline, and proceed without delay to the nearest hospital emergency department. After injection of the adrenaline, the person must go to the hospital, even if the symptoms appear to be improving. This apparent improvement is sometimes followed by a secondary phase of the response, which can prove fatal. Specific instructions for the use of the Epipen or Anakit should be obtained from the allergic person's doctor. Anaphylaxis-prone patients should also wear a MedicAlert® bracelet to expedite appropriate treatment if they become unconscious. Most experts agree that people who have asthma are at particular risk of a severe or fatal anaphylactic reaction. Refer to the accompanying box for a summary of these guidelines.

FOOD ALLERGY IN CHILDREN

Most studies indicate that 80% of children who are **atopic** (prone to allergy) are allergic to only one or two foods. Children tend to outgrow early allergies to certain foods, such as milk, egg, wheat, and soy, by about the age of five years. However, when food allergy shows up later than three years, the allergy is less likely to be outgrown. Allergies to some foods are less likely to be outgrown that others; those that are *most likely* to persist into adulthood include **peanuts, nuts, shellfish, and fish.** These foods may be a problem for a lifetime once a person has reacted to them, especially if the reaction was severe.

GENERAL GUIDELINES FOR AVOIDING FOOD ALLERGENS ASSOCIATED WITH ANAPHYLAXIS

◆ Avoid **all** sources of the food.

◆ Become familiar with **every** term on food labels that indicates the presence of the allergen. Many terms bear little resemblance to the original name of the food, so there must be careful education about these terms, especially with children who know how to read.

◆ Make sure that the food does not enter the home and that, as much as possible, all meals are "made from scratch" from basic ingredients.

◆ When manufactured foods are eaten, make sure that **all** ingredients are known.

◆ When eating outside the home or at restaurants, make sure that the ingredients in every meal are known.

RELATEDNESS OF ALLERGENS

When two or more foods are frequently found to cause allergic symptoms in the same individual, doctors often refer to them as **cross-reacting allergens.** In the past it was thought that foods from one botanic family would cross-react with others in that family. In other words, if a person was allergic to plums, it was assumed that he or she would also be allergic to apricots, cherries, peaches, nectarines, prunes, and almonds, all of which are classified in the plum family. However, newer research has shown that this was a false assumption. Cross-reactivity among foods in the same botanic or zoological family is in fact uncommon. For example, cross-reactivity between members of the legume family (peanut, soy, peas, beans, lentils, etc.) is very uncommon, and allergic people usually react to only one or two members of this group. Avoiding all members of a botanic family when a person is allergic to only one is unjustified and may lead to nutritional deficiencies. For example, because a person is allergic to peanuts, it is not necessary to eliminate all legumes from his or her diet. Each food needs to be tested separately. (For a more detailed discussion on cross-reacting allergens, refer to Chapter 7.)

Shellfish, however, tend to be exceptions to this generalization. People who are allergic to crustaceans such as crab, lobsters, prawns, shrimp, and similar shellfish do seem to suffer from a high degree of reactivity to others of the same group. In addition, there is evidence that people who are sensitive to crustaceans are also more likely to be allergic to the bivale group of shellfish, which includes mussels, clams, scallops, and winkles. People who are allergic to these types of shellfish should avoid **all** shellfish. The same restrictions usually do not apply to fin fish (free-swimming species, such as salmon, trout, and whitefish), which do not exhibit the same degree of cross-reactivity. Hypersensitivity to each bony fish appears to be limited to the specific species of fish to which the person is allergic. In most cases, it is wise for each type of fish to be "challenged" (reintroduced in a controlled fashion) separately.

INCIDENCE OF ALLERGY

Estimates of the incidence of true food allergy range from 0.7% to 7.0% of the population, with a male-to-female ratio of approximately 2:1. However, these statistics are based on a number of reports that use different criteria for their diagnosis. A recent estimate, based on reports in the current medical literature, indicates the prevalence of "adverse food reactions" to be approximately 2% to 8% in infants and 1% in adulthood. Reports of cow's milk protein allergy in infants range from 0.5% to 2.0% of the population under five years. A U.S. Department of Agriculture report in 1983 estimated the incidence of food allergy in the general population to be 15%. The public perception of the incidence of food allergy tends to be much higher. In studies from various countries, up to 50% of the population believe they or their children have some degree of sensitivity to foods or food additives.

For all allergies, including ingested (foods), inhaled (pollens, dust, animal dander, mold spores), injected (wasp or bee venom), or contact (dust, animal dander), the allergic tendency, or potential, is estimated to be

    5% to 15% if neither parent has allergies
    20% to 40% if one parent has allergies
    20% to 60% if both parents have allergies
    60% to 80% if both parents have the same allergy
    25% to 35% if one sibling has allergies

Allergy is an inherited tendency and current research is beginning to determine the specific genes that may be responsible for transmitting allergic potential. Hopefully, in the future, potentially atopic (prone to allergy) babies can be identified at birth and appropriate precautions taken for these children in order to avoid sensitization to, and expression of, allergy.

WHAT MAKES A PERSON ALLERGIC TO FOOD?

Merely inheriting appropriate genes for allergy will not necessarily lead to a person showing symptoms of food allergy. A number of environmental and lifestyle factors will determine which allergies he or she experiences. Some of these factors are discussed below.

Increased Permeability of the Lining of the Digestive Tract—the "Leaky Gut"

Permeability refers to the ease with which the molecules pass from the inside of the digestive tract (the gut lumen) through the dividing walls of cells known as the epithelium. The more permeable the epithelium, the quicker and easier it is for food molecules to pass into blood circulation. A very permeable epithelium allows food allergens to easily contact cells of the immune system, whereas the intact, less permeable lining may exclude the larger molecules. In other words,

the epithelium acts as a "sieve"; the size of the "holes" in the sieve will determine the size of the particles that pass through. The larger the holes (the more
permeable the epithelium), the larger the food molecules that get into the blood.
Once in the blood, allergens encounter immune cells. The size of the food molecules is very important in determining whether the immune system starts to
reject them or not and, therefore, whether an allergic reaction will occur. In
most cases, the larger the molecules, the more likely it is that the immune system will reject them.

   An increase in the permeability of the epithelium can be due to a number
of causes including the following:

IMMATURITY

The digestive lining is very permeable in the early months of life and gradually matures over the first three to four years. Infants under the age of six
months are particularly vulnerable to food allergies. The reason for this is the
way in which the immune system is exposed to the food and how it responds
to it. The first encounter of the immune system with a food can lead either to
tolerance or to *sensitization*. This is critical in determining whether the child will
be able to eat the food in the future without symptoms, or will be allergic to
it. In the vast majority of cases, the immune system is *tolerized* at the first
encounter; that is, it is programmed to accept the food as harmless. From then
on the immune system does not react to the food when the child eats it. In the
rare cases when *sensitization* occurs, the immune system is programmed to
reject the food. This is allergy, and when the child eats the food in the future,
the immune system will automatically reject it until the child "outgrows the
allergy." Outgrowing often involves a decrease in the permeability of the
epithelial lining of the digestive tract, so the food molecules can no longer pass
through into the blood system and encounter the sensitized immune cells.
Refer to Chapter 3 for more detail on the process of sensitization. Most sensitization to food allergens occurs within the first year of life and, to a lesser
extent, from one to five years. If the child avoids most allergenic foods during
this vulnerable period, he or she can avoid or reduce the chance of a great deal
of food allergies.

INFLAMMATION

An inflammatory reaction in the digestive tract (enteritis) can interfere with the
lining of the digestive tract and make it more permeable. Food allergens can
then come into contact with cells of the immune system more readily, and there
is a greater chance that the allergy will occur. Infection, or some other medical
condition in the digestive tract, can result in inflammation.

COMBINED ALLERGIC REACTIONS

When more than one allergic reaction takes place at the same time, inflammatory chemicals from each of the reactions can add up and reach a level higher than any single reaction alone. For example, an allergy to inhaled allergens, combined with a food allergy, may result in symptoms, whereas the response to the food alone might not be enough to cause symptoms. This may also explain the observation that certain foods eaten together result in a reaction, while the same foods eaten alone may not.

ENHANCED UPTAKE OF FOOD ALLERGENS

Anything that promotes food absorption through the lining of the digestive tract can increase the allergic response. Alcohol can increase the speed of uptake from the digestive tract as much as cutting in half the time it normally takes for absorption of certain food components. Therefore, having an alcoholic drink at the same time as eating an allergenic food will cause a dramatic rise in the levels of a food allergen. This may result in allergic symptoms, whereas eating the food alone does not.

Exercise

Vigorous exercise after eating an allergic food sometimes results in an allergic reaction, when eating the food without exercise does not. We do not really know the precise physiological mechanism that is responsible for this phenomenon. It may result from a faster rate of uptake of the food or from increased body temperature during exercise.

Changes in Hormone Levels

Changes in the levels of hormones such as estrogen, progesterone, and testosterone appear to affect the responsiveness of the immune system to allergens. The symptoms of food allergy seem to fluctuate depending on the level of estrogen and/or progesterone during the menstrual cycle (symptoms appearing more frequently at ovulation and just prior to and at the onset of menstruation). During pregnancy, many women report a significant improvement in their allergies, which often extends into the early period of lactation, but the allergies tend to recur as hormone levels return to normal. Both boys and girls sometimes experience a change in reactivity to allergens at puberty. Women's allergic responses sometimes change at menopause, and men seem to experience a change in their mid-thirties.

Stress

Many allergy sufferers notice that their symptoms appear, or seem worse, during periods of stress. This has been suggested to be due to the release of "stress hormones" which affect the degree of responsiveness of the immune system.

Frequency of Exposure to the Allergen

Allergenic foods are often those that we eat frequently. The reason for this is unknown, but it may be due to early exposure during infancy when the intestinal lining is very permeable, because the child's family eats the food as a part of their diet, rather than the number of times the child is exposed to the allergen. Definitive clinical trials have not yet been carried out on this topic.

Now that you are familiar with the different ways food sensitivities can affect people and how allergy can manifest itself in you and your family, you may be curious about just what is happening in your body when you experience a reaction to a particular food. In the next chapter, we will discuss the scientific background of food allergy and go into details of exactly what happens when the immune system goes into defensive mode and someone experiences an allergic reaction to food.

— CHAPTER 3 —

FOOD
ALLERGY

THE SIMPLE EXPLANATION

A simple definition of food allergy is "an inappropriate response of the immune system that results in symptoms." Our immune system keeps us free from disease by recognizing a "foreign invader" when it enters the body and responding to the presence of the invader by releasing defensive chemicals (called **inflammatory mediators**) into our body's tissues and its bloodstream to destroy the threat to our health. All the food we eat comes from the foreign material–plants and animals–that we consume as nourishment. Normally our immune systems see this material as "foreign but safe" due to a complex process of tolerance that occurs when we digest and absorb food. When something goes wrong in this process, a person becomes "sensitized" to the food, and from then on the immune system sees that food as "foreign and a threat." Whenever that food enters the body again, the immune system treats it as if it will cause disease. The symptoms that we experience as a result of our body's defense action are called allergy. Medical practitioners may also refer to allergy as *atopy* or a *hypersensitivity reaction*.

Unlike allergy, food intolerance does *not* involve a response of the immune system. The chemicals released by the immune response are not involved in an intolerance reaction. Most intolerance reactions that we understand (and there are many that we do not!) involve a defect in the processing of the food, either during digestion or later, after the food and its parts or components have been absorbed into the body. The symptoms are often caused by an excess of a food component that has not been digested completely (for example, lactose intolerance), or cannot be processed efficiently for some reason after it has entered the body.

27

These are the simple explanations for why we experience food allergies or intolerances. However, these processes are complex and diverse. For those readers who want a more detailed, scientific explanation of the mechanisms leading to food allergy and food intolerance, please read on. Understanding these processes will take some time and effort for the "nonscientist," but will be ultimately worthwhile. Not only will you understand–and appreciate–your own body more, you will be able to comprehend, and act on, information that you access from other sources of information on allergy.

THE SCIENTIFIC DEFINITIONS

Food allergy or atopy is caused by an inappropriate reaction of the immune system to a component of food. Food intolerance, on the other hand, is any reaction to a food or food additive (a chemical added in its processing or manufacture) that does not involve the immune system. The American Academy of Allergy and Immunology Committee on Adverse Reactions to Foods defines **food allergy** as "an immunologic reaction resulting from the ingestion of a food or food additive" and **food intolerance** as "a general term describing an abnormal physiological response to an ingested food or food additive which is not proven to be immunologic."

There are several different processes within each of these two categories of reactions. Because there are so many different ways the body can respond adversely to a food, it is sometimes very difficult for a doctor to pinpoint the precise cause of the reaction and determine whether it is caused by an allergy or an intolerance. To make things even more difficult, we often do not have any exact tests to determine some of these reactions. This chapter and the next will provide you with the scientific information that you need to fully understand these processes.

In order to understand the processes responsible for these different reactions, we first need to define a few terms that will be used throughout any discussion of adverse reactions to food.

Food Sensitivity

When doctors are not sure whether a reaction is caused by an immune-system-mediated reaction (allergy), or if it is due to a response that does not involve the immune system (intolerance), they tend to refer to the reaction under the general term **food sensitivity.** You will often encounter the term *food sensitivity* or *adverse reaction to food* in the place of either food allergy or food intolerance. They can mean either.

The terms food allergy and food intolerance are *not interchangeable* because they have very precise, well-defined meanings, as mentioned above, and that will become clear in the discussion that follows.

A **hypersensitivity reaction** refers to an immune-system-mediated reaction and therefore is synonymous with allergy or atopy (but, as you will see later, it can include other immune-mediated reactions *in addition* to allergy). It does not refer to food intolerance.

Food Allergy

Food allergy is the immune system's response to a component or part of a food that it recognizes as "foreign." The component of the food that triggers the immune response is almost always a protein, a **glycoprotein** (a protein linked with a sugar), or some other molecule linked to a protein. We call these protein molecules that the immune system responds to **antigens.** Not all antigens cause allergy. **Allergens** are a type of antigen that the immune system specifically responds to in an allergic reaction. All allergens are antigens, but not all antigens are allergens, just as all oranges are fruits but not all fruits are oranges.

The scientific term for food allergy is *food hypersensitivity;* the medical term is *atopy.* A hypersensitivity reaction of the immune system involves events that result in allergy symptoms. In the 1960s, immunologists realized that there are several different ways in which the immune system can respond to foreign molecules entering the body. Although most of the responses of the immune system are protective, and keep us free from illness by destroying the "foreign invader" (called a pathogen) that causes the disease, the new evidence showed that the immune system also responds to non-disease-causing (nonpathogenic) agents. The responses to nonpathogens were shown to be different from those that were triggered by bacteria, viruses, and other pathogenic microorganisms. These nonprotective responses were called hypersensitivity reactions and classified into four distinct types (Types I to IV) by their discoverers, Dr. Philip Gell and Dr. Robin Coombs. The hypersensitivity reactions are classified according to the way in which the immune system responds in each type. Each reaction type has a very specific function. Traditionally, the term *allergy* (or its medical equivalent, *atopy*) has been reserved for the Type I hypersensitivity reaction, while Types II, III, and IV may be referred to as "immune-mediated reactions." We shall discuss each of these reaction types, and its role in adverse reactions to food, later in this chapter. First of all, though, we have to talk about the immune system itself.

THE IMMUNE SYSTEM AND HOW IT WORKS

Allergy results from the immune system responding to foreign material entering the body as if that foreign material were a threat. Under normal (nonallergic) conditions, your body needs immune protection only when the foreign invader can cause disease. Viruses, bacteria, other pathogenic microorganisms, cancer cells, and other disease-causing agents cause your body to launch a protective response in an attempt to destroy the invader and maintain your health. Allergy is a similar response, but in this case the immune system is aiming its protective weapons at an invader that cannot cause disease. The symptoms of allergy are caused by defensive chemicals released by the immune system acting on body cells. Both defense against disease and defense against allergy are a result of an extremely complex interaction between the immune cells and their products. It really isn't possible to understand allergy unless you have some idea of how the immune system works. Let's set off on this journey toward coming to terms with food allergy by starting right at the beginning: let's take a look at the immune system.

Blood Cells

The most important cells of the immune system are found in blood (Figure 3-1). All blood cells start life as *stem cells* in bone marrow, which is present in the center of the larger bones of the body. **Stem cells** are immature cells that mature into different types of blood cells, each with a unique structure and function.

There are three main groups or classes of blood cells:

◆ Red blood cells give blood its color and carry oxygen from the lungs to the rest of the body.
◆ Blood **platelets** are responsible for the clotting of blood.
◆ White blood cells, or **leukocytes** (leuko = white; cyte = cell), are the most important agents of the immune system.

For our purposes, when we discuss the immune system in this chapter and in the rest of the book, we are referring to the white blood cells, or leukocytes, and their functions, so let's look at these cells in more detail.

White Blood Cells

Scientists divide the white blood cells, or leukocytes, into three separate groups, each with a distinct function (Figure 3-1):

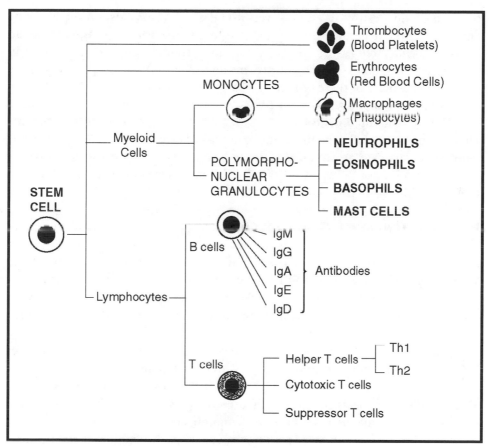

Figure 3-1
The Most Important Cells of the Immune System, Found in Blood

◆ Monocyte/macrophages
◆ Polymorphonuclear granulocytes (familiarity referred to as granulocytes)
◆ Lymphocytes

Each group of leukocytes has specific functions in the immune system. We will learn more about these functions now.

MONOCYTE/MACROPHAGES

Macrophages are principally phagocytes. **Phagocytes** are cells that engulf or "gobble up" a foreign particle, enclose it within a vacuole (a hole within the cell contents), and destroy it with powerful chemicals (enzymes). After breaking down the foreign particle into its separate parts, the **macrophage** acts as an *antigen-presenting cell* (APC). The APC has an extremely important function in the immune response. An antigen-presenting cell presents, or displays, all of the individual particles of the engulfed foreign particle on its surface. Special white blood cells, or lymphocytes called T cells (see below for more information on T cells), are circulating in the blood and detect anything foreign in the vicinity. These T cells carefully examine the material displayed on APCs and decide whether to activate an immune defense against it. This process is known as "antigen recognition." Just what the T-cell lymphocytes are and how they do their job will be discussed later under "Lymphocytes."

POLYMORPHONUCLEAR GRANULOCYTES

This group of cells, referred to as **granulocytes**, is characterized by their distinctively shaped nucleus. All of them contain granules (small vessels) that store very important defensive chemicals called *inflammatory mediators*. The inflammatory mediators released from these cells cause the symptoms we associate with infection, injury, and allergy. Their primary purpose is to defend the body against the effects of invading pathogens.

Most of the granulocytes can be found circulating in blood. But granulocytes called **mast cells** differ from the rest and are situated almost exclusively in tissues. We shall be talking a great deal about mast cells in our discussion of the allergic response, because mast cells are the most important source of the inflammatory mediators that cause the symptoms of allergy.

Granulocytes are subdivided on the basis of their function and can be identified by doctors and technicians by the way the granules in the cells respond to dyes applied in the laboratory. Neutrophils stain with neutral dyes; basophils stain with basic (alkaline) dyes; and eosinophils stain with a dye called eosin, a bromine derivative of fluorescein. We shall see later, in our discussions of the allergic response, that each of these types of granulocytes plays a different role in the reaction and in causing symptoms.

LYMPHOCYTES

The third category of white blood cells, or leukocytes, are the lymphocytes. **Lymphocytes** are the "control cells" of the immune system and are considered to be central to the immune response. Lymphocytes are divided into two important groups: B cells and T cells. As B cells and T cells are key topics in our discussion of the immune system, we will now focus our discussion on learning more about their function and their role in the allergic response.

B Cells

The main function of **B cells** is to produce antibodies. **Antibodies** are the complex molecules that the immune system produces in response to antigens. **Antigens** are foreign proteins, or glycoproteins (a sugar linked to a protein), that trigger the immune response. Every living cell (plant, animal, fungus, and microorganism) produces several different proteins, unique to its own cell type and species. If a protein triggers the immune system to produce an antibody, it is called an *antigen*. The antibody produced against the antigen is specific to that antigen and fits together with it like a lock and key, forming an antigen-antibody complex.

When the body is invaded by a microorganism like a bacterium or virus, the B cells will make antibody exactly designed to fit or couple with molecules of that specific bacterium or virus (microorganism) and no other. The reason why you become immune to a microorganism that has caused you to suffer from a disease, such as chickenpox, mumps, or "flu," and why you will not get the same disease again, is that the body has produced antibodies against the specific bacterium or virus that caused the disease while it was fighting the infection. When the microorganism enters your body the next time, the pre-made antibodies will couple with the virus or bacterium and immobilize it. Inflammatory mediators (destructive chemicals) will then be released by the granulocytes to destroy the microorganism. In summary, the B cells make antibodies in response to foreign antigens. The antibodies then cause the granulocytes to release inflammatory mediators and destroy the foreign invader.

The process of immunization (vaccination) exploits this response of the immune system. The virus or bacterium for mumps, measles, diphtheria, rubella, "flu," and so on, is introduced into the body in a noninfectious state (in a form that will not cause disease). The immune system then produces antibodies against it. If and when the microorganism in its infectious state (also called the "live state") does get into the body, it won't cause disease because the antibodies are waiting for it, and it gets destroyed before it can make you sick.

In allergy, antibodies are made by B cells against antigens in the pollen, animal dander, dust, insect venom, or food that are responsible for the allergic response. These antigens are then termed allergens, but they are essentially the same as the antigens of an infectious microorganism. The antibodies made against a specific allergen couple with that allergen, and inflammatory mediators (destructive chemicals) are then released by granulocytes in an effort to destroy the foreign invader (the allergen). The symptoms of allergy are caused by the inflammatory mediators when they act on tissues of the body. Once the antibodies have been made against a specific allergen, whenever that same allergen enters the body again, the antibodies are waiting. They couple with the allergen, granulocytes (particularly mast cells) release their inflammatory mediators, and the symptoms of allergy appear within minutes of the allergen entering the body. This is like developing immunity to a previous infection, or immunization against future infection by a microorganism. This process will be discussed in more detail later.

ANTIBODIES

The primary function of B cells is antibody production. The antibodies produced by B cells are of five distinct types called IgA, IgG, IgM, IgE, and IgD. The Ig stands for **immunoglobin.** Each antibody molecule is made up of a special protein called a globulin. Because this globulin is associated with the immune system, the prefix immuno- is attached to it. Each of these five antibodies has a specific role in immune protection and in the hypersensitivity reactions responsible for adverse reactions to foods.

IgM

IgM is the largest of the antibodies and is found circulating in blood. It acts by seeking out antigens and attaching them at the end of one or more of its five "arms." It has ten attachment sites (two per arm) and can mop up many antigens at a time. This is why IgM is produced by B cells as the first line of defense against a foreign molecule when it reaches the bloodstream.

IgA

IgA is found mainly in mucous secretions (secretions from all surfaces exposed to the outside world through orifices such as the mouth, respiratory tract, and vagina), where it is called "secretory IgA" (sIgA) to distinguish it from the IgA found in blood. IgA acts as the first line of defense against molecules in these areas, before they enter the bloodstream.

IgG

IgG is the most important antibody in the immune system's defense against invading disease-causing microorganisms. It is produced in the bloodstream after the first-line IgM has started to mop up the invader. In fact, the immune system first produces IgM, then "switches" to IgG once it has established that the invader is a real threat to the body. IgG remains long after the disease has been successfully suppressed, in order to make sure that the same microorganism is incapable of causing disease a second time. It is IgG that remains after an immunization shot, to defend the body when the real live virus or bacterium does get in. In addition to defending against pathogenic microorganisms, IgG is central to Type II and Type III hypersensitivity reactions. We shall discuss these in more detail later.

To complete the discussion of IgG, we should also mention that there are four different types of IgG antibodies, which function in different situations. Not surprisingly, these four types are called IgG1, IgG2, IgG3, and IgG4. IgG4, and to a lesser extent IgG1, are important in food hypersensitivity reactions that are called allergy by some practitioners, but "immune-mediated reactions" by others. This distinction becomes important in any discussion of blood tests for food allergy, which we deal with in more detail in Chapter 4.

IgE

IgE is the most important antibody in allergy of all types—the "classic allergy" of hay fever, asthma, skin reactions, and food allergy of the anaphylactic (life-threatening) type. It is central to Type I hypersensitivity reactions. The only role for IgE apart from the allergic reaction is in fighting parasites and intestinal worms. It is not produced against viruses, bacteria, and other disease-causing micro-organisms, and therefore an IgE-mediated reaction is generally not considered to be "protective." The term "protective" immune response is usually reserved for IgG-mediated and, to a lesser extent, IgA-mediated reactions.

IgD

The last antibody is IgD. This antibody's role is less well-defined and is usually associated with aiding other immune functions, such as "switching" from one class of antibody to another. It is mentioned here simply for completeness. Its role in allergy is minimal.

T Cells

The other type of blood cells in the lymphocyte group in addition to B cells are **T cells.** T-cell lymphocytes control almost every aspect of the immune response. They recognize a foreign antigen, decide whether the immune system should react to it, determine the type of response that would be most appropriate to the situation, direct all of the other immune components to proceed in a certain way, and, finally, end the response when the required results have been achieved. They tell the B cells to begin to produce antibodies and stimulate the granulocytes to release inflammatory mediators.

T cells are of three main types, each having very specific functions:

◆ T helper cells
◆ T cytotoxic cells
◆ T suppressor cells

The functions of these three T-cell types are quite different. Briefly stated, T helper cells recognize a foreign invader and direct the immune system's response to it; T cytotoxic cells release toxic, or poisonous, chemicals that aid in destroying the invader; and T suppressor cells stop the whole immune response once the invader has been destroyed. Let us look at the important parts of the T cells' function in the allergic response in more detail.

T HELPER (TH) CELLS

T helper cells recognize a foreign antigen by comparing it to the major histocompatibility complex (MHC) or "self" antigens (those antigens normally found in our own bodies). The MHC molecules define us as unique individuals; no two people have exactly the same MHC molecules on their cells. This uniqueness allows the T cells to identify what is part of our body, and what is foreign to it, by comparing the foreign antigen and the MHC. When the two are different, T helper cells then release **cytokines**—messenger molecules—that signal the immune system to defend the body against the foreign invader. T cells are able to compare "self" and foreign antigens using a process involving special cells called antigen-presenting cells (APCs). The APCs surround foreign material, such as food, when it enters the body. The APCs then proceed to break down the material into smaller and smaller parts by means of enzymes (similar to the way our bodies digest food in the digestive tract). Eventually, the small parts of protein in the food, called peptides, are moved to the surface of the APC and displayed on special structures beside the MHC molecules on the cell surface. The T cells are then able to compare the two–the peptides from the food and the "self" antigens (MHCs) of the APC. When the two are different, the T cell signals the immune system to mount a defense against this potential threat–the foreign invader. Cytokines are released and the whole immune response begins. (Figure 3-2).

CYTOKINES–MESSENGER MOLECULES

The specific types of cytokines–messenger molecules–released by the T cells depend on the nature of the antigen and the way it is presented by the APC and recognized by the T cell. Each cytokine has a specific role and function in directing the immune response. It is at this stage that we see very important differences in the way the immune system responds to an invading pathogen (disease-causing microorganism) and an allergen.

T HELPER CELL TYPES

There are two types of T helper cells, designated Th1 (Type 1) and Th2 (Type 2). They secrete different cytokines, and they are activated by different cytokines. They also have different effects on the immune system. (Figure 3-3).

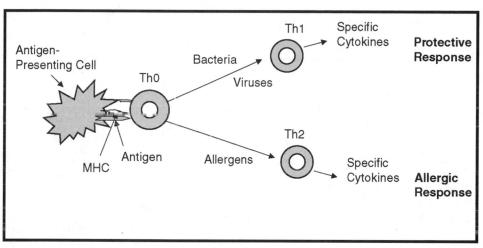

Figure 3-2
Release of Cytokines, Triggering An Immune Response

APC CELLS AND T CELL RESPONSE

◆ An immune response can begin only after a foreign antigen has been presented to a T cell by an antigen-presenting cell (APC).

◆ Each APC has markers on its surface that are "self" antigens, called major histocompatibility complex (MHC) molecules.

◆ When the T cell finds that the foreign antigen and the self antigen are different,
it signals the immune system to mount a defense response. In the case of a
microorganism, the response is "protective"; in the case of an allergen, the
response is a hypersensitivity (allergic) reaction.

CYTOKINES

◆ Cytokines are small proteins that regulate cellular growth and function.

◆ They signal between cells of the immune system.

◆ There are a number of cytokines, each with a specific function.

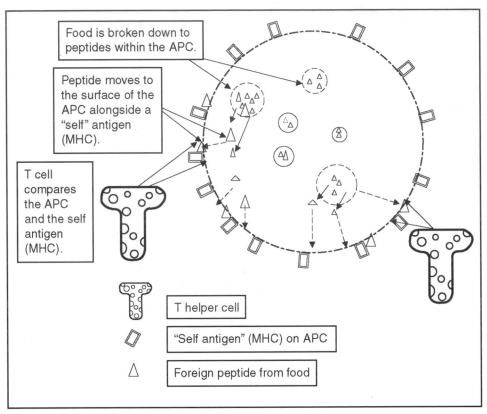

Food is broken down to peptides within the APC.

Peptide moves to the surface of the APC alongside a "self" antigen (MHC).

T cell compares the APC and the self antigen (MHC).

T helper cell

"Self antigen" (MHC) on APC

Foreign peptide from food

Figure 3-3
T-Helper Cells and Their Effects on the Immune System

PROTECTIVE RESPONSE

Th1 Cells:

◆ They are activated by, and initiate, the immune response to pathogenic microorganisms such as bacteria and viruses.

◆ Induce B cells to synthesize antibodies of the IgG type (this is explained in more detail in the text under "Antibodies".)

◆ This response is essentially a protective response.

◆ Th1 activity will continue until the response is terminated by T-suppresser cells.

ALLERGIC RESPONSE

Th2 Cells:

◆ They are activated mainly by allergens and also by parasites, especially intestinal worms.

◆ Cytokines secreted by Th2 cells are essential in inducing B cells to synthesize antibodies of the IgE type.

◆ Other cytokines from the Th2 cells also stimulate B cells to produce increased levels of IgE, mast cells, basophils, and eosinophils, all of which enhance the allergic response and increase the severity of the symptoms. These activities result in the Type I hypersensitivity reaction.

◆ Th2 activity will continue until the response is terminated by T suppresser cells.

The T helper cell is known as the Th0 type before it "commits" to the Th1 or Th2 response. The Th1 response produces cytokines against an invading pathogen (disease-causing microorganism); the Th2 type response produces cytokines against an allergen. Th0 cells can produce any of the T helper cell cytokines, but once the Th1 or the Th2 response has been selected, only those cytokines needed are produced. (Figure 3-3). Sometimes the two types of responses are referred to as the Th1 protective response and the Th2 allergy response.

THE "HYGIENE THEORY" OF ALLERGY

As well as determining which antibody type is produced, Th1 and Th2 cells and the cytokines they secrete interact with each other and with other leukocytes in a complex process of regulation. Under certain conditions, cytokines of the Th1 type can suppress production of (down-regulate) those involved in the Th2 response, and vice versa. This is an important point as this mechanism probably underlies the likelihood that allergies are increasing in the clean, "sanitized" environment of the developed world. Children in a clean environment are not exposed to the many microorganisms that would normally induce a Th1 (protective) response. This would allow an increased potential for a Th2 (allergy) response to develop, and to increase, as the Th1 is suppressed (down-regulated) and the Th2 is increased (up-regulated) the more the child is exposed to allergens. In other words, the less the protective (Th1) response is needed, the more likely the immune system is to mount a response (Th2) against allergens in the child's environment—of which there are many. This is the basis of the so-called "hygiene theory" of allergy.

THE IMMUNE SYSTEM'S ROLE IN FOOD ALLERGY

To review, the immunological response begins when the foreign antigen is identified in a series of steps known as *antigen recognition*. As we discussed earlier in the chapter, specific leukocytes (white blood cells) known as antigen-presenting cells (APCs), encounter the foreign protein antigen. The antigen is taken inside these cells and split into **peptides** (small fragments of proteins). The peptide fragments (still referred to as antigens) move to the surface of the APC and bind to major histocompatibility complex (MHC) molecules on the cell's surface, as described on page 36. We can visualize this as the antigens being exhibited on specially designed display structures, a process known as *antigen presentation*. Recognition of the foreign antigen, and regulation of the whole immune response to it, is then controlled by T-cell lymphocytes, as described on page 36. As we are about to learn, in food allergy there are a first signal and a second signal. The first will occur whenever a "foreign" food enters the body. This is the "recognition phase" described here. Only people whose immune systems respond to the "second signal" will be allergic to the food. The first signal is "tolerance" (no allergy); the second signal is allergy (or "sensitization" if it is the first reaction).

T Helper Cells and Antigen Presentation

The peptide fragments (antigens) on the surface of the APCs are presented to specific T helper cells. The antigens and the specific receptor on the T cell interact. This interaction of the APCs (antigen-presenting cells) with the T-cell receptor results in partial activation of the T cell. The T cell is not completely activated until it receives a *second signal*. After the second signal comes in, the now completely activated T cells instruct the B cells to produce antibodies, specifically designed to couple with the antigen. The second signal is supplied by the cell-surface molecules on T cells and antigen-presenting cells, or by cytokines (messengers). Full activation of T cells results in

- ◆ production of cytokines that control the rest of the reaction.
- ◆ multiplication of T cells that are involved directly in the reaction, and which produce more of the cytokines required in the response.
- ◆ activation of B cells, which produce antigen-specific antibodies.

In the absence of the second signal, T cells do not respond to antigen stimulation. What this means in the case of food is that the "foreign" material of the food will trigger an immunological response, but the recognition that the food is foreign to the body does not trigger a full immune system reaction. In simplistic terms, the food is recognized as "foreign," but in the absence of a second signal, it is deemed to be "safe" and the immune system proceeds no further. This is what happens in the body of a person who is *not* allergic to food.

THE TYPE OF T CELL DETERMINES THE RESPONSE

If the second signal *is* produced, however, the immune system then proceeds to "defend" the body against this potential threat. The type of response (allergy, Th2; or protection, Th1) is determined by which of the T helper cell types and their cytokines are activated.

TYPE I HYPERSENSITIVITY

When the Th2 response is selected, the immune system proceeds to a **Type I hypersensitivity reaction** (allergy). The Type I hypersensitivity response involves the production of IgE antibodies (see page 35), followed by the release of defensive chemicals (inflammatory mediators) from mast cells and other granulocytes (see page 32) in a process known as degranulation (described below). The release of these inflammatory mediators results in symptoms of allergy, such as skin reactions (hives, facial swelling); stuffy nose, itchy, watery eyes; digestive tract upset; and the most severe whole-body response of anaphylaxis.

The reaction can be divided into two phases, the early and the late response.

◆ The *early phase* results in the release of inflammatory mediators from granulocytes (mast cells in tissues and basophils in blood). This may be experienced as itching, swelling of tissues (sometimes in the throat), occasionally a feeling of being unwell, an increased heart rate, or digestive tract upset.

◆ The *late phase* results in the recruitment of additional granulocytes, which are drawn to the reaction site by chemicals called **chemotaxins**. The newly recruited granulocytes release their own inflammatory mediators, which enhance the allergic reaction by increasing the levels of the inflammatory mediators already there. This late phase is sometimes experienced as a "second wave" of symptoms. The second wave can be particularly dramatic in the case of an asthma attack. The first-stage response to the allergen sometimes seems to be getting better, but the late phase, which can happen several hours after the first, takes the person by surprise. This late phase of an asthma attack can often be more severe than the first phase. Several cases of death from asthma have been the result of the late phase not being recognized in time.

The Early Phase of Type I Hypersensitivity

As soon as IgE antibodies are produced by the activated B cells in the Type I hypersensitivity reaction, they move to the surface of specific white blood cells to couple with the antibody. The white blood cells have receptors on their surface to make this possible. These receptors can couple with the IgE type of antibody. Granulocytes such as mast cells in tissues, and basophils in blood (refer to Figure 3-1 for details of blood cells), have these IgE compatible receptors. The **mast cell** is the key granulocyte in the allergic response. It has been estimated that there may be as many as 500,000 receptors for antibody molecules on the surface of a mast cell.

DEGRANULATION TRIGGERS THE RELEASE OF INFLAMMATORY MEDIATORS

Mast cells, basophils, and other granulocytes manufacture and store inflammatory mediators in internal granules (vessels). The **inflammatory mediators** are the chemicals that protect the body in the process of inflammation. When required to defend the body against a potential threat, the inflammatory mediators are released in a complex sequence of reactions, called **degranulation.** It is the action of these chemicals (the inflammatory mediators) on your body tissues that causes the symptoms of allergy.

Degranulation begins when an allergen cross-links two IgE molecules on receptors that are next to each other on the surface of a mast cell. The allergen effectively forms a bridge between the IgE molecules. The allergen needs to be a certain size (estimated at 10 to 80 kilodaltons) to make this bridging happen. In addition, there needs to be a sufficient number of IgE molecules on the surface of the cell so that two potential "bridging" allergens would be close enough for the allergen to bridge them. When the bridge occurs, inflammatory mediators are released.

Often the first exposure to an allergen does not result in enough IgE antibody molecules to allow the allergen-bridges to form, and so a single exposure to an allergen rarely results in degranulation and the release of the inflammatory mediators that cause symptoms to appear. Consequently, the initial episode is usually symptom-free. This process, in which a person is exposed to an allergen but does not exhibit symptoms, is called the *sensitizing event.* On subsequent exposure, when enough IgE molecules are present on the surface of the mast cells, degranulation will occur and a person will experience symptoms.

Inflammatory Mediators from Mast Cells

Each of the inflammatory mediators released from the granules within the mast cells has a different and powerful effect on your body tissues. Let us look at a few of the most important of these inflammatory mediators so that you can understand what is happening when you experience their effects on your body.

HISTAMINE

Histamine is an extremely powerful inflammatory mediator that controls a number of different responses in your body. The most important include

◆ widening of small blood vessels (vasodilation).
◆ increase in the permeability of the membrane around the blood vessels, allowing fluids and protein to leak out.
◆ contraction of smooth muscle surrounding the lungs (bronchoconstriction).
◆ stimulation of nerves, resulting in itching.
◆ increased secretion of mucous.

ENZYMES

Several inflammatory mediators called **enzymes** (such as tryptase, kinino-genase, and phospholipases) result in further activation of inflammatory processes and can result in tissue damage. The visible signs of enzyme release are skin reactions and other sites of an allergic reaction that seem to take a long time to heal after the allergy has ended.

Phospholipase A1

Phospholipase A1 is the key enzyme that leads to the production of several different types of powerful inflammatory mediators in a series of enzymatic reactions. First, arachidonic acid is released from its position in the membrane of the cell. The arachidonic acid is then processed and forms *secondary mediators of inflammation* (known as eicosanoids). These secondary mediators, or eicosanoids, can be divided into two very important groups, **protaglandins** and **leukotrienes.** The enzyme systems responsible for the production of the prostaglandins and the leukotrienes are the cyclo-oxygenase pathway and the lipoxygenase pathway respectively.

The Cyclo-Oxygenase Pathway.

◆ The cyclo-oxygenase pathway produces prostanoids called PG_2. Some of these are PGD_2, PGF_2, PGE_1, and PGE_2. They include prostaglandins, prosta-cyclin, and thromboxane, which have important functions in many body systems. In allergy, an important mediator is PGD_2 that, like histamine, causes vasodilation, bronchoconstriction, nerve stimulation, and mucous secretion.

◆ $PGF_{2\alpha}$ stimulates mast cell degranulation, while PGE_1 and PGE_2 tend to inhibit mast cell degranulation.

The Lipoxygenase Pathway

◆ The lipoxygenase pathway produces the leukotrienes of the "4 series," written as LT_4. Some of the leukotrienes—LTB_4, LTC_4, LTD4, and LTE_4, for example–are powerful inflammatory chemicals.

◆ LTB_4 powerfully attracts granulocytes to move to the site of the reaction and thus is responsible for augmenting the allergic response when the newly recruited granulocytes release their own battery of inflammatory chemicals.

◆ LTC_4, LTD_4, and LTE_4 cause smooth muscle contraction and are key factors in the bronchospasm of asthma. They also mediate mucous secretion and mucosal swelling (edema), which are frequent symptoms of allergy.

The Late Phase of Type I Hypersensitivity

During the late phase of the allergic response, granulocytes like neutrophils, eosinophils, monocytes, and basophils are attracted to the reaction site by the **chemotaxins** produced in the early phase (chemotaxins are chemicals that cause cells to move from one place to another). When the new granulocytes release their own supply of inflammatory mediators, the allergic reaction is increased. This can be experienced in the late phases of an asthma or anaphylaxis attack when the initial reaction seems to be ending. Suddenly the attack becomes extremely bad and the victim is in serious danger. Sometimes the second phase of an anaphylactic reaction proves fatal. The second phase may occur several hours after the initial response, but usually happens within a maximum of 4–6 hours after the first phase.

CLINICAL EXPRESSION OF ALLERGY (ATOPY)

Type I allergy or atopy is a multifaceted disease that depends on both genetics and environmental influences. Even if someone inherits the potential to produce IgE antibodies, further genetic elements appear to be required for atopic disease (allergy) to appear. For example, the ability of granulocytes to release inflammatory mediators is likely determined by genetic factors, but exposure to the allergens that trigger the response is dependent on lifestyle events.

TYPE II AND TYPE III HYPERSENSITIVITY

Type II and Type III hypersensitivity reactions resemble the type of immune response that is triggered by an invading pathogenic virus or bacterium. As you will recall, this reaction is initiated by Th1 lymphocytes. The foreign antigen is processed by antigen-presenting cells (APCs) and recognized by T helper cells of the Th1 type. This leads to the production of antigen-specific antibody IgG. Unlike the antibody IgE, the antibody IgG does not directly initiate degranulation of mast cells. Instead, when IgG and its matching antigen couple together, it leads to a complex series of reactions. These reactions trigger something called the **complement cascade.** In the complement cascade, a unique sequence of proteins is activated. This sequence of proteins leads to the final destruction of the invader by a process of splitting (also called **lysis**) of the foreign cell.

Because of the activities of the proteins of the complement cascade, several newly formed proteins emerge. Two of these new proteins (C3a and C5a) are powerful agents called **anaphylatoxins,** which are able to degranulate basophils and possibly mast cells without the help of IgE. In addition, the new protein C5a attracts granulocytes to the reaction site and thus increases the amount of inflammatory mediators present.

You have probably heard of IgG-mediated "allergy" to drugs. For example, an allergic reaction to penicillin is a Type II hypersensitivity reaction. Type III hypersensitivity reactions (also IgG-mediated) to antibiotics, such as sulfonamides and penicillin, can result in symptoms such as rash, painful joints, and hives.

The Questionable Role of Type III (IgG-mediated) Hypersensitivity Reactions in Food Allergy

The role of IgG antibodies produced against a specific food in causing allergic symptoms has been suggested and debated for many years. Theoretically, release of inflammatory mediators, either by the action of the new proteins called anaphylatoxins or by direct bonding of anti-food IgG to IgG receptors on basophils, might occur. IgG-mediated allergy to egg white and fish has been reported, so it is likely that such allergy is valid. However, because the triggering of the complement cascade, and the release of the inflammatory mediators by this mechanism, is complicated, it takes much longer for the symptoms to appear. Therefore, IgG-mediated "allergic reactions" are characterized by a delay of up to eight or more hours after the food has been eaten. Because the effect is not immediate, it is much more difficult to identify the food responsible for the reaction than it is in an immediate IgE-mediated reaction.

It is relatively easy to measure the level of antigen-specific IgG in blood, and many laboratories now offer "food-allergy blood tests" that measure the antibodies IgE and IgG against specific foods (anti-food antibodies). However, the mere presence of anti-food IgG, even at high levels, does not necessarily indicate that the food is the cause of the reaction. We commonly find anti-food IgG anti-bodies circulating in blood, even in people who have no signs or history of adverse reactions to foods. In fact, an increase in anti-food IgG in some cases might indicate successful treatment of an IgE-mediated allergy in the past. IgG-mediated food allergy is extremely complicated. It remains for future research to determine the role of IgG, especially IgG4 anti-food antibodies in allergy. (Refer to page 35 for an explanation of IgG4 and other antibodies.)

TYPE IV HYPERSENSITIVITY

The Type IV hypersensitivity is commonly known as a *contact allergy*. It involves cell-to-cell contact between the antigen (allergen) and T-cell lymphocytes, usu-ally in the skin. Some of the T cells respond to the antigen by producing inflam-matory mediators, while others develop cytotoxicity. *Cytotoxicity* is the term we use to describe damage to the cell by toxic agents, which destroy cells in the tis-sues surrounding the site of their release. A common example of this type of response is the rash caused by poison ivy or contact with metal in jewelry. The reaction continues as long as the antigen is in contact with body cells. Because of this, it is often referred to as a cell-mediated response. No antibodies are pro-duced, although certain cytokines seem to be involved in the process.

The allergen involved in a Type IV hypersensitivity reaction is usually a sim-ple chemical that would normally not cause the immune system to respond. But by linking with a body protein (usually in the skin), the allergen becomes anti-genic. A Type IV hypersensitivity reaction is typically a delayed response that is visible 24–72 hours after skin-to-allergen contact. It is normally diagnosed by means of patch tests. In a patch test, the suspect allergen is applied to the skin and covered by an adhesive bandage. The site is examined after a delay of up to 72 hours for development of the characteristic reddened area (wheal).

CAN A TYPE IV REACTION HAPPEN INSIDE THE BODY?
Although damage to intestinal cells can be caused by a Type IV hypersensitivi-ty reaction in animals, there is no clear evidence that food can cause such a reaction in humans. However, a type of dermatitis on the hands of sensitized people who come in contact with raw foods such as potato, tomato, apple, watermelon rind, or carrot has been labeled as a Type IV hypersensitivity response. It follows that if such a reaction occurs on the hands, a similar response might be expected in the intestines when the food is eaten. At pres-ent, there is no good evidence for this because there are no methods available for assessing such a reaction.

ORAL ALLERGY SYNDROME (OAS) AND LATEX ALLERGY

Oral allergy syndrome (OAS) and latex allergy are examples of conditions in which contact with the offending allergen results in local reactivity. Both of these conditions can lead to severe allergic reactions, and latex allergy is becoming an increasing problem among health-care workers. Although latex allergy is thought to be initiated by a Type IV hypersensitivity reaction, IgE-mediated Type I hypersensitivity is the reaction responsible for the acute symptoms in both OAS and latex allergy. These conditions are discussed in greater detail in Chapter 7.

NICKEL CONTACT DERMATITIS AND FOOD ALLERGY

An association between food and contact allergy has emerged from observation of nickel-associated dermatitis. Contact allergy to nickel, often suspected when dermatitis develops at sites where nickel-containing jewelry, watch bands, and other metal objects touch the skin, occurs in approximately 10% of females and about 3% of males. Since the mid-1970s a number of reports have indicated that dermatitis, especially on the hands, can be aggravated by oral administration of nickel. Because nickel occurs in many foods to varying degrees, some practitioners assumed that a diet low in nickel might cure or reduce the severity of dermatitis in people who responded positively to oral nickel challenge. However, there seem to be differing opinions on what constitutes a low-nickel diet and on the degree to which symptom improvement can be achieved on such a regimen. Nevertheless, nickel-associated dermatitis serves as an example of the possible association between food constituents and the immune system that differs from the more familiar protein/glycoprotein antigen in an IgE-mediated reaction. Future research will no doubt shed light in the nature of the reaction and possibly uncover other, similar interactions.

ALLERGY IS AN INFLAMMATORY PROCESS

Regardless of the type of hypersensitivity reaction involved, the symptoms of allergy result from the release of inflammatory mediators that act on body tissues and cause the clinical condition. In other words, *allergy is an inflammatory process*, and each inflammatory mediator that is released has its own effect. We have already discussed some of these important inflammatory mediators and the role they play in the allergic response. Now we will look at what you can expect as far as symptoms linked to specific inflammatory mediators.

Histamine

High levels of histamine released in the allergic response result in symptoms such as

- Nasal congestion (rhinitis)
- Earache, sometimes with itching and fluid drainage
- Hives: urticaria in the skin and swelling, often in facial tissues (angioedema)
- Flushing or reddening
- Headache
- Drop in blood pressure (hypotension)
- Speed-up of the heart rate (tachycardia)
- Contraction of smooth muscle around the lung (bronchospasm)
- Swelling and irritation in mucous membranes (mucosal edema)

Other Inflammatory Mediators

Prostaglandins control both widening of blood vessels (vasodilation) and narrowing of blood vessels (vasoconstriction).
Leukotrienes cause contraction of smooth muscle and are largely responsible for the bronchospasm of asthma.
Bradykinin, in conjunction with prostaglandins, causes pain.

Allergy is the result of the combined effect of all of the inflammatory mediators. Treatment usually involves giving drugs to relieve symptoms. These drugs are designed to combat the effects of each type of mediator. For example, antihistamines control itching, swelling of tissues, and reddening and flushing of the skin caused by histamine. Inhaled drugs such as Ventolin and salbutamol are given to people with asthma to combat the effects of histamine and leukotrienes in contracting the smooth muscle around the lungs. Corticosteroids inhaled into the lungs, or applied to the skin in creams, stop the effects of many combined mediators in asthma and eczema. Analgesics such as aspirin and nonsteroidal anti-inflammatory drugs such as Ibuprofen stop the release of prostaglandins that cause pain.

WHEN ALLERGY-LIKE SYMPTOMS ARE *NOT* CAUSED BY ALLERGENS

The definition of allergy as an immune-system-mediated process becomes unwieldy when we realize that the degranulation of mast cells can occur without the initial stimulation of an allergen. Because the inflammatory mediators are released, the resulting symptoms are the same whether their release was allergen-mediated or not. The key event is the degranulation of the mast cell. Because the mast cell is an essential immune system component, these reactions should thus be included under the umbrella of immune-mediated reactions. Let us look at this process of "non-allergen-triggered" release of inflammatory mediators in more detail.

The Nervous System

It may come as no surprise to you that your immune system can indeed cause the release of inflammatory mediators from mast cells, even when you have not come into contact with any known allergen or eaten any food that could have caused the reaction. You always suspected that "stress" could cause you to experience symptoms of an allergic reaction, didn't you? Here is the evidence to show that this really can happen.

There are two important agents that have the ability to stimulate mast cell degranulation: substance P and vasoactive intestinal peptide (VIP). There are **neuropeptides** (small proteins made in the central nervous system) produced by nerve cells. They are frequently detectable in the gastrointestinal tract. It is possible that neuropeptides stimulate the degranulation of intestinal mast cells. When this happens, inflammatory mediators are released into the area and can cause chronic inflammation. This irritation and inflammation of the intestines may be experienced as irritable bowel syndrome.

Physical Factors

Physical factors can also lead to mast-cell degranulation. When your skin is irritated by pressure and becomes red as an object is drawn across the surface, we call it *dermatographia* (or *dermatographism*). Inhaling cold air into the lungs can bring on an asthma attack in sensitive individuals. Cold air passing across sensitive tissue in the nose can cause a runny nose.

Drugs and Medications

Some medications such as codeine and morphine can induce mast-cell degranulation. Biologically active chemicals such as interferon, phospholipase, chymotrypsin, certain serum factors, and basic polypeptides that are involved in other physiological processes can likewise release inflammatory mediators from mast cells.

A great deal of research is required in this field, which is presently poorly understood. However, the recognition that factors other than the well-known inhaled, ingested, and injected antigens can cause symptoms resembling allergy should alert practitioners to the fact that sometimes the search for an external allergenic cause for an adverse reaction may be futile.

ALLERGENIC FOODS

Every food contains potentially allergenic proteins, but some are more common allergens than others. This topic is dealt with in more detail in Chapter 6. Children under the age of five years are more vulnerable to the development of food allergies because of their immature immune and digestive systems. Cow's milk proteins, egg proteins (especially ovalbumin), and peanuts are the most common foods causing Type I hypersensitivity in children. Often, children "outgrow" early food allergies by the age of five years, but certain allergies to foods, specifically peanuts, nuts, shellfish, and sometimes fin fish, can last for a lifetime. These are also the foods that are most frequently implicated in life-threatening anaphylactic reactions.

Sometimes inflammatory mediators are released, or their levels are enhanced, by food components or food additives acting through mechanisms that are independent of the immune system: This is presently classified as food *intolerance* rather than allergy and is discussed in more detail in Chapter 4.

— CHAPTER 4 —

FOOD
INTOLERANCE

An adverse reaction to a food that results in clinical symptoms, but which is *not* caused by a reaction of the immune system, is called food intolerance. In contrast to food allergy, which is a response of the immune system to antigenic proteins, food intolerance is usually triggered by small-molecular-weight chemical substances and biologically active components of foods. The physiological mechanisms that cause adverse reactions to foods can be diverse and complex, and many are still poorly understood. In general terms, a **food intolerance** is defined as "a non-immunologically-mediated adverse reaction to a food or a food additive."

There are three main categories of non-immunologically-mediated adverse reactions to foods:

1. Toxic reactions (for example, food poisoning in response to a microbial toxin in a food)
2. Metabolic dysfunction (for example, enzyme dysfunction such as lactase deficiency causing lactose intolerance)
3. Pharmacologic responses (for example, a reaction to a pharmacologically active agent, such as tyramine, in food that causes migraine headache)

A tendency to react adversely to a component of food that causes no ill effects in the majority of the population is considered to be an idiosyncratic response. Therefore, food intolerance is usually defined as an idiosyncratic response to a food, or a component of food, that is not caused by a response of the immune system. Because toxins in foods will cause ill effects in anyone who consumes them, food poisoning is not usually considered to be food intolerance within this definition of the term.

Although convenient for classification purposes, the categories listed above are not easily separated in practice. Often, a reaction that may be classified in one category because of the symptoms (effect) may have its cause in another. For example, a response to a pharmacologically active agent such as tyramine may be caused by a reduced ability of an enzyme to break down the chemical—in the case of tyramine, a reduction in diamine oxidase. In other words, the cause is an enzyme deficiency; the effect is a pharmacological ("drug-like") response.

Many food intolerance reactions can be explained on the basis of metabolic dysfunction or pharmacologic responses to components of foods that may be naturally occurring, added to foods, or arise during their manufacture. In many cases the mechanism responsible for the adverse response is not known. The reactions discussed in this chapter provide an overview of the research findings and current understanding of a few of the more common causes of food intolerance. These include intolerance of carbohydrates, including lactose intolerance; intolerance of biogenic amines such as histamine and tyramine; intolerance of salicylates; intolerance of artificial food colors such as tartrazine and preservatives such as benzoates, BHA, BHT, and sulfites, and flavoring agents such as MSG. A summary of this information for quick reference is provided in Table 4-1 at the end of this chapter.

INTOLERANCE OF CARBOHYDRATES

Carbohydrates in food need to be first digested in the small intestine by digestive enzymes. The result of digestion (products) are then absorbed through the lining of the digestive tract and taken into the blood circulation. These are two distinct processes, and both need to be functioning efficiently to ensure normal digestion. When either or both of these processes are impaired by absence of, or immaturity in development of, any component of the system, trouble results. Symptoms of abdominal bloating, pain, excessive gas, diarrhea, and constipation are common signs of a disturbance in these processes.

Impaired digestion and absorption of carbohydrates may result from a variety of causes including

◆ Enzyme deficiencies such as lactase deficiency and sucrase-isomaltase deficiency
◆ Enteropathies (pathology of the intestinal tract) such as cow's milk and soy-protein-sensitive enteropathy and gluten-sensitive enteropathy
◆ Infections with microorganisms such as *E.coli*, salmonella, and related bacteria, parasites such as *Giardia lamblia* (giardiasis), and viruses such as the rotavirus group

In infants, additional causes may include immaturity in development of, or an inherited absence of, enzymes for digestion, and of components of the transport systems needed to absorb the products of digestion into the blood stream.

In all of these examples, the symptoms of abdominal discomfort or pain and diarrhea will result when a person with such problems consumes carbohydrate-containing foods. Thus, the effect will be intolerance of one or more carbohydrate: the cause in each case differs, and the treatment will be dictated by the underlying cause. However, in all cases, identification and removal of the offending carbohydrate from the diet will lead to resolution of the gastrointestinal symptoms.

Carbohydrate Digestion

Carbohydrates are consumed as starches, sugars, and nonstarch polysaccharides, which are complex in structure. In order to cross the digestive barrier and pass into circulation, all dietary carbohydrates must be broken down to their simplest and smallest components, called **monosaccharides** (mono = one; saccharide = sugar). These are mainly glucose, galactose, and fructose. This breakdown is carried out by **enzymes** in the digestive tract.

During digestion the complex carbohydrates are reduced first to **oligosaccharides** (less complex carbohydrates), then to **disaccharides** (two sugars) by enzymes (amylases) in saliva and pancreatic secretions in the small intestine. The disaccharides are further split into monosaccharides (single sugars) at the surface of the absorptive cell in the small intestine by locally produced enzymes called disaccharidases (Figure 4-1). Many of the adverse reactions that are classified as carbohydrate intolerance and treated by food exclusion are due to a deficiency of enzymes responsible for the breakdown of disaccharides. The most well-known, because of its high incidence in the population, is lactose intolerance.

INADEQUATE CARBOHYDRATE DIGESTION

Any carbohydrates, sugars, starches, and polysaccharides that are *not* digested in the small intestine and absorbed into circulation pass into the large bowel. Here they cause an imbalance in the concentration of water and sugar. This leads to an increase in fluid and electrolytes (such as sodium and potassium) in the bowel because the water that is usually withdrawn from the bowel at this stage remains inside. In addition, extra water is drawn into the bowel in order to dilute the high sugar content. The extra load of undigested carbohydrates in the bowel also stimulates growth of intestinal microorganisms, which produce gases and other irritating substances. The result is watery diarrhea, abdominal

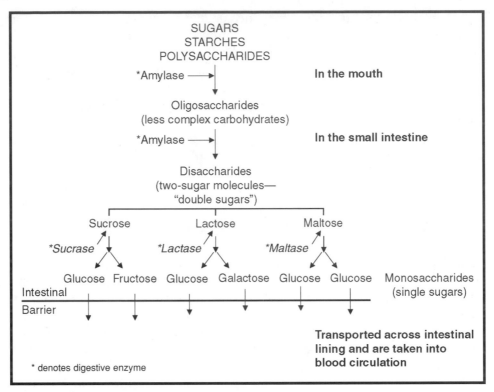

Figure 4-1
Carbohydrate Digestion in the Mouth and Small Intestine

distention, and flatulence. Disaccharides that may be responsible for this condition include lactose from milk, sucrose from fruits, vegetables, table sugar, and syrups, and maltose and isomaltose from dietary starches. Lactose is the most common disaccharide responsible for disaccharide intolerance.

Lactose Intolerance

Lactose (present in the milk of animals, including humans) is broken down to its constituent monosaccharides glucose and galactose by the enzyme **lactase** in cells at the border of the lining of the small intestine. When there is not enough of the enzyme to split all the molecules of lactose, some remain intact and pass into the large bowel. The result is an imbalance in the concentration of water and sugar in the bowel, an increase in fluid, and increased microbial fermentation of the undigested lactose.

A deficiency in lactase may be due to several causes:

CONGENITAL LACTASE DEFICIENCY

Congenital lactase deficiency is extremely rare. It is an inherited, genetically determined condition that is present at birth and is evident as a watery diarrhea when the infant is first given milk in any form, including its mother's breast milk. Treatment is lifelong avoidance of lactose.

ADULT-ONSET PRIMARY LACTASE DEFICIENCY

This condition is due to the gradual loss of lactase after weaning and is in the adult population of most countries. Persons of Northern European descent tend to have the lowest incidence (less than 20% of the population), while more than 80% of people of all other ethnic groups tend to have some degree of lactose intolerance. Usually, lactase production does not cease entirely–some lactase continues to be produced–so a person producing less than an adequate amount of lactase can usually consume a limited quantity of lactose without getting sick. However, consumption of excessive quantities of lactose that overwhelm the enzyme's capacity to digest the milk sugar will result in digestive tract symptoms.

SECONDARY LACTASE DEFICIENCY

A *temporary* lactase deficiency often results from intestinal damage due to infection by bacteria, viruses, and sometimes parasites; inflammation due to food allergy, especially to milk; and a variety of pathological situations that harm the enzyme-producing cells in the lining of the small intestine. It is much more common in infants and children than in adults, because children tend to be prone to more intestinal infections and food allergies in comparison to adults. Management of the condition involves restricting the intake of lactose until the infection clears up or the cause of the inflammation is removed, when the enzyme-producing cells return to normal. Lactose restrictions can be gradually removed as the intestinal damage is repaired.

A discussion of lactose intolerance and its management can be found in Chapter 8, page 123.

Intolerance of Other Disaccharides

Abdominal distress and pain with diarrhea can result from deficiencies in disaccharidases other than lactase, but much more rarely. Extensive damage to the enzyme-producing cells can result in deficiencies in the enzymes called sucrase, isomaltase, and other alpha-dextrinases as well as lactase. Consequently, consumption of any disaccharide, or polysaccharide will result in digestive tract symptoms as long as there are not enough enzymes for their digestion. The damage may be due to a temporary or treatable condition such as an infection, in which case the level of the enzymes will increase as the enzyme-producing cells return to normal. As long as the damage persists, all disaccharides, (including sucrose, lactose, and maltose); starches, and other complex carbohydrates must be avoided in order to avoid abdominal distress.

CONGENITAL (INHERITED) SUCRASE-ISOMALTASE DEFICIENCY

Congenital sucrase-isomaltase deficiency is reported to be more common than congenital lactase deficiency. The condition is especially prevalent in Greenland and Canadian Eskimos in whom the incidence has been reported to be as high as 10% of the population. When sucrose is fed to a sucrase-deficient infant, usually in the form of fruit or fruit juice, watery diarrhea, abdominal bloating, and gas occur. Treatment is avoidance of all foods containing sucrose.

The lactose-restricted diet is discussed in Chapter 8; the disaccharide-restricted diet is discussed in Chapter 18.

INTOLERANCE OF BIOGENIC AMINES

There are varying opinions on the significance of **biogenic amines** (a biologically active group of compounds) in non-immunologically-mediated reactions to foods that may be termed "food intolerance" in contrast to "food allergy." Because the effects of biogenic amines result in symptoms sometimes indistinguishable from those due to allergy, there is often debate and confusion surrounding the definition of the reaction mechanism and the foods responsible for it. Histamine is probably the most well-studied of the biogenic amines because of its central role in causing inflammation and allergy. However, histamine is present in a number of foods and beverages, such as those fermented in manufacture such as cheese, processed meats, alcoholic beverages, and soy sauce. In sensitive individuals it can be an important direct cause of symptoms of food intolerance.

Histamine

Because **histamine** is the most important mediator responsible for the symptoms of "classical allergy" in the Type I (IgE-mediated) hypersensitivity reaction (see Chapter 3), it is difficult to distinguish between reactions due to allergy and those resulting from excess histamine in the body, because the symptoms may be the same in both cases. However, histamine sensitivity, or intolerance, is becoming increasingly recognized as a cause of a disease that is distinct from allergy. Histamine intolerance may be suspected when an allergic cause for the symptoms has been ruled out.

High doses of histamine are toxic for all humans, but *individual tolerance* determines reactivity to small quantities. Just about everyone who ingests histamine from a food in which microorganisms are active in producing a level of histamine of more than 2.7 milligrams per kilogram of body weight will show symptoms of "histamine poisoning," but at lower concentrations only a few sensitive persons will experience an adverse reaction. Differences in levels of tolerance are probably inherited, but tolerance can be reduced by disease and by certain medications.

Research indicates that the cause of histamine intolerance is most likely a defect in the enzymatic breakdown of histamine. In humans, enzymatic inactivation of histamine occurs through the operation of two enzymes, diamine oxidase (DAO) and histamine methyltransferase (HMT), that have different characteristics. When these enzymes are unable to rid the body of excess histamine, the sensitive person has symptoms that include tissue swelling, especially of facial areas, nasal congestion, hives, itching, and headache.

FOOD SOURCES OF HISTAMINE

Histamine is present in most *fermented* foods. Microbial enzymes convert the amino acid *histidine* (present as a constituent of all proteins) to histamine. Any foods that have undergone microbial fermentation in the manufacture of the food–such as cheeses, fermented soy products, fermented foods (sauerkraut), alcoholic beverages, and vinegars–contain histamine. Foods that have been exposed to microbial contamination (spoilage) will contain histamine; the level is determined by the rapidity of microbial activity and replication. Histamine levels will rise to a reactive level long before any signs of spoilage occur in the food. This is particularly true in fish. Bacteria in the gut will start to convert histidine to histamine as soon as the fish dies. The longer the fish remains ungutted, the higher the level of histamine in the flesh. Some foods, such as eggplant, tomato, and spinach, contain high levels of histamine naturally.

Histamine may be released by certain foods, by a mechanism that is still poorly understood. Foods such as strawberries, egg white, shellfish, and alcohol appear to have this ability. In addition, a number of food additives, such as azo dyes (e.g., tartrazine), and preservatives (e.g., benzoates) mediate the release of histamine from mast cells (see Chapter 3, page 32, for an explanation of mast cells and their function). Some of these chemicals (such as benzoates) occur naturally in foods, especially fruits, and may have the same effect as the food additive in releasing histamine. The histamine-restricted diet is discussed in Chapter 19.

Tyramine

Sensitivity to **tyramine** is probably caused by low levels of the enzyme *monoamine oxidase*, which normally breaks down tyramine and rids the body of the excess. People taking monoamine oxidase inhibiting drugs (MAOs) such as the antidepressants tranylcypromine (Parnate), phenelzine (Nardil), and moclobemide (Manerix), and some drugs used in the treatment of Parkinson's disease (e.g., selegiline and Eldepryl), are especially at risk for tyramine toxicity. Tyramine releases norepinephrine from tissues, where it is stored for use in important body functions. The effect of the neurotransmitter norepinephrine at high levels is to constrict blood vessels, which is a cause of migraine headaches in sensitive people.

Tyramine is formed from the amino acid *tyrosine*, a component of protein. Microbial fermentation is responsible for the high levels of tyramine in some fermented foods such as aged cheeses, wines, and vinegars. People who have chronic hives or migraine headaches that are suspected to be due to tyramine sensitivity would benefit from a tyramine-restricted diet. The response to tyramine is dose-dependent, and the amount of tyramine in foods that causes an adverse reaction will depend on individual tolerance.

FOOD SOURCES OF TYRAMINE

Tyramine is present in a number of foods, particularly aged cheeses (especially Camembert and Cheddar), yeast extract, wines (especially red), beer, other fermented beverages, vinegar, and foods containing vinegar such as pickles and relishes. Tyramine occurs naturally in some foods, especially raspberries, bananas, red plums, eggplant, tomatoes, and chicken liver. Details of the tyramine-restricted diet can be found in Chapter 19.

INTOLERANCE OF SALICYLATES

The only **salicylate** proven to cause an adverse reaction is aspirin (acetylsalicylic acid). Sensitivity to aspirin is more common among asthmatics than in the nonasthmatic population. Up to 25% of aspirin-sensitive individuals also react adversely to the azo dye *tartrazine*. However, it is not known whether aspirin and tartrazine act in the same way in the body to produce adverse reactions. Aspirin sensitivity has also been linked to sensitivity to benzoates and sulfites, but research studies have not yet confirmed such cross-reactivity.

Salicylates (but not acetylsalicylic acid) occur naturally in a large number of foods of different types. However, research studies have not proven that this source of salicylates causes adverse reactions even in aspirin-sensitive persons. The level of salicylic acid may be the determining factor in salicylate sensitivity. The daily dietary consumption of salicylate is estimated to be 10 to 200 milligrams. One dose of extra-strength aspirin provides 600 to 650 milligrams of acetylsalicylic acid, which is far more than consumed even in a meal made up of many salicylate-containing foods.

Aspirin sensitivity has been implicated in urticaria (hives), angioedema (swelling), and in triggering an asthmatic attack in asthmatics. People with asthma who are sensitive to aspirin can usually ingest the salicylates in foods without difficulty. There are no well-controlled research studies to indicate the dietary reduction of salicylates has any important effects on the course of asthma.

How Salicylate Works in the Body

Acetylsalicylic acid inhibits the cyclo-oxygenase pathway of arachidonic acid metabolism (refer to Chapter 3, page 43, for a discussion of this pathway and its importance in allergy). Prostaglandins are produced by this pathway in the allergic response. Some types of prostaglandins are responsible for causing the sensation of pain. Aspirin reduces the production of these prostaglandins, which explains the pain-reducing properties of aspirin and other analgesics that act in a similar fashion. A result of this inhibition is that the lipoxygenase pathway leading to leukotriene production may be enhanced. It is the leukotrienes that mediate the smooth muscle contraction that is the cause of bronchospasm (narrowing of the bronchi) in people who have asthma, thus explaining why many aspirin-sensitive individuals tend to be asthmatic. (Again, see Chapter 3 for a discussion of the mediators released in the allergic response.)

Symptoms of Salicylate Sensitivity

Wheezing, hives, and tissue swelling have been associated with salicylate sensitivity. Some investigators have suggested that hyperactivity in certain allergic children has been triggered or enhanced by salicylates. However, the role of salicylates in attention deficit hyperactivity disorder (ADHD) has not been proven by controlled studies. Currently, investigators are looking into the role of food components and additives in attention deficit hyperactivity disorder.

Some practitioners in the field of food intolerance recommend that although avoiding foods high in salicylates is unlikely to improve the symptoms of most aspirin-sensitive individuals, a trial on a salicylate-restricted diet might be of benefit for those who have a pronounced sensitivity to aspirin and have found no relief from other treatments. Details of the salicylate-restricted diet can be found in Chapter 20.

Intolerance of Artificial Colors: Tartrazine and Other Food Dyes

One of the most important aspects of making food appealing to the consumer is *color*. Food is unlikely to be eaten unless it has the right color. To ensure acceptance and consumption of a manufactured or processed food, the most appropriate color must be added. Ten artificial coal-tar-derived colors are allowed in foods by the U.S. Food and Drug Administration (FDA) under the Food Dye and Coloring Act (FD&C). Many other countries, including Canada, tend to follow these guidelines. Most of these colors are "generally regarded as safe" (GRAS) and have not been cited as a cause of adverse reactions. However, **tartrazine** and some of the other **azo** dyes have been implicated in some adverse reactions in highly sensitive people. "Azo" indicates that the dyes have nitrogen in their structure; the term is used in chemistry and food manufacture to distinguish these dyes from others. In the United States, tartrazine is required to be listed separately on foods or medications containing it. In Canada at the present time, this is voluntary. Other azo dyes have also been implicated in adverse reactions on a number of occasions.

Adverse Reactions Caused by Tartrazine in Sensitive People

FD&C #5 (Tartrazine) can cause symptoms resembling those of an allergic reaction. Some people who are sensitive to aspirin (acetylsalicylic acid) also may experience an adverse reaction to tartrazine. It is unclear whether dietary salicylates, which are naturally present in a large number of foods (especially fruits and vegetables), also are involved in this cross-reactivity.

Symptoms that have been reported to be caused or made worse by tartrazine and other azo dyes include asthma, urticaria (hives), nausea, migraine headaches, allergic rash (vasculitis or purpura), hyperkinesis (hyperactivity disorder), and contact dermatitis. However, none of these conditions have yet been *conclusively* proven to be caused by tartrazine in carefully controlled research studies.

How Tartrazine Works in the Body

Evidence indicates that tartrazine may initiate the release of histamine from mast cells. Because tartrazine seems to affect individuals in a manner similar to that of salicylic acid, some investigators think that it might have an inhibitory effect on the cyclo-oxygenase pathway of arachidonic acid conversion to prostanoids, but this has not been proven. See Chapter 3, page 43, for details of this pathway in releasing mediators of allergy. Chapter 21 discusses tartrazine intolerance in detail.

INTOLERANCE OF PRESERVATIVES

Any food that is required to have a shelf-life of more than one or two days will need to be treated with–or, in the case of a manufactured food, to contain–a preservative. Many foods would not be safe for human consumption after only a few hours, if preservatives were not used; for example, bread becomes moldy in 2 to 3 days without preservatives. Without preservatives, food poisoning from microbial toxins would become a vast problem. Most of the preservatives in our foods and beverages have been extensively tested for safety, after which they are granted the GRAS status. However, occasionally a sensitive individual will react adversely to a common preservative. The mechanisms responsible for sensitivity to preservatives are as yet poorly understood. The following are a few of the probable mechanisms of sensitivity to preservatives suggested by current research.

Benzoates

BENZOIC ACID AND SODIUM BENZOATE

Use in Manufactured Foods
Both benzoic acid and sodium benzoate are used to prevent spoilage by microorganisms in a wide variety of processed foods, beverages, and pharmaceuticals, thus extending their shelf life.

Benzoic acid is used up to a level of 0.1% in processed foods. It is commonly used in chocolate, lemon, orange, cherry, fruit, nut, tobacco, and other flavorings for carbonated and noncarbonated beverages, ice cream, ices, candies, baked goods, pie and pastry fillings, icings, and chewing gum. It may also be used in pickles and margarines.

Natural benzoic acid occurs in most berries (especially strawberries and raspberries), prunes, tea, spices (such as cinnamon, cloves, and anise), cherry bark (often used as a natural cherry flavor in beverages and ice creams), and cassia bark (used as a natural flavor in cola and root beer and a spice flavoring in beverages, ice cream, candy, and baked goods). It occurs in other foods at lower levels.

Sodium benzoate is often used as a preservative in margarine, codfish, bottled soft drinks, maraschino cherries, mincemeat, fruit juices, pickles, fruit jelly preserves, and jams. It may be used in the ice for cooling fish, in skin preparations such as eye creams and vanishing creams, and toothpastes.

Absorption and Excretion in the Body

Benzoic acid and sodium benzoate are rapidly absorbed in the body, combine with glycine (a component of protein) in the liver, and are excreted without any remaining in the body. The success of this process depends on a healthy functioning liver and on sufficient glycine, which is usually in abundant supply in the body.

BENZOYL PEROXIDE

Use in Manufactured Foods

Benzoyl peroxide is an effective bleaching agent that is used in the manufacture of white flour and some cheeses (especially white cheeses such as feta and blue cheeses such as Gorgonzola). Lecithin is used as an antioxidant (a substance that keeps oxygen from changing a food's color and flavor) in many prepared foods such as breakfast cereals, candies, chocolates, bread, rolls, buns, and margarines. It is commercially extracted from eggs, soybeans, and corn. Benzoyl peroxide, hydrogen peroxide, acetic or lactic acids, and sodium hydroxide are reacted with lecithin to produce hydroxylated lecithin, which disperses more readily in water and acts as a better emulsifier (an agent that allows two dissimilar ingredients to mix, e.g., oil and water) than pure lecithin.

Certain vitamins can be destroyed by benzoyl peroxide, so U.S. government regulations require that the vitamin be added when benzoyl peroxide is used in the manufacture of a food that contained the vitamin originally. An example of this is the destruction of beta carotene in milk, which is replaced when vitamin A is added to cheese made from bleached milk.

Absorption and Excretion in the Body

Benzoyl peroxide degrades almost completely to benzoic acid by the time the food is consumed. Only a small fraction of the bleach is ingested, most of which is converted in the intestine to benzoic acid or to a form that is readily excreted in the urine.

How Benzoates Cause Symptoms in Benzoate-Sensitive People

The actual way benzoate works in the body is unknown, but evidence suggests that the cyclo-oxygenase pathway of arachidonic acid metabolism (see Chapter 3, page 43) may be affected. Persons sensitive to aspirin are particularly vulnerable to benzoate sensitivity.

Adverse Reactions Due to Benzoates

Conditions reported to be triggered or made worse by benzoates include asthma, urticaria (hives), angiodema (tissue swelling), rhinitis (nasal congestion due to hay fever), and headaches. Persons with existing Type I hypersensitivity reactions (atopic allergy) may be particularly vulnerable to benzoate sensitivity. Benzoic acid can be a mild irritant to the skin, eyes, and mucous membranes. Its adverse effects can increase when it is combined with other additives.

Recommendations for Persons Sensitive to Benzoates

Each individual differs in their sensitivity to chemicals such as benzoates. Consequently, it is not possible to define a limit of benzoate intake that will apply to every benzoate-intolerant person. The general directive is to restrict or avoid as much as possible any foods known to contain benzoates.

BENZYL AND BENZOYL COMPOUNDS

A large number of benzyl and benzoyl compounds are allowed in foods. Examples of these include benzyl acetate, alcohol, ether, butyrate, cinnamate, formate, propionate, salicylate, among others. On food labels, the ingredient will include the words *benzyl* or *benzoyl*. Most of these compounds are used as synthetic flavorings and perfumes in a wide variety of processed and manufactured foods, beverages, chewing gum, soaps, hair sprays, hair dyes, skin creams, sunscreens, perfumes, and cosmetics.

Some benzyl compounds are skin irritants and can cause hives and contact dermatitis. Others are digestive-tract irritants and can cause intestinal upset, vomiting, and diarrhea. In very high concentrations they can have a narcotic effect. A few benzyl compounds cause irritation of the eyes when applied to the face and respiratory symptoms when inhaled.

PARABENS

Paraben compounds are sometimes used as preservatives in foods to prevent the growth of molds and yeast. They are used in baked goods, sugar substitutes, and in artificially sweetened jams, mincemeat, milk preparations, soft drinks, packaged fish, meat, and poultry, and fats and oils. They are also used in frozen dairy desserts and many milk products. Persons who are sensitive to benzoates might also react to parabens because paraben's metabolism may mimic that of benzoate in the later stages. There are no naturally occurring parabens; they are manufactured in the laboratory for use as preservatives in a variety of processes.

On food labels, parabens are indicated by the words *methyl p-hydroxybenzoate* or *propyl p-hydroxybenzoate*. Parabens are used in processed vegetables, baked goods, fats, oils, and seasonings. They may be present in foods such as cakes, pies, pastries, icings, fillings, fruit products (sauces, juices, salads, syrups, preserves, jellies), syrups, olives, and pickles, and in beverages such as beers, ciders, and carbonated beverages.

Management of benzoate sensitivity and the benzoate-restricted diet are discussed in Chapter 22.

Intolerance of Butylated Hydroxyanisole (BHA) and Butylated Hydroxytoluene (BHT)

BHA and BHT are antioxidants that are used as preservatives to prevent or delay fats, oils, and fat-containing foods from becoming rancid and developing objectionable tastes and odors. They are often used with other antioxidants in a variety of manufactured foods.

Role of BHA and BHT in Adverse Reactions to Foods

Controlled trials have indicated that these chemicals may induce urticaria (hives). Extremely high doses of BHA and BHT have consistently resulted in considerable enlargement of the liver in experimental animals. They may affect both kidney and liver functions. There is evidence of an adverse effect on the brain of experiment animals, resulting in abnormal behavior patterns. These additives have been implicated in trials on hyperactivity behavior in children, but several investigators question the result of these studies. The precise mechanism of the physiological response in sensitivity to BHA and BHT is still unclear. Individuals with food allergies are reported to be the population most sensitive to these chemicals.

The United Nations Joint FAO/WHO Expert Committee on Food Additives suggested that daily ingestion of BHA and BHT should not exceed a total of 0.5 milligrams per kilogram of body weight (34 milligrams for a 150-pound adult). Individuals who are sensitive to BHA and BHT should limit their daily intake to a much lower amount than this. The directive is to *avoid these preservatives completely* by careful reading of food labels.

Use of BHA and BHT in Foods

BHA and/or BHT are frequently used as preservatives in vegetable oils and foods cooked in or containing vegetable oils such as potato chips, nut meats, doughnuts, pastries, pie crusts, breakfast cereals, baked goods, dehydrated potatoes, dried fruits, and dry yeast. Other foods that may contain the preservatives include canned and bottled beverages, lard, shortening, ice cream, animal fats, candies, unsmoked dry sausage, chewing gum, enriched rice, gelatin desserts, cake mixes, soup bases, glacé fruits, potato and sweet potato flakes, and dry dessert mixes.

INTOLERANCE OF SULFITES

Sensitivity to sulfites, which are used as food preservatives, is most common in asthmatics. Steroid-dependent asthmatics are the population most at risk for sulfite sensitivity. Although adverse reaction to sulfites is estimated to be as high as 1% of the U.S. population, sulfite sensitivity in nonasthmatics is quite rare. Symptoms have been reported to occur in most organ systems, including the lungs, gastrointestinal tract, and the skin and mucous membranes. Very rarely, life-threatening anaphylactic reactions in asthmatics have been recorded. There is no evidence that avoiding all sources of dietary sulfites improves asthma. For individuals who are *not* sensitive to sulfites, exposure to sulfiting agents poses very little risk. Toxicity studies in volunteers showed that ingestion of 400 milligrams of sulfites daily for 25 days did not produce any adverse effects.

How Sulfites Cause Symptoms

Respiratory symptoms are thought to be caused by sulfur dioxide, which acts as a direct irritant on hypersensitive airways. Sulfur dioxide is formed from sulfuric acid when the sulfite dissolves. Asthmatic subjects can experience significant bronchospasm after inhaling as little as 1.0 part per million of sulfur dioxide. There are published reports of observations that wheezing, flushing, and other symptoms of asthma have been induced in a person who inhaled vapors from a bag of dried apricots; dried fruits are usually treated with sulfite in order to preserve the color.

An IgE-mediated reaction has been suggested, in which the sulfite acts as a hapten combining with a body protein to form a neoantigen that elicits antigen-specific IgE. (Refer to Chapter 3, page 42, for an explanation). However, because levels of IgE, eosinophils, and histamine are normal in most people who show sulfite sensitivity, IgE-mediated reactions are considered to be unlikely or at least very rare.

A deficiency in the enzyme *sulfite oxidase,* which converts sulfite to the inert sulfate, has been suggested as a possible cause of abnormally high levels of sulfites in the body, which may lead to an adverse reaction. However, this hypothesis has not yet been substantiated.

Use of Sulfites in Foods and Medications

Sulfites are used as preservatives in beverages, fruits, vegetables, prepared and presliced foods, and packaged snack foods where they prevent multiplication of harmful microorganisms. They are used to control browning in foods such as potatoes, apples, coconut, dehydrated vegetables, dried fruits, white wines, white grape juice, and some vinegars. Sulfites are used to texturize dough, especially frozen pizza doughs and pie shells. They act as bleaching agents, particularly in the production of maraschino cherries, glacé fruits, and citron peel. In addition, sulfites occur naturally in many foods, including wines, because of their presence in grapes, and they are used to terminate fermentation in the production of wines and other alcoholic beverages that depend on careful control of the fermentation process.

Some medications, including inhalable and injectable drugs, contain sulfites, where they act as antioxidants. Some forms of epinephrine (adrenaline) contain sulfite as a preservative. However, epinephrine's role in controlling a potentially life-threatening anaphylactic reaction is more important than the possibility of an adverse reaction to the sulfite. Therefore, administration of epinephrine in anaphylactic emergencies is advised despite the risk of an adverse reaction to the sulfite in the medication.

Avoiding Food Sources of Sulfites

Sulfites in foods are *not destroyed by cooking.* Because sulfites can bind to several substances in foods, such as protein, starch, and sugars, they *may not be removed by washing.* Therefore, a person sensitive to sulfites is advised to avoid **all** food sources of sulfites, whether they are washed or not. A test kit is available commercially for the detection of sulfites in foods (Sulfitest). However, there are problems in the sensitivity of the test and frequent false negative reactions make its use risky. Sulfite-sensitive people need to be aware of this.

Sulfates

Sulfates do not cause the same adverse reactions as sulfites. They are inert in the body and need not be avoided by persons who are sensitive to sulfites. Information on the management of sulfite sensitivity and the sulfite-restricted diet can be found in Chapter 23.

INTOLERANCE OF MONOSODIUM GLUTAMATE (MSG)

Monosodium glutamate (MSG), a flavoring common in Chinese cooking, is increasingly being used to flavor Western foods. In addition, some foods, such as tomatoes, mushrooms, and cheese, contain *natural* glutamate, which can have the same effect as MSG in sensitive persons. People who are sensitive to MSG report a variety of symptoms that are usually classified as "Chinese restaurant syndrome" (also known as Kwok's syndrome).

Symptoms Reported to be Caused by MSG

The symptoms reported to be caused by sensitivity to MSG are many and varied. They include tightness around the face, jaw, and chest, numbness of the face, tingling and burning of the face and chest, rapid heartbeat, nausea, diarrhea, stomach cramps, headache (especially at the back of head and neck), weakness, dizziness, balance problems, staggering, confusion, slurred speech, blurring of vision, difficulty focusing, seeing shining lights, chills, shakes, excessive perspiration, difficulty in breathing, asthma (in asthmatics), water retention, thirst, depression, paranoia, insomnia, sleepiness, stiffness, heaviness of arms and legs, and mood changes (such as irritability and depression).

Skepticism is understandable on the part of practitioners who are confronted with such a vast array of seemingly unrelated, and sometimes apparently subjective, symptoms. Experts are widely divided on the subject of MSG sensitivity. A recent review suggests that the result of a number of research studies "leads to the conclusion that 'Chinese Restaurant Syndrome' is an anecdote applied to a variety of postprandial [occurring after a meal] illnesses: rigorous and realistic scientific evidence linking the syndrome to MSG could not be found."[1] On the other hand, other clinicians have estimated that the prevalence of "Chinese restaurant syndrome" may be as high as 1.8% of the North American adult population.[2]

---

[1] L. Tarasoff and M.F. Kelly, "Monosodium L-glutamate: A Double-Blind Study and Review." *Food Chemistry and Toxicology* 31, no.12 (1993): 1019-1035.

[2] G. Kerr, M. Wu-Lee, and M. El-Lozy, "Prevalence of the 'Chinese Restaurant Syndrome.'" *Journal of the American Dietetic Association* 75 (1979): 29-33.

How MSG Causes Symptoms

MSG is made up of sodium and the amino acid *glutamic acid*. Glutamate ions are the active ingredients in MSG. One gram of glutamate is equivalent to 1⅓ grams of MSG. Glutamate usually enters the body as part of a food protein where it is linked to a number of other amino acids. Before glutamate is incorporated into the body, the linkages to other amino acids (peptide bonds) have to be broken by enzymes. This is a gradual process, and the level of free glutamate in the body is thus kept at a tolerated level at all times. However, if the glutamate enters the body already free from other amino acids, which happens when MSG is consumed, it is rapidly absorbed and passes easily into circulation. Consequently, the level of glutamate in the body rises to levels much higher than that from food sources not containing MSG.

One of the most creditable theories put forth to explain the mechanism of action of MSG suggests that because glutamate acts as a precursor (building block) for the neurotransmitter acetylcholine (as well as a number of other physiological chemicals in the body), the symptoms ascribed to MSG sensitivity may be caused by excessively high levels of neurotransmitters, which reach toxic levels in a very short period of time. According to this theory of "neurotransmitter toxicity," when MSG is eaten, free glutamate enters the bloodstream at a high level and very rapidly because no peptide bonds need to be broken by enzymes. Biochemical studies have shown that after a dose of MSG (0.1 gram per kilogram of body weight) in water, glutamate can increase to peak concentrations greater than 15 times that of the usual level of glutamate in blood (there is always a small quantity there) in approximately one hour. Because acetylcholine acts on the brain and central nervous system, the symptoms of the Chinese restaurant syndrome may be explained on the basis of an abnormally high level of acetylcholine. However, a correlation between the level of glutamate in the blood and symptoms has not been demonstrated, so this theory still requires validation.

Some practitioners have noticed a vitamin B6 (pyridoxine) deficiency in a number of their MSG-sensitive patients; this may be an additional factor contributing to a less efficient metabolism of glutamate.

MSG-sensitive individuals are advised to restrict their intake of this flavor additive. Alcohol seems to increase the rate of absorption of many foods, including MSG, so drinking alcoholic beverages at the same time as eating foods containing MSG increases the severity and rate of onset of the symptoms considerably. Eating foods containing MSG on an empty stomach also seems to increase the adverse effects of MSG. Symptoms are usually reported to occur about 30 minutes after eating a meal high in MSG. Asthma has been reported to occur 1 to 2 hours after MSG ingestion and even as long as 12 hours later.

Sources of MSG

A number of flavorings owe their taste enhancement to MSG and may be indicated on labels as Accent, Zest, Vetsin, Ajinomoto, Kombu extract, Subu, Mei-jing, Wei-jing, Gourmet powder, Chinese seasoning, Glutavene, RL-50, Glutacyl, hydrolyzed vegetable protein (HVP), hydrolyzed plant protein (HPP), natural flavoring (may be HVP), or simply "flavoring." Glutamate is also present in *monopotassium glutamate, monoammonium glutamate, calcium glutamate,* and other salts of glutamic acid. Some sensitive individuals may react to these salts also. Many prepared foods contain MSG or one of the above flavorings, and they may be used in restaurant meals under any of the above names.

Dietary management of MSG sensitivity is discussed in Chapter 26.

Table 4-1

EXAMPLES OF THE FACTORS MOST FREQUENTLY IMPLICATED IN FOOD INTOLERANCE REACTIONS

Intolerance Factors	Site of Action	Symptoms Associated with Intolerance	Types of Foods Represented	Discussion and Management
Carbohydrates: Disaccharides: Lactose Sucrose Maltose	Digestive tract	Excessive gas Abdominal bloating, abdominal pain Diarrhea, loose stool Occasional nausea	Sugars Starches Polysaccharides	Disaccharide intolerance: Chapter 18 (pages 000–000) Lactose intolerance: Chapter 8 (pages 000–000)
Biogenic Amines Histamine	May be circulating in blood (systemic) but can affect tissues as it settles in one area or one organ system (localized)	Skin (hives, angioedema, itching, reddening) Mucous membranes (itching, swelling), reddening) Headaches Digestive-tract disturbances	Fermented foods Alcoholic beverages Some fruits Some spices Some artificial colors	Chapter 19 (page 233)

Table 4-1 (continued)
EXAMPLES OF THE FACTORS MOST FREQUENTLY IMPLICATED IN FOOD INTOLERANCE REACTIONS

Intolerance Factors	Site of Action	Symptoms Associated with Intolerance	Types of Foods Represented	Discussion and Management
Tyramine		Migraine headache Hives Itching	Fermented foods Alcoholic beverages (e.g., red wine) Vinegars Yeast extract Some vegetables and fruits Chicken liver	Chapter 19 (page 233)
Salicylates	Systemic: Inhibition of cyclo-oxygenase pathway and imbalance in inflammatory mediators	Hives Angioedema Asthma in asthmatics People sensitive to aspirin at particular risk for developing symptoms of intolerance	Most naturally occurring in a variety of foods, including Many fruits and vegetables Some spices	Chapter 20 (page 255)

Table 4-1 (continued)

EXAMPLES OF THE FACTORS MOST FREQUENTLY IMPLICATED IN FOOD INTOLERANCE REACTIONS

Intolerance Factors	Site of Action	Symptoms Associated with Intolerance	Types of Foods Represented	Discussion and Management
Artificial Colors Tartrazine and other azo dyes	Systemic: Inhibition of cyclo-oxygenase pathway and imbalance in inflammatory mediators Release of histamine	Asthma in asthmatics, especially in aspirin-sensitive asthmatics Hives Nausea Headaches Rashes Hyperactivity in a few sensitive individuals	Manufactured foods Do not occur naturally	Chapter 21 (page 265)
Benzoates	Unknown Suggested to be due to inhibition of the cyclo-oxygenase pathway and imbalance in inflammatory mediators	Asthma in asthmatics Hives Angioedema Nasal congestion Headache Skin irritation (contact dermatitis) Digestive-tract disturbances	Manufactured foods as: Antimicrobial preservatives Color preservatives Bleaching agent Naturally occurring in foods such as: Berries Cinnamon and a few other spices Tea Prunes	Chapter 22 (page 277)

Table 4-1 (continued)

EXAMPLES OF THE FACTORS MOST FREQUENTLY IMPLICATED IN FOOD INTOLERANCE REACTIONS

Intolerance Factors	Site of Action	Symptoms Associated with Intolerance	Types of Foods Represented	Discussion and Management
Butylated hydroxyanisole (BHA) Butylated hydroxytoluene (BHT)	Unknown	Usually skin reactions, such as hives	Manufactured foods as Antioxidants for delaying rancidity in fats, oils, and fat-containing foods Often used in treatment of food packaging materials (e.g., cereal packaging)	Chapter 24 (page 301)
Sulfites	Systemic and local	Asthma in asthmatics Reactions in skin and mucous membranes Anaphylaxis in asthmatics	Manufactured foods as Antimicrobial preservative, especially on grapes where mold occurs naturally Color preservative, to control browning especially in dried fruits, cut potatoes, apples, coconut	Chapter 23 (page 287)

Table 4-1 (continued)

EXAMPLES OF THE FACTORS MOST FREQUENTLY IMPLICATED IN FOOD INTOLERANCE REACTIONS

Intolerance Factors	Site of Action	Symptoms Associated with Intolerance	Types of Foods Represented	Discussion and Management
Sulfites (continued)			Bleaching agent in maraschino cherries, glacé fruits, and citron peel Texturizer, especially for frozen uncooked dough Fermentation control in manufacture of wine and other alcoholic beverages	
Monosodium glutamate (MSG)	Systemic	Suggest involvement of the central nervous system, such as Flushing Facial numbness Tingling and numbness in hands and feet Tightening of the chest	Manufactured foods with "added flavor" Added as a flavor enhancer to cooked natural foods	Chapter 26 (page 313)

| | | | Table 4-1 (continued) | |
EXAMPLES OF THE FACTORS MOST FREQUENTLY IMPLICATED IN FOOD INTOLERANCE REACTIONS				
Intolerance Factors	Site of Action	Symptoms Associated with Intolerance	Types of Foods Represented	Discussion and Management
Monosodium glutamate (MSG) (continued)		Dizziness Balance problems Blurring of vision Visual disturbances "Psychological" reactions Asthma in asthmatics Digestive-tract disturbances	Glutamates occur naturally in some foods, such as Cheeses Mushrooms Tomatoes	

— CHAPTER 5 —

DIAGNOSIS OF
FOOD SENSITIVITIES

One of the most difficult problems faced by both doctors and patients is the diagnosis of food sensitivities. The patient is aware that whenever he or she eats, symptoms develop–sometimes immediately–often several hours later. The symptoms may be severe, especially if they happen immediately after eating, or quite mild, which is a common experience if they are delayed for an hour or more after the meal. The symptoms can vary considerably from patient to patient. Some people experience tingling in the mouth, throat tightening, and perhaps a tightness in the chest and breathing difficulty. Others may have swelling of tissues of the face and around the mouth, often accompanied by itching and hives. An asthmatic may have an asthma attack. Other people may experience digestive-tract upset, with nausea, abdominal pain, bloating, and diarrhea. Someone else may develop a migraine headache, and another will have rather vague symptoms of being unwell, feeling light-headed and "out of it." And what can be most confusing is that *all of these people could be reacting to the same food*. Furthermore, the same symptoms, perhaps facial swelling and hives, could be caused by quite different, unrelated foods in different people. This is indeed a dilemma because we are all used to diseases in which one cause results in the same symptoms in whomever is affected: for example, the influenza virus causing common symptoms of "flu," the rubella virus causing German measles, or the pertussis bacterium causing whooping cough.

Having read Chapters 2, 3, and 4, you are now aware that foods, components of foods, and food additives are all capable of causing symptoms in susceptible people. You are also aware that the processes in the body that are responsible for the symptoms–whether they are due to a reaction of the immune system or to intolerance mechanisms not related to immune responses–are diverse and different. It should therefore not surprise you to learn that a single test would be incapable of diagnosing all of these reactions. And there is the dilemma. How can a doctor determine precisely which food or foods are causing your symptoms, if he or she does not have the tool to do the job–the test that will tell you exactly what it is you are reacting to? The answer is that many tests have been developed to identify the food components that are triggering your symptoms, but all of them have the drawback that they are looking for only one mechanism each. Your symptoms could be caused by other processes that are not being tested, or could be caused by a combination of several distinct mechanisms. This chapter will discuss the tests available to clinicians who are trying to diagnose your sensitivity to food, and then we shall discuss the limitations of each test in identifying the precise components and additives that are giving you problems.

After reading this chapter you will realize, as each of us working in this field has to do, that any test needs to be confirmed by the seemingly simple but often complex process of eliminating the suspect foods from your diet to see if your symptoms disappear, and then reintroducing each of them separately, to prove that they are triggering your symptoms. This is the primary purpose of this book–to allow you and your medical team to correctly identify the food components that are making you sick. Only after you have identified your culprit foods can you proceed to the correct, safe management of your food sensitivities.

Restrictive diets can place an enormous burden on food-allergic individuals and their families, in terms of both physical and emotional stresses. *No food should be restricted unless there is a very good reason for doing so.* Elimination of large numbers of foods from the diet is rarely necessary. Every effort must be made to diagnose food allergy exactly, and a person must replace each eliminated food with a food of equivalent nutrient value. Merely avoiding the culprit food(s) is not sufficient to maintain health. It is essential to eat a well-balanced and nutritionally complete diet. This requires a careful and systematic approach. Any number of foods or food additives could be responsible for the reactions, and symptoms can be various, occurring in different parts of the body. It is important to remember that symptoms of food allergy and intolerance, especially those in the gastrointestinal tract, can be mistaken for a variety of other abnormal conditions, so before food allergy is considered as the reason for a person's symptoms, all other causes must be ruled out.

THE IMPORTANCE OF CORRECTLY IDENTIFYING FOODS RESPONSIBLE FOR ADVERSE REACTIONS

There are several important reasons why the correct identification of the food(s) responsible for symptoms should be made:

◆ **All** the foods and food additives responsible for symptoms must be removed from the diet to control symptoms. This requires precise identification of the culprit foods.

◆ It is particularly important that the food responsible for an anaphylactic reaction be correctly identified, because all forms of the food must be strictly avoided.

◆ Restriction of foods that are *not* involved in the elicitation of symptoms is unnecessary and may be harmful in many ways. For example:
  — There are numerous reports of serious nutritional deficiencies and disease in patients who follow overly restricted diets.
  — Because food plays such an important and integral role in normal family and social life, over-restriction of the diet may seriously threaten a person's quality of life and emotional health.
  — Inappropriate reinforcement of food avoidance may lead to obsessions with food as a "threat." In extreme cases this may lead to food phobia and possible *anorexia nervosa* in vulnerable persons.

UNNECESSARY FOOD AVOIDANCE

In the past, whole groups of foods have been restricted unnecessarily because of the perception that botanical, or zoological, relatedness implied antigenic relatedness, or "cross-reactivity." The first classification of foods into botanically related families for the purpose of diagnosis of food allergy was published in 1929, and to this day many allergists continue to advise their food-allergic patients to avoid all members of a botanic family when allergy to one representative is demonstrated. In fact, most allergy textbooks still perpetuate this myth. It is common to see statements to the effect that if peanut allergy is diagnosed, all members of the *Leguminoseae* (legume family) should be carefully avoided.[1] Fortunately, modern research, using more sophisticated methods, demonstrates

---

[1] National Institute of Allergy and Infectious Diseases Task Force Report, *Adverse Reactions to Foods,* NIH publications no. 84-2442 (Bethesda, MD, 1984), p.7.

that a person is rarely allergic to more than one or two foods and, furthermore, that there is often a greater degree of antigenic relatedness between *non-botanically-related* plants than between those within the same botanic family. Research into oral allergy syndrome and latex allergy has helped expand our knowledge in this area (see Chapter 7). Each food must be assessed individually before it is identified as allergenic for each person.

LABORATORY TESTS FOR IDENTIFYING FOOD ALLERGENS

In reviewing the wide range of immunological and physiological mechanisms that are responsible for the clinical symptoms of adverse reactions to food, it is obvious that any single laboratory test cannot identify the specific food components responsible for all types of reactions. Laboratory tests are of little value on their own and can result in an incorrect diagnosis if the patient's clinical history is not considered at the same time. All tests must be confirmed by careful **elimination and challenge** of the indicated foods before the final identification is made.

The following is a summary of the tests most commonly used in the diagnosis of food allergy, with a brief appraisal of their diagnostic value.

Tests for Food-Specific IgE

The majority of tests used by allergists in the diagnosis and treatment of food allergy detect the presence of **antibodies** against foods, in particular, food-specific IgE (see Chapter 3 for a discussion on antibodies). They depend on the concept that when antibodies specific to food antigens are present, an allergic state exists. Tests for allergen-specific antibodies work well for respiratory allergy to inhaled allergens such as plant pollens, animal dander, dust and dust mites, and mold spores. Foreign antigens continuously enter the respiratory tract in each breath. The inhaled antigens in their natural state encounter cells of the immune system and are recognized as foreign. The immune system is able to distinguish between "foreign and a threat" (potentially pathogenic microorganisms) and "foreign but safe" (inhaled allergens). In allergic individuals, the former situation may trigger a Th_1 response (protection), the latter a Th_2 response (allergy); in both situations the body rejects the foreign antigen (refer to Chapter 3 for a detailed discussion of this response and its importance in allergy).

However, a similar type of response in the digestive tract, where foreign material enters with every mouthful of food or beverage, would greatly impair its functions. Antigens from foreign plants and foreign animals not only are *not* rejected, but they are allowed into the body to become an integral part of its structure and to participate in essential biochemical and physiological functions. If all foods were rejected as "foreign," starvation and death would result. At the same time as it allows foreign material into the system as food, the digestive tract must protect the body from pathogens entering with the food. In this case the immune system must reject the foreign invader. In the digestive tract therefore, the immune system functions not only as a protective barrier, but also as a selective mechanism where "foreign but safe" and "foreign and a potential threat" are clearly defined and instantly acted upon. When the distinction between the two different responses within the same system becomes disturbed for some reason, things go wrong. Scientists cannot yet explain precisely what this difference is nor what causes it to malfunction. In fact, the mechanism that is responsible for tolerance of foods is itself poorly understood. At present, tolerance is perceived as suppression of the "normal" protective immune rejection of foreign antigens.

Skin Tests

The skin test is designed to detect any **IgE** that has been made by the immune system in a previous response to the allergen. The allergen-specific IgE is sitting on the surface of **mast cells** in the skin. When the test allergen comes into contact with the IgE and bridges two adjacent molecules, inflammatory mediators are released into the surrounding skin. This results in a small swollen area at the site of application of the allergen (wheal) and spreading of histamine into an area surrounding it (flare). This is the **wheal and flare** reaction that is the cornerstone of skin testing for allergy.

The allergen may be introduced into the skin by several methods:

◆ **Prick test**—A drop of commercial allergen extract is placed onto the surface and the skin underneath is pricked with a lancet.
◆ **Scratch test**—The skin is scratched and a drop of allergen is deposited onto the site.
◆ **Intradermal test**—The allergen is injected into the skin from a syringe.

In each case, two controls without allergen are included: the positive control is a measured amount of histamine; the negative control is the medium in which the allergen is suspended, usually saline. If the negative control triggers a reaction, or if the response to the histamine control is less than 3 millimeters in diameter, all of the tests are invalid.

Although intradermal tests are considered by some practitioners to be slightly more sensitive than prick tests, they also cause more nonspecific positive responses (responses not caused by the food allergen) and may induce systemic reactions; for the latter reason, many allergists strongly advise against the use of the intradermal test because of the danger of inducing an anaphylactic reaction, which can be life-threatening.

A *positive* skin test is indicated by the development of a raised central area at the site of the reaction (called the *wheal*), surrounded by a flattened reddened area (called the *flare*). The diameter of each area is measured in millimeters and graded on a reaction scale:

◆   The most common measurement indicates the diameter of the total reaction, usually on a scale of 1+ (mild reaction) to 4+ (strong reaction).
◆   Other practitioners consider that a wheal size of not less than 3 millimeters in diameter (not including the erythema, or flare) greater than the negative control is positive; they consider anything less to be negative.
◆   Some practitioners favor different scales of measurement, resulting in values of 30, 40, or above.
◆   Others measure both wheal and flare and report the numbers separately (for example, 15 x 10 mm or 8 x 12 mm.

Estimated Accuracy of Skin Tests

Negative skin tests for IgE-mediated allergy to the highly allergenic foods such as egg, peanut, wheat, milk, fish, and tree nuts are considered to be accurate about 95% of the time. However, negative reactions to other food allergens, such as soy, have a significantly reduced rate of accuracy, and some practitioners rate them no higher than 30-50%–that is, only 30-50% of the reactions are true! *Positive* skin tests have an even lower predictive value; the most optimistic clinicians rate positive skin tests to foods at less than 50% accuracy.

Overall, routine skin tests for food allergens may be unreliable or misleading for a number of reasons. Some of the causes of *false positive* tests include the following:

◆   Patients may have IgE antibodies, but no symptoms: There is a positive skin test, but the food causes no symptoms when eaten. Some practitioners refer to this as "latent food allergy."
◆   The commercial allergen extract itself contains histamine, which elicits a positive response when introduced into the skin. Histamine release from

skin mast cells is the basis of a positive test (see page 82). This poses a particular problem with intradermal skin tests in which the histamine in the extract is actually injected into the skin and is thus more likely to elicit a wheal and flare response independent of the allergen itself.

◆ The food can cause a nonspecific ("irritant") positive skin reaction.

◆ Skin mast cells release inflammatory mediators in response to a much wider range of both immunologic and nonimmunologic stimuli compared to mast cells in other types of tissue, especially in the digestive tract. As a result, many positive skin test reactions are due to factors other than food allergen-specific IgE.

◆ In many cases, the food is eaten in a processed or cooked form that changes the nature of the proteins that make up the allergen molecules.

The form in which food molecules reach the immune system in the lining of the digestive tract (the gut associated lymphoid tissue of GALT) is in many ways quite different from that of the intact food from which allergen extracts used in tests are derived. For example, digestive processes start immediately when food enters the mouth, and they continue throughout the length of the digestive tract. This means that the food molecules are changed, and new potential antigens are uncovered, as the food progresses through the system where it encounters digestive secretions and enzymes.

It is estimated that only about one-third of patients with positive skin prick tests show clinical symptoms during food challenge. Intradermal skin tests in particular are considered to have very little value when positive. Some clinicians rate their accuracy no higher than 10%. The British pediatrician Dr. T. J. David states that "it is difficult to see a place for skin testing in the general diagnosis or management of intolerance to food or food additives."[2]

Other practitioners, especially in the United States, rate the accuracy of skin tests higher. Negative skin tests, especially, are considered to be of greater value than positive skin tests. However, there are a number of reasons for *false negative* skin tests, including:

◆ The reaction may not be mediated by IgE antibodies.

◆ The commercial allergen extract contains none of the specified allergen.

◆ The allergen has been denatured in the preparation of the extract.

---

[2] T. J. David, "Skin Tests," in *Food and Food Additive Intolerance in Childhood* (Oxford: Blackwell Scientific Publishers, 1993), pp. 244-292.

The third reason, in particular, poses a problem in the identification of plant foods that are responsible for oral allergy syndrome, or OAS. In OAS, people with known respiratory allergy to plant pollens (pollinosis) develop irritation, swelling, and reddening in oral and perioral tissues (tissues around the mouth) when eating certain raw fruits and vegetables, which, in most cases are botanically unrelated to their allergic pollen-producing plants (see Chapter 7, page 113). Commercial allergen extracts were found to be unsuitable for skin tests of the culprit food in these cases for two important reasons:

1. Unlike pollen allergens, glycoprotein food antigens are often denatured by treatment with heat, acid, and proteases (enzymes that digest proteins).
2. When plant tissues are crushed, chemicals called phenols are released to prevent microbial invasion of the damaged tissues. This leads to rapid protein denaturation, which changes the nature of the natural antigen, that is, of course, a protein.

Consequently, during preparation of the antigen for tests, the antigen is no longer in its natural form and does not elicit an immune response. To overcome this problem, the prick-to-prick skin test was developed.

Prick-to-Prick Skin Test for Raw Foods

◆   A sterile needle is inserted into the raw fruit or vegetable.
◆   The skin (usually the arm or back) of the patient is pricked with the same needle. Thus, the antigen is transferred to the skin.
◆   The site of antigen application is observed for the wheal and flare response for up to half an hour.
◆   A positive response (graded from 1+ to 4+) indicates release of inflammatory mediators from mast cells and histamine release.

Patch Tests for Delayed Hypersensitivity Reactions

There are two types of patch tests in general use for the identification of allergens responsible for distinct types of allergic reactions:

◆   Type IV (T-cell mediated) hypersensitivity reaction in contact dermatitis
◆   Delayed reactions in which prick and scratch tests for food-specific wheal and flare reactions may or may not be positive

TYPE IV HYPERSENSITIVITY

This method is commonly used to test reactivity to chemicals such as nickel and other metals; preservatives such as thimerosol, benzalkonium chloride, and parabens; constituents of medications and cosmetics, such as Balsam of Peru; detergents; perfumes; latex; and any number of materials that trigger a dermatitis on the skin surface after contact.

◆ The test material is applied to the surface of the skin in an impregnated patch, *or* an adhesive bandage is placed over the test material which is applied directly onto the skin surface.

◆ The skin is not scratched or pricked.

◆ The site is examined *twice* for an inflammatory response, typically 24 and 48 hours after application of the allergen.

◆ The patch usually remains in place for up to 72 hours. If there is no response after this time, the test is considered to be negative.

PATCH TESTS FOR DELAYED REACTIONS TO FOODS:
THE DIMETHYLSULFOXIDE TEST (DIMSOFT)

Patch tests have been in use since the 1970s in situations where conventional skin tests (prick, scratch, or intradermal) are negative, but symptoms occur after consumption of a food.

◆ The food extract is suspended in 90% dimethylsulfoxide.

◆ Dimethylsulfoxide is thought to aid in skin penetration by the food antigen.

◆ It has been suggested that the DIMSOFT allows detection of all four Gell and Coombs hypersensitivity reactions.

The tests have been employed especially with symptoms in the skin (atopic dermatitis) and in the digestive tract. Such tests have proven useful in identifying the role of foods such as cereal grains and milk in childhood gastroenteritis and eczema. The results of a study reported in 1996[3] seem to be representative of the type of responses observed: In a study of cow's milk allergy in 183 children ranging in age from 2 to 36 months:

◆ 54% of children developed symptoms following ingestion of milk, either immediately or after a delay of several hours.

---

[3] E. Isolauri, and K. Turjanmaa, "Combined Skin Prick and Patch Testing Enhances Identification of Food Allergy in Infants with Atopic Dermatitis," *Journal of Allergy and Clinical Immunology* 97, no. 1, part 1 (1996): 9-15.

◆ Skin prick tests were positive in 67% of the cases with acute onset of symptoms after milk challenge, while patch tests were generally negative.
◆ Patch tests were positive in 89% of children with delayed onset symptoms,
and skin prick tests were mostly negative in this group.

The significance, mechanism of activity, and reliability of such patch tests in the
diagnosis of delayed-onset food allergy have not been confirmed by well-controlled investigations.

Blood Tests for Food-Specific Antibody

A number of tests for detecting antibodies in blood against food allergens are
being used extensively for the diagnosis of food allergy. These include the
enzyme-linked immunosorbent assay (ELISA; see Figure 5-1) for allergen-specific IgE and IgG, particularly IgG4; the radioallergosorbent test (RAST; see Figure
5-2) for allergen-specific IgE; and FAST (fluorescence allergosorbent test). (For a
discussion of the role of IgE, IgG, and IgG4 in allergy, refer to Chapter 3, page 34.)

◆ A patient's blood serum is tested for the presence of anti-food antibodies.
◆ Since anti-food antibodies are frequently present in normal blood, the level
of antibody to each food is graded according to the laboratory standards,
usually on a scale of
— non-reactive
— low reactivity
— moderate reactivity
— high reactivity
◆ The patient is usually instructed to avoid the foods in the moderate and high
categories.
◆ Some laboratories use the Phadebas scoring method for IgE, in which case a
score of 3 or greater is considered positive.

Value of Blood Tests in Practice

There is a great debate among practitioners about how much reliance should be
placed on blood tests in identifying allergenic foods. Some argue that the tests
will not determine which foods will lead to clinical symptoms when consumed
by an individual and therefore must be followed by careful elimination and challenge of the foods that test positive before a definite diagnosis can be made.

- Known food antigen is attached to a solid base, usually in a plastic well.
- The patient's serum is poured into the well.
- If IgE antibodies matching the food antigen are present, they attach to the food antigen.
- Unattached serum is washed away.
- The "marker" unit is then added as a solution; this consists of antibody to IgE attached to an enzyme.
- If the IgE is attached to the food antigen, the anti-IgE with its attached enzyme will link to it.
- Any unattached IgE is washed away.
- The substrate on which the enzyme acts is now added to the well.
- If the enzme is in place in the well, it will act on the substrate and change it to a known product.
- This change will be identified by a change in color of a dye which is then added to the well.
- If the dye does not change color, the enzyme is not present, and it can be assumed that there is no anti-food IgE in the patient's serum.

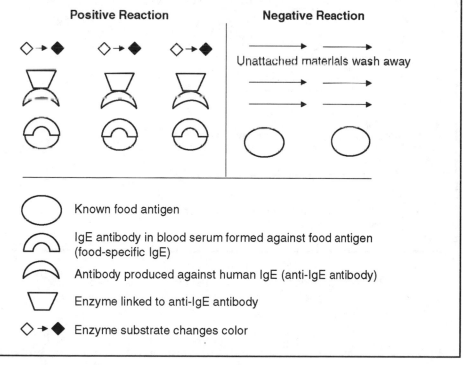

Positive Reaction   Negative Reaction

Unattached materials wash away

◯ Known food antigen

IgE antibody in blood serum formed against food antigen (food-specific IgE)

Antibody produced against human IgE (anti-IgE antibody)

Enzyme linked to anti-IgE antibody

◇ → ◆ Enzyme substrate changes color

Figure 5-1
Enzyme-Linked Immunosorbent Assay (ELISA) for Allergen-Specific IgE and IgG

- ELISA employs essentially the same "sandwich" technique as RAST.
- A known food antigen is immobilized in a plastic well.
- The patient's serum, suspected to contain anti-food IgE, is added to the well.
- If food-specific IgE is present, it will attach to the food antigen.
- Unattached IgE is washed away.
- Anti-IgE antibody is added: instead of being linked to an enzyme as in the ELISA, the "marker" in RAST is a radioactive molecule.
- If the anti-IgE antibody links to IgE, the radioactive isotope stays with it in the well after non-attached antibody and radioactive isotope are washed away.
- The radioactivity remaining in the well is then measured.

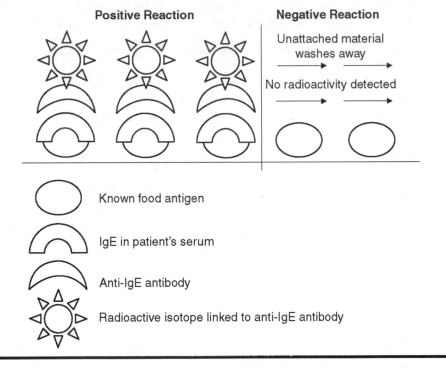

Figure 5-2
The Radioallergosorbent Test (RAST) for Allergen-Specific IgE

Laboratory tests for specific antibodies are considered by some practitioners to be of little if any practical value in the management of food intolerance unless followed by confirmation of symptoms by the suspect food.

Blood tests have traditionally been considered to be slightly less accurate than skin tests in determining IgE-mediated food reactions; however, some practitioners rate the two types of test about the same. The newer methods such as Phadebas RAST and CAP-RAST are considered to be much more sensitive than the older blood tests, and practitioners are now relying more frequently on these for identifying their patients' food allergies, especially in children.

Although percentage risk of allergy based on IgE levels has been estimated by several practitioners, most authorities agree that many atopic individuals exhibit an IgE with normal values, so no IgE level, no matter how low, rules out a food allergy diagnosis. Many practitioners have attempted to rate the risk of a food allergy by basing their estimation on the level of IgE in the blood. However, because some people have normal IgE levels in their blood, but do have "true" allergy, most authorities agree that even a low IgE might indicate allergy to food. This may be because most of the IgE is sitting on the surface of mast cells and therefore will not be circulating in the blood. It is the *IgE circulating in the blood* that is measured in the allergy blood tests.

Any positive tests should always be followed by elimination and challenge of the incriminated foods because everyone is likely to have circulating antibodies to food antigens, but only a few people will develop symptoms of allergy. Because anaphylactic reactions are mediated by IgE, many allergists believe that *any* food-specific IgE might bring on a life-threatening situation. For this reason, consumption of food in a challenge test to confirm allergy when moderate or high levels of IgE have been detected is always conducted under medical supervision in the United States. In most other countries, if the food has been eaten in the past with only mild or no symptoms, and if there is no history of anaphylaxis-like symptoms in the patient, such precautions are considered to be excessive. However, in the interests of safety, most food challenges in infants and young children should be carried out under medical supervision in an appropriately equipped facility.

Total Serum IgE

Elevated total serum IgE indicates allergy when parasitic infection has been excluded, but it does not incriminate any specific allergens and does not indicate the organ system in which symptoms (if any) are likely to occur.

Other Circulating Anti-Food Antibodies

Frequently, antibodies to several different milk proteins are commonly found in nonatopic people. Their presence does not necessarily indicate allergy, and they may be absent in persons with documented food hypersensitivity.

The presence of IgM, IgG, IgA, and IgE plasma cells that can give rise to antibodies can be detected by immunofluorescence techniques. However, because IgG, IgA and IgM, and sometimes IgE antibodies directed against food antigens can be found in the serum of food-tolerant subjects, the significance of both the plasma cells and the antibodies arising from them remains to be determined. (For a description and discussion of these antibodies, refer to Chapter 3, page 34). Currently, the presence of these cells is not considered to be of any diagnostic value on their own.

EOSINOPHIL COUNT

About 50% of patients with allergic eosinophilic gastroenteritis show the presence of eosinophils in circulating blood. **Eosinophils** are white blood cells containing the chemicals that when released cause inflammation and the symptoms of allergy (refer to Chapter 3 for a discussion of these cells).

Eosinophils may be detected in the stool of patients with

◆ dietary protein-induced enterocolitis (inflammation in the small intestine and colon)
◆ dietary protein-induced protocolitis (inflammation of the colon and rectum)
◆ allergic eosinophilic gastroenteritis (inflammation of the lining of the stomach and intestines with symptoms of nausea, diarrhea, abdominal pain, and weakness)

The presence of eosinophils in blood, tissue, or stool suggests that an allergic reaction is taking place (atopy), but it does not provide any clue as to the identity of the allergen.

INTESTINAL SIGMOIDOSCOPY AND BIOPSY
BEFORE AND AFTER FOOD CHALLENGE

These invasive techniques are used to rule out gastrointestinal pathology unrelated to food allergy, such as celiac disease, colitis, and Crohn's disease. Inflammation, villous atrophy (damage and flattening of the *villi*, protrusions that extend from the lining of the small intestine), and other injuries in the lining of the digestive tract can be identified by these methods. Microscopical examination of biopsy samples is often used in confirming a diagnosis, but will not identify the foods responsible for the reaction.

Researchers are investigating a variety of more sophisticated methods for measuring changes in intestinal cells and the products of their activity (by measurement of "tension" or pressure of liquids or gases in cells by use of an instrument called a *manometer*) in an attempt to identify ways to make a definitive diagnosis and identify the causes of diseases in the digestive tract. However, the value of these procedures has yet to be assessed and at the moment they remain within the realms of research, not clinical practice. Few researchers have investigated their use in identifying food allergy, and their value in diagnosis has yet to be determined.

Controversial Tests

A number of scientifically unproven tests are becoming very popular in the often frustrating search for a diagnosis in adverse reactions to foods. In the absence of a definitive diagnosis, many patients with chronic, recurrent complaints seek alternative care. A large number of scientifically unproven methods of detection of "food allergies" have been developed to satisfy the demand for a "quick and easy" diagnosis. Two of the most popular "noninvasive" tests include the electroacupuncture (Vega) test and biokinesiology.

VEGA TEST
The Vega test is a method of electroacupuncture that utilizes "energy waves" to indicate a person's reactivity to foods and other allergens in a vial within an electrical circuit that includes a meter to measure the degree of reactivity. Allergy to food is measured by a drop in electric current when the detection device is applied to the skin at points considered suitable for detecting food allergy (usually on a finger). By this method, practitioners also attempt to measure the activity of organ systems and endocrine glands.

BIOKINESIOLOGY OR APPLIED KINESIOLOGY
The basis of the biokinesiology test is the assumption that muscles become weak when influenced by the allergens that are causing the patient's symptoms. The allergen, contained in a vial, is held in one hand while the practitioner tests the strength of the other arm in resisting downward pressure. A weakening of resistance indicates a positive (allergic) reaction.

OTHER ALLERGY TESTS
Two excellent reviews on the current scientific status and value of other types of diagnostic tests, such as subcutaneous, intracutaneous, and sublingual provocation and neutralization, cytotoxic testing, autologous urine injections, and immune complex assays, have been published in the last decade.[4,5]

---

[4] B. J. Goldberg and M. S. Kaplan, "Controversial Concepts and Techniques in the Diagnosis and Management of Food Allergies," *Immunology and Allergy Clinics of North America* 11, no. 4 (1991): 863-884.

[5] C. Ortolani, C. Bruijnzeel-Koomen, U. Bengtsson, C. Bindslev-Jensen, B. Bjorksten, A. Host, M. Ispano, R. Jarish, C. Madsen, K. Nekam, R. Paganelli, R. Poulsen, and B. Wuthrich, "Controversial Aspects of Adverse Reactions to Food," *Allergy* 54 (1999): 27-45.

Tests for IgG

"Conventional" doctors and allergists tend to consider that the only "real" allergic reaction is the IgE-mediated immune response of a Type I hypersensitivity reaction (see Chapter 3, page 41), which they term "atopy" or "atopic allergy." However, more liberal allergists, and practitioners of what is considered alternative or complementary medicine, consider that IgG-mediated (Type III) hypersensitivity reactions (Chapter 3, page 44) may also be the cause of allergic reactions. This has led to a great deal of heated debate and disagreement among practitioners—and much confusion for patients who have consulted both types of practitioners. Because of this, we will discuss this topic in more detail so that you will have a clear idea of what the tests for IgG mean in practice and how valid they may be in identifying your "allergenic foods."

A **Type III hypersensitivity reaction** involves the production of IgG by the immune system against antigens that are not disease-causing (refer to Chapter 3, page 44 for a detailed discussion of this reaction). IgG may be produced against antigenic molecules of food when they cross from inside the intestines into blood circulation through the intestinal lining, or epithelium. The immune system is then treating the food antigens as if they might be a threat to the body. In most cases, the low level of the food and the immune system's tolerance of these harmless molecules prevent the immune system from mounting a full-scale attack on them. As a result, we often have low levels of IgG against food antigens in our bloodstreams, but we are unaware of this because we do not experience symptoms as the immune system does not react to them: In other words, the "second signal" is not received and the immune system remains quiescent (see Chapter 3, page 40 for a full discussion of this process, known as tolerance). Antibodies of both IgM and IgG types are frequently seen in babies and young children, whose intestinal linings are more highly permeable than adults', and food molecules pass through into circulation more easily.

However, because IgG can trigger a powerful immunological protective response, it is possible that some of the food-induced IgG will cause the release of inflammatory mediators as the immune system attempts to protect the body from what it now perceives to be a threat. These inflammatory mediators then act on body tissues and cause symptoms. This reaction involves the triggering of the **complement cascade,** a chain reaction involving a series of highly reactive proteins (see Chapter 3, page 45). This response takes some time, so, typically, a reaction to a food that triggers it occurs several hours after the food is eaten—sometimes 8 to 12 hours afterward. As a result, it is often extremely difficult to pinpoint the food responsible for this type of reaction because many foods have been eaten in the meantime. In contrast, a **Type I IgE-mediated**

hypersensitivity reaction (atopic allergy) occurs immediately; it may start while you are eating the meal or within a few minutes afterward. It is difficult to miss a Type I hypersensitivity to a food.

There are four subtypes of IgG; IgG1, IgG2, IgG3, and IgG4. IgG4 is considered to be the most likely antibody to induce this type of reaction to food, so, typically, blood tests for food-related IgG antibodies test for IgG4. When your doctor orders tests for anti-food antibodies, many laboratories report the level of both IgE and IgG (usually IgG4) antibodies against all the foods it is testing for. However, it is the *interpretation* of these tests that is crucial to identification of your particular food allergens. Because we all have circulating IgG to foods in our blood from time to time, but don't show any signs of it, the mere presence of the anti-food antibody is not significant. Nevertheless, if the level is high, your doctor may consider it to be a likely cause of your symptoms. However, different laboratories and doctors rate low, medium, and high at differing levels of antibody, so one clinician may interpret this differently from another.

Another confusing factor comes into play when we consider some new research. This seems to suggest that the appearance of IgG to foods in the blood may indicate a recovery from a Type I hypersensitivity reaction, particularly in people who have had previous tests indicating that they have high levels of anti-food IgE. Instead of producing IgE in an immediate Type I IgE-mediated hypersensitivity reaction (atopic allergy), the patient's immune system is now producing IgG. What this means is that their immune system has switched from an allergic (atopic) Th2 response to a more "normal" Th1 reaction (again, refer to Chapter 3, page 41 for a discussion of this topic and an understanding of the significance of these reactions). This can be an indication that the patient is no longer at risk of a potentially life-threatening IgE-mediated anaphylactic reaction. In children, it may indicate that the child has outgrown their early food allergy. Their immune system has matured, and they are now responding with a Th1 rather than the "allergic" Th2 response (page 44).

So, what is the answer? What is the significance of anti-food antibodies, and should people have these tests? The answer is the same as all others in this book: The only way to accurately determine if the food is causing your symptoms is to remove it from your diet for a period of time, and see if your symptoms disappear. Reintroduce (challenge) it in the controlled fashion that you will learn later, and see if it causes your symptoms to reappear. Allergy tests may help you in choosing the most likely candidates, but elimination and challenge is the *only* way to determine the validity of any allergy test and to find out exactly what is causing your particular adverse reactions to foods.

Status of Tests for Food Allergy and Intolerance: Current Opinions

The current opinion among European allergists is summarized in a position paper published in 1999.[6] These clinicians and researchers indicate that many doctors rely on tests such as skin, blood (antibody) tests, and others, for the diagnosis of adverse reactions to foods. They state: "In reality, no test designed to establish allergy/intolerance carried out on a patient (*in vivo*) or in the laboratory (*in vitro*) will of itself allow one to formulate this diagnosis with certainty. The diagnostic accuracy of currently available tests is low, and for some tests there are no studies on diagnostic sensitivity and specificity." They conclude that the only reliable way to determine that a patient's symptoms are caused by an adverse reaction to a food, food component, or food additive is elimination and challenge. This conclusion is supported by American allergists,[7] who agree that diagnostic tests indicate which foods are likely to be the cause of the allergic symptoms, but that elimination and challenge is necessary to support the diagnosis.

The *only* definitive diagnostic test presently available for the detection of specific foods, food components, and food additives that are responsible for food sensitivity reactions is the **elimination and challenge procedure.** The process involves the use of a diet diary or food record, followed by exclusion diets and oral provocation. The oral provocation test is the "gold standard" due to the fact that we cannot make the diagnosis only with a skin test or a blood test. Even in some immediate-onset (anaphylactic type) allergies, both tests may be negative.

Elimination and Challenge Procedure

Suspected foods and additives are eliminated from the diet for a specific period of time. The restricted foods are selected on the basis of food-intake diaries, medical history, and appropriate tests. When improvement is achieved (usually within 4 weeks), a sequential incremental dose challenge is instituted to identify the specific food components responsible for the reactions. The flow chart in Figure 5-3 summarizes this process. Finally, a diet is developed that restricts the

---

6 C. Ortolani, et al., "Controversial Aspects of Adverse Reaction to Food," *Allergy* 54 (1999): 27-45.
7 H.A. Sampson, "Food Allergy, Part 2: Diagnosis and Management," *Journal of Allergy and Clinical Immunology* 103 (1999): 981-989.

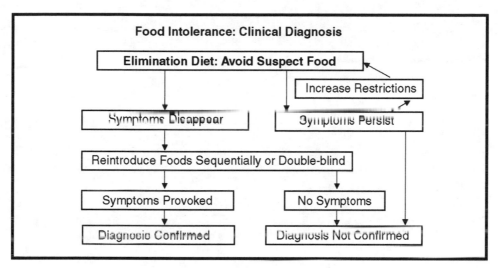

Figure 5-3
Flow Chart

intake of the "reactive foods" and provides complete, balanced nutrition from alternative sources. Detailed instructions for this procedure are provided in Chapters 27 and 28.

Ultimate Goal

The final goal is always the same: The food responsible for the symptoms must be correctly identified and avoided, and foods of equivalent nutrient must be substituted. This may require major adjustments in lifestyle and certainly in food choices, but the ultimate reward of improved health and quality of life will justify all the time and effort that has gone into detecting foods that cause adverse reactions and developing a nutritionally balanced and satisfying diet.

— CHAPTER 6 —

THE ALLERGENIC POTENTIAL OF FOODS

To what extent should a person who has a known food allergy avoid the culprit food? For example, if someone is allergic to soy, should he or she eliminate *all* forms of soy from the diet, including hydrolyzed soy protein, lecithin made from soy, fermented soy (soy sauce), and so on? This is a question that few practitioners can answer with certainty. So, for safety, the allergic person is usually advised to avoid all forms of the food, even when this may lead to a great deal of work, possible nutritional deficiency, social and economic stress, annoyance, and fear, especially when foods are inadequately labeled as to the source of the ingredients.

Authorities in the field seem to agree that someone who is *mildly* allergic to a food needs to take less stringent precautions in detecting the food as a "hidden ingredient" than if the food is likely to cause a life-threatening anaphylactic reaction. The degree to which an allergic person will react to a food allergen depends on a number of factors, especially the atopic (allergic) potential of the person and the allergenic potency of the food. **Egg, cow's milk, soy, and peanut proteins** in babies and young children; **peanut, tree nuts, shellfish, and fin fish** in adults tend to be the foods that are most likely to cause a severe, and sometimes anaphylactic, reaction in hypersensitive people. *All sources of these foods should be strictly avoided if the allergic person has shown signs of an anaphylactic reaction to them.* What about other foods that may not have triggered an anaphylactic reaction, but are known to cause symptoms of allergy, albeit mild ones? How do we determine the degree of vigilance required in avoiding the food, and how do we assess its potential to trigger a life-threatening reaction in the future? Before we can answer these questions, we need to know exactly what a food allergen is.

WHAT IS A FOOD ALLERGEN?

This is a question that many scientists have tried to answer, but at the present time we do not have a precise definition, only that a **food allergen** is "an antigen present in a food that causes an allergic reaction." (Just a reminder to the reader that an **antigen** is the part of the food that triggers the immune system to respond as if the food were capable of causing a disease.) Several controversial aspects of food allergy present difficulties in reaching consensus on a precise definition:

◆ There is a lack of agreement about the frequency, severity, and symptoms caused by foods.

◆ Some food-induced reactions persist for years, whereas others do not. The majority of children outgrow most of their early food allergies by the age of five years.

◆ The target organ for many food allergies varies from person to person: The same food can induce a reaction in entirely different organ systems in different people. For example, cow's milk protein may induce digestive tract symptoms in one child, atopic dermatitis (skin rash) in another, and an anaphylactic reaction in a third child.

◆ Some foods are more common in provoking allergic reactions than others that are very similar. For example, peanut has a greater allergic potential than lentil, although both are legumes.

◆ Immunological processes other than Type I hypersensitivity (IgE-mediated) reactions can trigger allergy to food. Many clinicians restrict their definition of allergy to those reactions that can be proven to be triggered by IgE (refer to Chapter 3, page 41, for a discussion of these reactions).

Because most traditional allergists define food allergy as an immediate-onset IgE-mediated reaction, a food allergen is usually defined as "a food component that induces the production of, and reacts with, IgE antibodies to cause mediator release from mast cells and basophils resulting in an immediate hypersensitivity reaction" (for details, again refer to Chapter 3). These characteristics allow scientists to identify, separate, and study the food component. Once they isolate the antigen/allergenic component, they can determine its structure and molecular characteristics.

Scientists are beginning to determine the structure of some specific molecules that cause the immune system to produce IgE antibodies. This is certainly increasing our understanding of what an allergenic food component looks like. However, there is still not enough scientific data to determine why one particular molecule rather than another will trigger an allergic reaction or why one person will respond to the molecule while another does not.

CHARACTERISTICS OF FOOD ALLERGENS

Chemical Structure

Most food allergens are either proteins or glycoproteins. **Glycoproteins** are proteins in which a carbohydrate chain is attached to the protein or peptide structure. Another frequent characteristic of allergens is that they tend to be soluble in water. Although huge numbers of different proteins and glycoproteins are consumed in the diet, only a few are capable of causing an allergic reaction. In addition, only *sensitized* persons will show symptoms of allergy. A person who is **sensitized** to an allergen is one whose immune system has responded to that same specific allergen in the past and treated the food as if it were going to cause disease in the body—in other words, the food is deemed "foreign and a threat." Most food is considered "foreign but safe," and the immune system leaves it alone. The latter situation is called **tolerance.**

Haptens

A few nonprotein molecules can cause an allergic response; these are called **haptens.** Haptens are small molecules and may even be inorganic compounds or elements such as nickel. Haptens become allergens when they attach to a protein. The "carrier protein" with its attached molecule forms a new antigen, or **neoantigen.** The carrier protein may be part of the food in which the hapten exists, or it may be a protein from the body, to which the hapten attaches itself after it is consumed. The neoantigen is then capable of triggering a Type I hypersensitivity response, leading to allergy. The IgE antibodies are specific to the hapten part of the new antigen; therefore, if the hapten is nickel or sulfite, the IgE is produced against the nickel or sulfite, not against the protein to which it is attached.

Attributes of Food Allergens

In order for a molecule to initiate a Type I hypersensitivity reaction (allergic response), it must have the following attributes:

◆ The molecule must be the appropriate *size* to bridge two adjacent IgE molecules on the surface of the mast cell. The **mast cell** is the key to allergy: It contains the **inflammatory mediators** that are responsible for the symptoms of allergy. These are released in the process called **degranulation**

when the mast cell is activated by IgE attached to its own allergen. The molecule must have a molecular weight of between 10,000 and 80,000 daltons. However, much smaller molecules may be allergenic when they act as haptens. The neoantigen formed when the hapten combines with a carrier protein is the correct size to bridge two IgE molecules.

◆ Two or more antigenic sites along the length of the protein molecule must be available for attaching to two adjacent IgE molecules. This may depend on the *shape* of the allergenic molecule because it needs to form a bridge between the two IgE molecules. The wrong shape would not fit properly.

◆ The molecule must pass the barrier of the intestinal lining in order to reach cells of the immune system. Proteins over 80,000 daltons in molecular weight are unlikely to pass through a healthy mucosa. The increased mucosal permeability resulting from certain conditions (e.g., intestinal inflammation; immaturity in young infants), however, may allow much larger molecules to pass through.

◆ The molecule must retain its allergenicity through various food-processing treatments. Many food allergens are heat- and acid-stable.

◆ The molecule must survive the digestive process and reach the intestinal lining in an immunogenic form. This means that it must be resistant to the effects of digestive **enzymes** that would break it down in the acidic environment of the stomach.

Function of Allergenic Molecules in Foods

Many laboratories are studying the molecule structure and characteristics of food allergens after they have been separated from the whole food. By a variety of analytical methods, researchers have determined the size (measured in kilodaltons, kD) and the activity of the antigenic component of the food. Based on this data, they have been able to assume or suggest the possible function of the molecule in the food. Several important allergens have been separated and studied in this way. These will be discussed in more detail in Chapter 7. This type of research has become important in recent years because of the growing number of novel, genetically engineered foods being produced all over the world. Because of the potential for incorporating allergens into, or developing new allergenic molecules within, the new species, methods for their detection need to be available to scientists. Most of the research into the function of the allergenic molecules has been carried out on plants.

Proteins consist of amino acids linked together to form the specific protein coded for in the DNA of the plant or animal. Up to 22 different amino acids combine in numerous different sequences to form all of the proteins in nature.

Based on the amino acid structure of the allergenic molecules, current research indicates that a surprisingly small number of amino acid sequences within the enormous range of proteins in plant foods can initiate a hypersensitivity response of the immune system. Furthermore, the functions of these proteins within the plant seem to be restricted to a very small number of categories. These include

◆ Seed storage proteins, especially in nuts, seeds, and cereal grains. These are proteins that are stored in seeds to allow them to germinate and grow.

◆ Enzyme inhibitors that may be destructive to storage components. For example, inhibitors of alpha amylase, the enzyme that breaks down plant starch, might break down starches, and the enzyme trypsin might destroy proteins in cereal grains.

◆ Structural proteins–the proteins that make up the structures of plants and allow them to keep their shape (in contrast to storage proteins).

◆ Regulatory proteins, such as profilins, that are important in plant fertilization.

◆ Pathogenesis-related proteins, which are involved in the defense-related activities of the plant and allow it to combat plant-destroying microorganisms and some chemicals.

It appears that many of the food allergens belong to the class of proteins called **albumins.** Albumins tend to be storage proteins in animals, fish, and plants. Eggs of all species contain ovalbumin; milk of all species contains lactalbumin; fish contain parvalbumin; and plants contain seed storage albumins. Because a great deal of our plant foods come from seeds (grains, flour, peas, beans, lentils, nuts, seeds), many plant albumins are consumed by most of us daily. Albumins from different species are distinct, so allergy to one species does not predict allergy to another even within the same genus. Albumins are resistant to a variety of adverse conditions. For example, they tend to resist enzymes that break down proteins, such as trypsin, chymotrypsin, and pepsin, which are released in the digestive tract to digest food proteins. They also tend to be highly resistant to heat and survive cooking temperatures as high as 88°C (190°F). For more information on allergenic proteins in plants, refer to Chapter 7.

FOODS MOST FREQUENTLY ASSOCIATED WITH ALLERGY

Although any food protein can be potentially allergenic, relatively few are known to cause most allergic reactions. In addition, *an allergenic protein can induce an allergic reaction only in an atopic person who has been sensitized to it.* Most of the severe allergic reactions to food occur in response to a surprisingly small number of foods. The foods most commonly associated with allergic reactions in **children** are **milk, egg, wheat, soy, peanut, tree nuts, fish, and shellfish.** Allergies to milk, egg, wheat, and soy are usually outgrown in early childhood. **Adults** tend to experience allergic reactions to foods that persist as allergens beyond infancy; these are **peanuts, tree nuts, shellfish, and certain species of fish.**

Lists of the most common allergenic foods vary according to the source of the data. In general, the "top eight" allergenic foods include

1. Peanut and peanut products
2. Soy and soy products
3. Egg and egg products
4. Milk and milk products
5. Tree nuts and tree nut products, the most allergenic of which are
   — Almond
   — Brazil nut
   — Cashew
   — Filbert (hazelnut)
   — Macadamia
   — Pecan
   — Pine nut
   — Pistachio
   — Walnut
6. Fish and fish products (not all species have the same allergic potential)
7. Shellfish: crustaceans (shrimp, prawn, lobster, crab, crayfish or crawfish) and mollusks (clam, mussel, oyster, scallop)
8. Wheat and wheat products

However, the *severity* of reactions associated with these foods varies. For example:

◆ Peanuts, tree nuts, shellfish, fish, milk, and egg account for most reported cases of anaphylactic reactions in children and adults.

◆ Soy is less frequently reported as a highly allergenic food, although it is often associated with severe cases of allergy and atopic dermatitis (eczema) in childhood.

◆ Gluten-sensitive enteropathy, more frequently known as celiac disease, is a chronic disorder of the intestines. It is caused by an immunologically-mediated reaction to gluten, an important protein that occurs principally in wheat, rye, barley, and to some extent in oats. A person who has celiac disease develops a number of symptoms that may include digestive-tract upset such as diarrhea, abdominal cramping and distress, and inadequate absorption of food. In children, this may cause inadequate growth, and in adults an inability to gain weight. Other symptoms may include anemia, infertility, recurrent sores in the mouth, and sometimes skin rashes known as dermatitis herpetiformis. Celiac disease is a distinct medical condition, unrelated to allergy, and has its own diagnostic tests. Treatment is strict avoidance of wheat of all forms, rye, barley, and oats.

Other allergenic foods, present on some lists, absent on others, include

◆ Sesame seed and products containing sesame seed
◆ Mustard seed
◆ Corn
◆ Kiwi fruit

Food additives rarely cause IgE-mediated hypersensitivity reactions and therefore do not appear on allergen lists. The exception is sulfite, which is included on many food allergen lists. (Refer to Chapter 4, page 65, for a discussion of sulfite sensitivity and the foods in which it may be found.)

The Allergen Scale

Every allergic person will react differently to foods, with diverse symptoms of varying severity, and will develop symptoms in response to various portions of foods. However, it is possible to summarize the more commonly allergenic foods in the form of a scale of "relative reactivity." The scale in Table 6-1 summarizes data and information from many published articles as well as individual allergists from several countries who have kindly shared their experiences in food allergy management of patients with the author.

A scale of this type has several advantages:

◆ Used as a "reactivity chart" it allows people to see the number of foods that are available to them after their allergens have been crossed off. So often patients are overwhelmed when told that they must avoid a number of staple foods (e.g., wheat, milk and milk products, and eggs), and the common response is "But there is nothing left to eat!" A glance at the remaining foods on the chart reassures them, and counseling can proceed in a less anxiety-provoking fashion.

◆ The foods most likely to cause an allergic response (the "top eight") are apparent in this scale. This is useful for the atopic individual because so often chronic reactivity to these foods in particular seems to lead to "hidden food allergy." *Hidden food allergy* is a term doctors use to refer to symptoms that disappear when foods are removed and appear when the food has been reintroduced, but were not apparent when the food was eaten regularly. Often the symptoms of hidden food allergy are chronic and mild and usually ignored until they become very noticeable during a food challenge. As people begin to make alternative choices, their symptoms are more readily identifiable when they eat the culprit food less frequently.

◆ If there is a risk of severe or anaphylactic reactions, the culprit foods can be marked in red on the scale. This makes family members more aware of the allergic individual's needs and alert to sources of the problem food. Many people like to keep a copy of the scale on the fridge; for this reason, the printed scale is limited to a single page.

The allergen scale in Table 6-1 is based on the typical experience of persons eating a Western diet. In cultures where significantly different foods are commonly eaten, this chart may not reflect the degree of allergenicity of the foods, but it is still useful when marked according to the person's own allergies.

HOW MUCH FOOD CAUSES AN ALLERGIC REACTION?

The amount of food that needs to be eaten in order to cause an allergic reaction depends on the potency of the allergen and how sensitive the person is to it. Unfortunately, data is scarce on this topic and rarely reported in the literature. A few studies have attempted to define a threshold level for a variety of food allergens. For example, tests have shown that

◆ 10 milligrams of ovalbumin was required to elicit symptoms in egg-allergic children.
◆ 6 milligrams of cod was required to elicit symptoms.
◆ 0.1 to 0.2 milligrams of peanut was required to elicit an allergic reaction.

The Food and Drug Administration (FDA) Ad Hoc Committee on Hypersensitivity to Food Constituents attempted to define "allergenic levels" of foods in their 1986 report[1]:

◆ The usual amount of food that causes an allergic reaction in a sensitized adult is 20 grams (0 to 7 ounces).
◆ Shrimp allergy will be produced by 1 to 2 grams (0.03 to 0.07 ounce) of shrimp.
◆ Peanut allergy can be caused by as little as 25 milligrams (0.0009 ounce) of peanut.

---

[1] FDA Ad Hoc Committee on Hypersensitivity to Food Constituents. Report. Washington, D.C.: U.S. Food and Drug Administration, 1986.

However, there are reports that *inhaling* food components (such as being in a room where fish is being cooked) or merely *handling* the food can cause a reaction in highly sensitive individuals.

As more sophisticated analytical tests become available, more data on this important subject will be collected. In the meantime, the directive is that **all** *sources of the most highly allergenic foods, especially those that have previously caused a severe or anaphylactic reaction in an individual, should be completely avoided.* To achieve this, a sensitive person must be aware of

◆ all types of natural foods that would be expected to contain the allergen,
◆ all terms in a food ingredient list that would indicate the presence of the allergen or its derivatives (refer to Chapter 4 for complete details), and
◆ foods and nonfood products that are likely to contain the culprit allergen.

ADDITIVES DERIVED FROM POTENTIALLY ALLERGENIC FOODS

In a number of cases, ingredients in processed and manufactured foods are derived from natural food sources, but their origins are somewhat obscure. Table 6-2 provides examples of common ingredients and their food origins. This is by no means exhaustive, and highly sensitive people should obtain information from food manufacturers concerning "hidden sources" of their particular allergens. They should also become familiar with terms on food ingredient labels that would indicate the presence of their allergens.

Table 6-1
FOOD ALLERGEN SCALE

Grains/ Flours	Vegetables	Fruits	Nuts/ Seeds	Meats/ Alternates	Milk/ Milk Products

Wheat
Triticale
Semolina
Bulgur
Spelt
Kamut
	Tomato
	Spinach
	Celery (raw)
		Strawberry
		Raspberry
		Orange
		Fig
		Mango
		Watermelon
			Peanut
			Nuts:
			  Hazelnut
			  (Filbert)
				Egg white
				Egg yolk
					Ice cream
					Cow's milk:
					  Homogenized
					  Raw milk
					  1% 2%
					  Skim

Rye
 	
Corn
	Carrot (raw)
	Green pea
	Lima bean
	Broad bean
	  (fava bean)
	Cabbage (heart)
		Apple (raw)
		Apricot (raw)
		Peach (raw)
		Date
		Cantaloupe
		
		Pineapple
		Raisin
		Apple (cooked)
			Walnut
			Pecan
			Brazil nut
			Almond
			Sesame seed
			
			Cocoa bean
			Chocolate
			Coconut
				Shellfish:
				  Crab
				  Lobster
				  Prawn/shrimp
				  Clam
				  Oyster
				  Scallop
					Cheese:
					  Fermented:
					    Cheddar
					    Camembert
					    Blue
					    Swiss
					    Edam
					    Mozzarella
					    Goat cheese

Oats
Barley
	Cauliflower
	Brussels sprouts
	Green bean
	Yellow wax bean
		Kiwi
		Cherry
		Plum/prune
		Apricot (cooked)
			Cashew
			Pistachio
			Macadamia
				Fin fish:
				  Cod
				  Sole
				  Other white fish
					Cottage cheese
					Cream cheese

White rice
Brown rice
Wild rice
 	
Millet
	Avocado
	Cabbage
	  (outer leaves)
	
	Onion
	Green onion
	Garlic
		Loganberry
		Boysenberry
		
		Plantain
		Banana
		Grape
			Legumes:
			  Soy
			  Dried peas
			  Lentils
			Dried beans:
			  Navy
			  Pinto
			  Garbanzo
			  Carob
			  Sunflower seed
			  Flax seed
				Tuna
				Salmon
				
				Processed
				meats:
				  Pepperoni
				  Salami
				  Bologna
				  Wieners
				  Ham
				  Bacon
					Cream
					Sour cream
					
					Canned milk
					(evaporated)
					
					Goat milk
					Sheep milk

Buckwheat (kasha)	Celery (cooked) Green/red peppers	Grapefruit Lemon Lime			
Amaranth	Potato Cucumber Lettuce	Currants (red/ black)	Pumpkin seed	Pork	Processed cheese
Tapioca Cassava	Asparagus Broccoli Beets	Peach (cooked/ canned)	Bean sprouts	Chicken Beef Veal Turkey	Soft cheese (Philadelphia)

Sago
Arrowroot
Quinoa
	Squashes
	(all types)
		Cranberry
		Blackberry
		Blueberry
			Poppy seed	Wild meats:
				  Deer
				  Elk
				  Moose
				  Bear
				  Buffalo
					Yogurt
					Buttermilk
					
					Butter

	Carrot (cooked) Parsnip	Pear			
	Turnip Sweet potato Yam	Rhubarb		Rabbit Lamb	Clarified butter

Note: Foods are listed from the highest to the lowest allergenicity, based on reports from a variety of sources. People vary in their reactivity to foods and show a different pattern of reactivity depending on their individual characteristics. The scale is based on the typical Western diet. Persons following ethnic diets tend to show a different order of allergenicity.

Table 6-2
SOURCES OF ADDITIVES IN COMMON FOODS:
PRESENCE OF POTENTIAL ALLERGENS

Name of Additive	Sources (Potential Allergen)	Foods Likely To Contain Additive	Function in Foods
Lecithin	Egg Egg yolk Soybeans Corn	Boxed breakfast cereals Candy Chocolates Bread Rolls Buns Margarines	Antioxidant and emollient. Lecithin is composed of choline, phosphoric acid, fatty acids, and glycerin
Starch	Wheat Potatoes Rice Corn Beans Other plants The plant source is not usually identified on an ingredient label.	"Thickened" or "creamed" products	Thickening agent in a number of manufactured foods. Usually used in its "modified" form.
Modified Starch	Derived from plants (above) Modified with acid to make it more digestible	Baby foods Nonfood products such as dusting and face powders, baby powders, and bath salts	Present in foods as bleached starch; acetylated distarch adipate; distarch phosphate; and others with "distarch" in the name.
Carotene	Carrots	Margarines, butter Shortening Skim milk Buttermilk Cottage cheese Beet juice A number of red-colored foods	Coloring agent. Source of vitamin A in "enriched" foods.

Table 6-2 (continued)
SOURCES OF ADDITIVES IN COMMON FOODS:
PRESENCE OF POTENTIAL ALLERGENS

Name of Additive	Sources (Potential Allergen)	Foods Likely To Contain Additive	Function in Foods
Annatto	Extract from the seed of a tropical tree	Dairy products (cheese, butter) Breakfast cereals Baked goods Margarines	Coloring agent (yellow to pink).
Hydrolyzed Vegetable Protein (HVP) **Hydrolyzed Plant Protein (HPP)**	Soybeans Peanuts Wheat Corn (Soybeans are most frequently used source)	Soups Meat-based entrees Stews Flavoring and seasoning mixes	Flavor enhancer. Plant protein is hydrolyzed (broken down) by enzymes or acids. High glutamate and salt content (high MSG).
Carrageenan	Algae (seaweed) "Irish moss"	Milk products Pressure-dispensed "whipped cream" Cheese spreads Ice cream Custards Sherbets Salad dressings Sauces Chocolates Artificially sweetened jams and jellies	Emulsifier (blender) and stabilizer. Prevents separation of ingredients. Thickening agent; gelling agent.
Malt Extract	Germinated barley	Beers Meat and poultry products Ice cream Flavored milks Sour cream Chocolate syrup Candy Cough drops Condiments Salad dressings Breakfast cereals	Flavoring agent.

Name of Additive	Sources (Potential Allergen)	Foods Likely To Contain Additive	Function in Foods
Table 6-2 (continued)			
SOURCES OF ADDITIVES IN COMMON FOODS:			
PRESENCE OF POTENTIAL ALLERGENS			
Xanthan Gum	Product of the fermentation of dextrose (derived from corn syrup) by the micro-organism *Xanthomonas campestris*	Dairy products Salad dressings May replace starch, sugar, and oil in low-calorie products Xantham gum is not digested by the body and passes out mostly unchanged.	Thickener, stabilizer, emulsifier, suspending agent. Prevents ingredients from separating.
Locust Bean Gum	Carob seed	Ice creams Sauces Salad dressings Sausages (acts as a binder)	Thickening and stabilizing agent. Used to blend ingredients and prevent separation. Binding agent. Texture modifier.

— CHAPTER 7 —

CROSS-REACTIVITY
OF ALLERGENS

In the management of food allergy, the subject of cross-reactivity of allergens is becoming increasingly complex. The term "cross-reacting" antigens or allergens suggests there is a relationship between antigens such that sensitization to one leads automatically to reactivity to another. The two cross-reacting antigens are related in some way–perhaps they belong to the same botanic or zoologic family or have the same structures.

Cross-reactivity between botanically related *inhaled* allergens such as grass pollens has been known for many years. However, there is a great deal of uncertainty about the degree of clinical cross-reactivity between members of botanically related food plants. It is not always valid to assume that because plants belong to the same family, they are related antigenically. Furthermore, a person who is allergic to one member of a botanic or zoologic family may not show symptoms of allergy to other members of the same family when they are eaten.

This chapter will discuss the types of antigenic relatedness that are important in the management of food allergy and how the allergic person can be aware of the foods that are most likely to cause problems in his or her particular case.

CROSS-REACTIVITY BETWEEN PLANTS OF THE SAME FAMILY

Prior to the 1980s, the popular assumption was that a person allergic to the edible part of one plant (fruit, vegetable, nut, or seed) would be, or would shortly become, allergic to other plants within the same botanic family. Many diets were limited unnecessarily under the assumption that an allergy to one member of a

111

botanic family equaled an allergy to all plants from that family. For example, someone allergic to peanut and perhaps also allergic to soy was advised to avoid all members of the Leguminosae family (legumes such as peanut, soy, peas, beans, lentils, alfalfa, acacia, licorice, carob, gum arabic, tamarind). A person allergic to potatoes was told to avoid all other foods of the nightshade family (bell pepper, cayenne pepper, paprika, eggplant, tomato, tobacco); someone allergic to peaches was instructed to avoid all fruits and nuts of the plum family (almonds, apricots, cherries, nectarines, plums, prunes); and so on. Charts of botanic families were standard reference for anyone involved in management of food allergy. It was a fairly simple matter for allergists to provide patients with lists of foods to avoid, based on the results of skin tests. Not surprisingly, a person entering an allergist's office for skin-testing for foods would leave with an extensive list of "foods to avoid," and when the symptoms failed to disappear, he or she was often accused of lack of diligence in following instructions. Happily, modern immunological techniques have demonstrated the errors in such simplistic thinking.

Research in immunology is beginning to explain why a person may experience an allergic reaction to several foods that are unrelated, and yet tolerate many within the same botanic or zoologic family. The answer lies in the molecular structure of the antigen that is responsible for triggering the allergic response, usually caused by antigen-specific IgE (Type I hypersensitivity; see Chapter 3). Briefly, **T-cell lymphocytes** (the "control cells" of the immune system) recognize specific structural characteristics of the antigen, and if prior sensitization has occurred, they respond by producing **cytokines** ("messenger molecules"). Cytokines lead to the immunological events that will eventually result in release of the inflammatory mediators which cause the clinical symptoms of allergy. Because the molecular structure of the antigens in each living cell is unique, relatedness based on botanic families or even genera does not determine identity at the cellular level. Sibling relatedness within a human family provides a simple analogy. All the siblings belong to the same genetically related family group, but their bodies differ, which can be observed clearly in the differences in color of hair and eyes, facial features, and body characteristics. These observable differences are based on differences at the cellular level, which also lead to differences in the way the siblings' bodies respond to drugs, foods, and potential for the development of diseases. Such differences occur in each living species, whether animal or plant. Thus, plants within a single botanic family will differ at the cellular level and therefore will have the potential to trigger quite different responses depending on the structure of their antigens. Only very few, and quite specific, antigenic structures can cause an allergic response.

CROSS-REACTIVITY BETWEEN PLANTS OF DIFFERENT FAMILIES

Oral Allergy Syndrome

Recent research into food allergen structures and their function within plants has focused especially on allergens in foods that cross-react with those in botanically *unrelated* trees and grasses. The reason for the interest in these particular allergens is that increasing numbers of people are reporting the symptoms of **oral allergy syndrome (OAS).**

Oral allergy syndrome is a combination of clinical symptoms in the mouth and throat resulting from direct contact with food allergens in a sensitized person who also has a respiratory allergy to an *inhaled* allergen. The inhaled (airborne) allergens are usually tree, weed, or grass pollens that cause hay fever symptoms in the allergic person. It seems that after several years, oral tissues, which are near the mucous membranes of the upper respiratory tract, also become sensitized to these antigens. However, the symptoms in the mouth do not occur in contact with the tree pollens; instead, they occur after exposure to structurally similar antigens in unrelated plant foods such as fruits, vegetables, and sometimes nuts. Oral symptoms following ingestion of specific fruits, vegetables, and nuts have been described in patients with co-existing allergy to trees of the birch/alder group, weeds such as mugwort and ragweed, and grasses.

Symptoms of oral allergy syndrome include itching and irritation of oral tissues, swelling of the lips and tongue, and sometimes papules or blisters. Persons who have this allergy begin to show symptoms usually within a few minutes after eating the offending food. Most patients show symptoms within 5 minutes, and almost all patients within 30 minutes, after contact with the food. Swelling and "tightening" in the throat (glottic edema) is probably the most severe reaction.

An interesting variation of oral allergy syndrome occurred in a woman whom I saw in the clinic. She complained of watery, itchy, swollen eyes while peeling potatoes and apples. She had also recently experienced irritation of oral tissues and throat tightening while eating a raw apple, and milder symptoms in the mouth after eating a raw carrot. She had a twenty-year history of hay fever to alder and birch pollens, but had been experiencing the eye, mouth, and throat symptoms only for the past year. The important association here is that raw potato, apple, and carrot contain structurally similar antigens to the birch and alder trees to which the woman is allergic. She remains free from these symptoms as long as she carefully avoids contact with raw potato, carrot, and apple. The association to oral allergy syndrome is that in peeling raw potato and raw apple, the antigens become aerosolized in small droplets that spray the eyes and can also be brought to the eyes by the contaminated hands. Wearing gloves will not solve this problem, but washing the hands carefully after peeling will reduce the transfer of allergen by this route.

Allergens Associated with OAS

All allergens are components of the living organism in which they occur. Some are structural components, others are regulatory factors, agents that control various processes within the cells of the organism. When we consider that some cell components, such as cytochrome c (which allows the cell to use oxygen from the atmosphere in important metabolic processes), are present and active in many organisms, it is not surprising that the same factor, with the same function, even in unrelated organisms, should arouse the same antibody when it enters the human system.

Plant Allergens' Function and Cross-Reactivity

As scientists learn more about the antigens that can cause the production of IgE, they may be able to predict cross-reactions between similar proteins within unrelated plant species. However, because allergy is individual, allergenic potential will not necessarily predict the effect of the food when consumed by any given person. Scientists have used statistical methods to measure the probability that a person sensitized to one edible plant will demonstrate significant cross-reactivity to other, unrelated plants. However, elimination of the suspect food from the diet and reintroducing it under controlled conditions (challenge) still remains the only reliable method of demonstrating individual reactivity to each suspect plant food.

An allergen's characteristics often suggest a probable function within the plant. For example:

◆ The birch pollen component named Bet v 2 and the 15 kd antigen in celery have been identified as profilins, which are regulatory proteins associated with the reproductive processes in plants, hence their association with pollens. Pollens are the agents that fertilize a plant in the process of reproduction.

◆ The birch antigen Bet v 1 and the apple antigen Mal d 1 are proteins that plants make during times of environmental stress. It is possible that the plants make these proteins in response to environmental pollution. This might explain the apparent surge of patients exhibiting oral allergy syndrome in the past few years as pollution levels, especially in cities, increase.

◆ Other antigens such as the allergen named Art v 1 from mugwort, which shows antigenic relatedness to antigens in a number of pollens and food plants (birch, timothy grass, celery), is described as trypsin resistant (a characteristic of allergens; see Chapter 6, page 101), but this allergen's function in the plant has not been identified.

Avoiding OAS

Frequently, high temperatures will destroy the antigen in the food that causes oral allergy syndrome. People who suffer from oral allergy syndrome after eating raw fruits and vegetables often can eat the same food when it is cooked without having an allergic reaction.

The ripeness of the fruit or vegetable may influence its allergic potential: the riper the fruit or more mature the vegetable, the greater the chance that it might cause an allergic response (compared to the unripe or less mature form).

If you have symptoms of an IgE-mediated allergy (for example, rhinitis, allergic conjunctivitis, asthma) to pollens of plants usually associated with oral allergy syndrome (birch, mugwort, ragweed, timothy grass, other grasses), you should avoid the foods known to have similar antigens when:

◆ The foods have caused immediate reactions in and around your mouth
◆ You have had positive indications of allergy to the foods, based on skin tests or immunological analysis such as RAST or ELISA (see Chapter 5).

When people are pollen-allergic but do not have oral symptoms, and skin tests and/or immunological tests are negative for the associated foods, it is probably unnecessary to avoid the foods. However, some allergists feel that as a safety measure it is wise to provide the patient with information on the types of foods likely to trigger OAS if he or she has shown signs of allergy to the pollens sharing common allergens with foods in OAS.

Table 7-1 lists the potential allergenic cross-reactivity between plant species that can be used as the basis of an elimination diet for detecting the triggers of allergic reactions. However, hypersensitivity to these plants is an individual idiosyncrasy. *Even if species are shown to have common antigens, people who are allergic to one species in an antigenically related group do not necessarily experience reactions to others in the same group.* As in all allergy management, the triggering of the allergic response when the food is reintroduced in a controlled fashion (challenge) is the only reliable way to identify the allergen responsible for the reaction.

Table 7-1
CROSS-REACTING FOODS, POLLENS, AND OTHER ALLERGENS

Nonfood Allergens	Fruits and Vegetables	Legumes and Grains	Nuts and Seeds	Other Foods
Birch pollen Mugwort pollen Grass pollens Timothy grass	Apple Apricot Carrot Celery Cherry Fennel Kiwi fruit Melon Nectarine Orange Peach Potato Tomato Watermelon	Peanut	Hazelnut "Tree nuts" (unspecified)	Spice (unspecified)
Ragweed	Banana Cantaloupe Cucumber Honeydew Melon Watermelon Zucchini			
	Kiwi fruit	Rye	Hazelnut Sesame seed Poppy seed	

LATEX ALLERGY

Allergy to natural rubber (latex) is an increasing and clinically important problem. It was first recognized in health care workers, who are in frequent contact with latex in surgical gloves. However, many items in everyday use are made from latex, and sensitization to the antigens responsible for allergy in latex has led to latex allergy becoming more common in the general population. People allergic to latex may experience sometimes severe, even anaphylactic, reactions, both to latex itself and to the foods containing similar antigens. Car and bike tires, clothing with elastic and other rubberized materials, children's toys, balloons, and other articles in the home and workplace are made from latex. An additional concern regarding latex allergy is that some of the allergens that are responsible for triggering the allergic response can be found in a number of, mostly unrelated, food plants.

Latex Allergens

Scientists have identified more than twelve antigens in natural latex that might be responsible for triggering an allergic response to latex. Some of these are structurally similar to antigens in some fruits and nuts, which could explain the reactivity to these foods when consumed by a person allergic to latex.

The fresh fruits that commonly cause such allergic reactions in people allergic to latex are **banana, avocado, and chestnut.** Foods less commonly associated with latex allergy are kiwi, mango, peach, and walnut. Table 7-2 lists the foods that are known to contain antigens similar enough to the allergens in latex

Table 7-2 FOODS WITH ANTIGENS RELATED TO LATEX			
Nonfood Allergens	**Fruits and Vegetables**	**Legumes and Grains**	**Nuts and Seeds**
Latex	Avocado	Peanut	Chestnut
	Banana	Soybean	Walnut
	Celery		"Nuts" (various
	Citrus fruits		species,
	orange,		unspecified)
	grapefruit,		
	lemon,		
	lime		
	Fig		
	Grapes		
	Kiwi fruit		
	Mango		
	Papaya		
	Passion fruit		
	Peach		
	Pineapple		
	Tomato		

to trigger an allergic reaction in latex-sensitive people. As in all cases of potential cross-reactivity, not everyone with latex allergy will develop symptoms when exposed to these foods; clinical expression of an allergy is an individual idiosyncrasy. However, many practitioners advise their patients with known latex allergy to avoid all foods that contain the allergens associated with latex allergy because of the real risk of an anaphylactic reaction–and an increase in the risk the longer the allergic person is exposed to the antigens.

OTHER FOOD ALLERGENS AND CROSS-REACTIVITY

Milk

Milks from unrelated animal species have been shown to frequently be cross-reactive. In one study, 22 out of 28 infants with cow's milk allergy were shown to be allergic to milk from goats as well, and studies with laboratory animals clearly demonstrate that 100% of the animals allergic to cow's milk appear to be allergic to goat's milk also. The strong antigenic similarity between cow and goat milk proteins suggests that goat's milk is unlikely to be tolerated by most people with genuine cow's milk protein allergy. The figure of 80% is usually quoted as the likelihood of a person allergic to cow's milk becoming allergic to goat's milk if it is substituted for cow's milk in the diet.

According to the results of the few studies that have been carried out on allergens in sheep's milk proteins, there appears to be an even greater antigenic similarity between certain cow and sheep milk antigens than between cow and goat milk antigens, suggesting that anyone who is allergic to cow's milk has a significant risk of being allergic to sheep's milk also. Apparently, cow milk proteins and human milk proteins are not cross-reactive, so a baby allergic to cow's milk will not be allergic to human milk. Recent research is being directed to mare's milk as a substitute for cow's milk, especially in infant formula. Mare's milk is nutritionally more similar to human milk than it is to cow's milk and shows very little evidence of containing allergens similar to those of cow's milk. Buffalo milk is a common food in many countries and has become more readily available in North America in recent years. So far it seems to be well tolerated by people with cow's milk allergy. As more people consume buffalo milk, undoubtedly its value as a milk substitute for cow's milk allergic people will become evident.

Eggs

Eggs from a variety of birds (chicken, turkey, duck, goose, seagull) have been reported to be cross-reactive. The major allergens in egg white, ovalbumin, ovomucoid, and ovotransferrin, are in eggs of all bird species tested, including turkeys, ducks, geese, and seagulls. The egg whites of chickens and turkeys are very similar immunologically and seem to differ somewhat from those of ducks and geese; the egg whites of ducks and geese may be less potent as allergens. Seagull's eggs seem to be the least potent of the bird species tested and seem to be the least similar to hen's eggs. However, because of the close similarity in the structure of the antigens, *it is advisable for anyone who is allergic to egg white of any bird species to avoid eggs from all birds.*

Fish

Allergic reactivity to one species of fin fish does not usually lead to allergy to other fish. In most studies, subjects were allergic to one, only occasionally to two, and very rarely to more than two species of fish. Other studies indicate that allergy to multiple fish species is uncommon and that restricting all fin fish from the diet based on an allergy to a single fish species is not necessary. However, because all fish contain the potentially allergenic proteins known as parvalbumins, some practitioners feel that allergy to one fish species means a risk of allergy to all. *People who have had a potentially life-threatening* **anaphylactic reaction** *to a fish are usually advised to avoid contact with all fish in the interest of safety.*

Shellfish

In contrast to fin fish allergy, people who are allergic to crustaceans (shellfish) are often allergic to **all** species, including **crab, lobster, shrimp, prawn and crayfish.** The degree of clinical cross-reactivity between crustaceans and mollusks (**clam, mussel, oyster, octopus, squid, scallop, snail, abalone**) is still unclear, although some reports indicate that allergy to *both* types of shellfish does not often occur in the same people.

Nuts

The question as to whether a person who is allergic to specific nuts should avoid nuts of all species is as yet unanswered. The incidence of cross-reactivity between nuts from unrelated trees is not known. A 1989 study on 14 nut-allergic children indicated that allergy to one species of nut did not necessarily indicate allergy to all species of nuts. In the study, one child reacted to five nuts, one child to two nuts, and the other twelve children reacted to only one nut each.

However, *individuals who have had an* **anaphylactic reaction** *to one type of nut should avoid nuts of* **all** *types* in the interest of safety. The likelihood of people reacting to tree nuts if they are anaphylactic to peanuts is also unknown; to ensure that accidental exposure to peanut is avoided, people who are anaphylactic to peanuts should avoid all tree nuts as well.

The warning to avoid all nuts and peanuts is based not on the concerns about antigenic cross-reactivity as much as it is on the interest of safety. *Because many of the life-threatening anaphylactic reactions occur in response to* **nuts**, *this group of foods is considered the greatest risk to the greatest number of allergic people, especially children.* Nuts are unique in that their small size and uniform color make it difficult to distinguish individual types of nuts within a mixture. In addition, the common practice of putting different species of nuts in the same container for sale in stores, using scoops in multiple bins of nuts where they are sold in bulk, and the danger of cross-contamination between nuts in food manufacture, increases the risk. Because only a tiny amount of a potentially lethal food allergen is required to trigger a fatal reaction, precautions in the at-risk population tend to be extreme, but necessary. Therefore, *most people with proven allergy to peanuts or any species of tree nut are usually advised to carefully avoid exposure to all nuts, nut-containing foods, and derivatives of nuts such as oils.* Because all of the nutrients in nuts are readily available from other dietary sources (protein, vitamins such as vitamin E, and the minerals niacin, amnganese, chromuim, and panlothenic acid), complete avoidance of peanuts and nuts will not normally lead to nutritional deficiency.

— PART II —

DIETARY MANAGEMENT OF FOOD ALLERGIES AND FOOD INTOLERANCES

In this section you will find detailed information for following a diet when you know exactly which foods to avoid. The first part provides information for avoiding the eight most common food allergens: milk, egg, wheat, soy, peanut, tree nuts, fish, and shellfish. It also includes a combination diet for eliminating the "top ten" allergens, which excludes the eight common allergens, plus corn and chocolate. You should follow these diets when skin tests, blood tests, and possibly elimination and challenge tests have clearly identified your culprit allergens. You can follow the diets for the long term. If appropriate substitutes are made, there is no risk of nutritional deficiency.

The second part of Part II takes us into a field of practice that is a little more controversial. Traditional allergists are comfortable with avoidance of IgE-related food allergies, such as those listed above. However, the field of food intolerance is more controversial because we lack the definitive tests that demonstrate specific responses, whether immunological, that the scientific practitioner relies upon. Nevertheless, management of food intolerances is extremely important for the person who is dealing with them. Even if skin and blood tests may be negative, the sufferer knows that when they eat certain foods, they become unwell. We are beginning to learn a lot about the different ways in which food components, both natural and artificial, can impact the body. Mostly, we identify the culprit food components by the tedious process of elimination and challenge–this is the subject of Part III.

In Part II you will find a discussion about each of the "intolerance triggers" that seem to cause the greatest grief for the largest number of people. Intolerance of disaccharide sugars, especially lactose, is not uncommon. Avoidance of disaccharides is not difficult, and can provide a great deal of relief for the person with this dysfunction of the digestive tract. This is an example of a situation where symptoms occur, but allergy tests are of no value, because the immune system is not involved. Certain invasive tests involving intestinal biopsy can be used to identify this condition. However, when we move into the realm of less-understood reactions, particularly those involving chemicals that occur naturally in food (for example salicylates, benzoates, glutamates), and those that are added to food (preservatives, colors or flavoring agents), the lack of definitive tests makes the matter difficult. It is hard to identify the culprit food component, and even more difficult to convince the "traditionalist" that the reaction is valid. Nevertheless, the sufferer obtains so much relief from their symptoms when the components are removed from their diet, that the process of determining the culprit, tedious and time-consuming as it may be, is more than worth the effort. Part II provides all the information you will need to follow a diet that eliminates your own personal food demons and yet supplies all the nutrients your body requires.

— CHAPTER 8 —

MILK ALLERGY AND LACTOSE INTOLERANCE

An adverse reaction to milk and milk products is not uncommon, especially in children, and results in a variety of symptoms. The most frequent reactions are in the skin, where eczema, hives, and angioedema (tissue swelling) may occur and in the gastrointestinal tract with abdominal bloating, pain, gas, diarrhea, constipation, nausea, vomiting, and occasionally blood loss in the stool (occult blood). In some people, upper respiratory tract symptoms and asthma may be caused or made worse when they consume milk or milk products.

Occult blood loss associated with cow's milk allergy can cause iron-deficiency anemia, especially in children, because blood is the most important source of iron in the body. Another effect of cow's milk allergy currently being investigated in children is an inability to fall asleep and restless, disturbed sleep. In an infant, inadequate growth and weight gain (failure to thrive) may be a result of milk allergy. The allergic reaction results in inflammation in the intestines, and absorption of nutrients may be impaired as a result of damage to the transport mechanisms in the intestinal cells. Transport mechanisms are processes that transport nutrients from the intestines into blood circulation.

The diagnosis of milk allergy is not a simple matter. Although any adverse reaction a person has after drinking milk is often ascribed to "milk allergy," when the symptoms are in the gastrointestinal tract the problem may be lactose intolerance, not an immunologically mediated allergy to milk proteins.

123

◆ **Milk allergy** is caused by an immune reaction against milk *proteins;* more than 25 distinct proteins are identifiable; any number of these may trigger an immune response.

◆ **Lactose intolerance** is due to the body's inability to produce enough of the digestive enzyme, called *lactase*, which splits lactose into its constituent mono-saccharides (single sugars), glucose and galactose.

WHAT CAUSES MILK ALLERGY?

Milk allergy results when the immune system produces antibodies against milk allergens. (For a discussion of the immunology of allergy please refer to Chapter 3).

◆ Milk allergens are proteins; more than 25 distinct milk proteins have been identified in the various fractions of milk. The fractions include casein, whey, serum, and certain additional ingredients (see Table 8-1).

◆ Most milk-allergic children and adults react to more than one milk protein.

◆ The potential of individual milk proteins to cause allergy has been studied by skin tests and oral challenge. Casein proteins produced the highest number of positive skin tests in children with milk allergy, whereas beta-lactoglobulin produced the highest number of positive oral challenges.

◆ More than 25 proteins in cow's milk can induce antibody production in humans.

◆ Beta-lactoglobulin (in whey); alpha, beta, and kappa caseins; and bovine serum albumin are the most important allergens.

◆ Clinical reactions to all the major cow's milk antigens have been documented.

Heat will change the nature of some milk proteins (they are described as heat-labile), but others remain unaffected (they are heat-stable). Serum proteins and beta-casein are the most labile and are readily denatured by heat, whereas beta-lactoglobulin and alpha-lactalbumin are the most heat-stable. This means that persons who are allergic to the heat-labile proteins will be able to drink boiled or cooked milk; those who are allergic to proteins unaffected by heat (heat-stable proteins) will not be able to drink either boiled or unboiled milk.

Table 8-1 INDIVIDUAL PROTEINS IN COW'S MILK			
Casein Fraction	**Whey Fraction**	**Serum Fraction**	**Others**
alpha caseins	beta-lactoglobulin	albumin	lactoferrin
alpha s_1	alpha-lactoglobulin	immunoglobulins	lactoperoxidase
alpha s_2	proteose peptones		alkaline phosphatase
beta-caseins			catalase
kappa-caseins			
gamma-caseins			

Antibodies produced against milk proteins may be IgE, IgM, IgG, or sometimes IgA (refer to Chapter 3, page 34, for a discussion of antibodies). Coupling of the milk protein antigen with its homologous (matching) antibody leads to the release of inflammatory mediators, which act directly on body tissues and cause inflammation. The tissues may be in the digestive tract, the skin, or the respiratory tract. Symptoms typical of allergy result in the affected tissues.

Milk allergy is much more common in young infants and children than in adults, so it is considered a condition of childhood rather than adulthood. More than 90% of cases of IgE-mediated allergy occur within the first year of life, the majority of these within the first six months. However, in most cases children "outgrow" IgE-mediated allergy to cow's milk by the age of 18 months to 2 years, due to the maturing of their immune system and the lining of the digestive tract.

It is necessary to differentiate between lactose intolerance (lactase deficiency) and milk protein allergy as some symptoms, such as abdominal pain, diarrhea, and vomiting, may be common to both conditions. However, in some cases, sensitivity to milk protein may cause inflammation of the gastrointestinal tract and may lead to a lactase deficiency, so it is possible for a person to have *both* conditions. Symptoms in other organ systems such as the respiratory tract and the skin are *not* symptoms of lactose intolerance. Management of lactose intolerance is discussed in further detail later in this chapter (page 141).

In order to successfully manage adverse reactions to cow's milk constituents, whether it is an IgE-mediated allergy to cow's milk proteins or an inability to tolerate lactose, a diet free from all sources of milk proteins and lactose is necessary. When the culprit components have been identified by appropriate challenge, the tolerated milk fractions can be reintroduced into the diet.

MILK-FREE DIET (TABLE 8-5)

People who have a known allergy to cow's milk proteins or are unable to tolerate lactose need to *eliminate* the following from their diet:

◆ All milk and milk-containing foods, including liquid and evaporated milks
◆ Fermented milks (yogurt, buttermilk)
◆ All cheeses (hard cheeses, cottage cheese, cream cheese)
◆ Ice cream and ice milk
◆ Any foods containing milk solids such as cream, butter, and margarines containing whey
◆ All foods or beverages containing components of milk such as casein, whey, lactoglobulin, and hydrolysates of these (Table 8-2)

Table 8-2
LABEL-READING GUIDELINES FOR A MILK-FREE DIET

Terms Indicating the Presence of Cow's Milk Components Butter

Butter fat	Acidophilus milk	Hydrolyzed casein
Butter-flavored oil	Lactaid® milk	Ammonium caseinate
Butter solids	Lacteeze® milk	Calcium caseinate
Whipped butter	Condensed milk	Potassium caseinate
Artificial butter flavor	Evaporated milk	Sodium caseinate
Natural butter flavor	Cultured milk	Rennet casein
Buttermilk	Milk solids	Whey
Buttermilk solids	Malted milk	Whey protein
Cheese	Milk powder	Whey powder
Cottage cheese	Cream	Sweet dairy whey
Processed cheese	Whipped cream	Whey hydrolysate
Cream cheese	Half-and-half	Hydrolyzed whey
Feta	Light cream	Delactosed whey
Ricotta	Ice cream	Demineralized whey
Quark	Ice milk	Lactose
Curd	Sherbet	Lactulose
Homogenized; 1%; 2%; skim; whole; low-fat; non-fat milk	Yogurt Casein	Lactoglobulin
	Casein hydrolysate	Lactalbumin

Ingredients That May Contain Milk Proteins

Brown sugar flavoring	Margarine	Simplesse®
Caramel flavor	Chocolate	High-protein flour
Natural flavor		

Note: Lactic acid, lactate, and lactylate do not contain milk and do not need to be eliminated from the diet.

Alternate Sources of Nutrients When Milk and Milk Products are Removed from the Diet

Adequate **protein** is readily available from meat, fish, soybeans and other legumes, nuts, grains, and vegetables, so removing milk and milk products from the diet is not usually a problem.

CALCIUM

Milk is the most abundant and readily available source of calcium in the normal diet. One cup of milk contains 290 milligrams of calcium. Table 8-3 gives the dietary reference intake (DRI) values for calcium and vitamin D.

Table 8-3 DIETARY REFERENCE INTAKE (DRI) VALUES FOR CALCIUM AND VITAMIN D		
Life Stage Group Male[a] and Female	Calcium AI (mg/day)	Vitamin D AI (mcg/day) [b,c]
0 to 6 months*	210	5
6 to 12 months	270	5
1 to 3 years	500	5
4 to 8 years	800	5
9 to 13 years	1,300	5
14 to 18 years	1,300	5
19 to 30 years	1,000	5
31 to 50 years	1,000	5
51 to 70 years	1,200	10
> 70 years	1,200	15
Pregnancy[a]		
18 years or younger	1,300	5
19 through 50 years	1,000	5
Lactation[a]		
18 years or younger	1,300	5
19 to 50 years	1,000	5

a Female-only for pregnancy and lactation values
b As cholecalciferol (1 microgram (mcg) = 40 IU vitamin D)
c In the absence of adequate exposure to sunlight
AI = Adequate intake
* Source of calcium is mother's milk.

Source: Health and Welfare Canada Nutrition Recommendations 1990

**IMPORTANT MICRONUTRIENTS
IN MILK**

Milk and milk products are an important source of calcium, phosphorus, vitamin D, vitamin B12, riboflavin, pantothenic acid, potassium, vitamin A, and vitamin E (vitamins D and A are added as fortification).

These nutrients must be obtained from other foods and supplements when all milk is removed from the diet.

CALCIUM ABSORPTION

◆ The percentage of the calcium contained in foods that is actually absorbed, used, and retained by the body is variable, depending on age, level of calcium intake, type of food eaten, and other nutrients eaten at the same time.

◆ An average adult will absorb approximately 40% of the calcium in their diet. This is increased during growth, pregnancy, and lactation, and it is reduced during aging. In general, the lower the intake, the more calcium is retained in the body (i.e., less calcium is excreted when intake is low).

◆ In order to efficiently absorb calcium, an adequate level of vitamin D in the body is necessary. Vitamin D is obtained from some foods (milk, liver, egg yolk), but the best source is the action of sunlight (UV light) on the skin.

◆ A diet high in phosphorus and protein (a traditional high-protein American diet) tends to reduce the amount of calcium retained in the body.

Alternative calcium sources include (Table 8-4):

◆ Canned fish such as sardines and salmon, *with bones.* (The calcium is in the bones; the canning process softens them, making them more easily digested.)
◆ Green leafy vegetables such as arugula, kale, beet and turnip greens, collards, mustard greens, and broccoli. However, the calcium in vegetables is not so readily absorbed by the body as that from animal sources.
◆ Some nuts and legumes also contain significant levels of calcium.

Table 8-4
NONDAIRY SOURCES OF CALCIUM

NOTE: Do not eat any food which causes you to have an allergic reaction.
Listed according to calcium content.   Ca = calcium

FOOD	PORTION	
	Metric	**Imperial**
More than 300 mg Ca		
Sardines, with bones, canned	85 g	3 oz
Rhubarb, frozen cooked*	270 g	1 cup
Wheat flour, artificially enriched	125 g	1 cup
Collards, frozen, cooked*	170 g	1 cup
Arugula (rocket kale)	170 g	1 cup
250 to 300 mg Ca		
Sockeye salmon, with bones, canned	100 g	½ can
(213 g/can) (7.5 oz can)		
Rhubarb, cooked, fresh*	270 g	1 cup
Spinach, cooked*	190 g	1 cup
200 to 250 mg Ca		
Almonds	125 mL	½ cup
Pink salmon, with bones, canned	100 g	½ can
(213 g/can) (7.5 oz can)		
Oysters, raw, meat only	250 g	1 cup
Sugar, brown, packed down	220 g	1 cup
Turnip greens, cooked *	165 g	1 cup
150 to 200 mg Ca		
Beet greens, leaves and stems, cooked*	145 g	1 cup
Kale, frozen, cooked	130 g	I cup
Amaranth (cooked grain): uncooked weight	100 g	(cooked) 1 cup
100 to150 mg Ca		
Baked beans, canned	250 mL	1 cup
Brazil nuts	125 mL	½ cup
Scallops		7 medium
Sesame seeds	125 mL	½ cup
Soya beans, cooked	250 mL	1 cup
Tofu	(8 x 6 x 2 cm)	1 piece
Shrimp, meat only	113 g	4 oz
Molasses, cane, blackstrap	20 g	1 tbsp
Dandelion greens, cooked *	105 g	1 cup
Mustard greens *	140 g	1 cup
Okra pods, cooked	160 g	1 cup
Brussels sprouts*	156 g	1 cup
Broccoli, cooked	250 mL	1 cup

Table 8-4 (continued)
NONDAIRY SOURCES OF CALCIUM

FOOD	PORTION	
	Metric	Imperial
50 to 100 mg Ca		
Asparagus, fresh, cooked, drained	240 g	1½ cups
Lima beans, cooked	180 g	1 cup
Green beans, cooked	125 g	1 cup
Yellow or wax beans, cooked	125 g	1 cup
Cabbage, fresh, cooked *	217 g	1½ cups
Chinese cabbage (bok choy)*	76 g	1 cup
Sauerkraut *	235 g	1 cup
Carrots, cooked	234 g	1½ cups
Parsnips, cooked	155 g	1 cup
Onions, cooked	210 g	1 cup
Tomatoes, canned, solids and liquid	241 g	1 cup
Chili con carne with beans	250 mL	1 cup
Red kidney beans, cooked	250 mL	1 cup
White beans, cooked	250 mL	1 cup
Beans, dry, cooked and drained	180 g	1 cup
Lentils, cooked	200 g	1 cup
Garbanzo beans (Chickpeas) (cooked)	250 mL	1 cup
Wheat germ	113 g	1 tbsp
Oats, puffed	50 g	2 oz
Orange, raw		1 medium
Orange sections	180 g	1 cup
Hazelnuts, chopped	28 g	1 oz
Cereal, All-Bran	250 mL	1 cup
Cereal, 100% Bran	250 mL	1 cup
Cereal, Branbuds	250 mL	1 cup
Cereal, Granola	150 mL	⅔ cup
15 to 50 mg Ca		
Cereals		
Bran flakes and raisins	250 mL	1 cup
Corn bran	250 mL	1 cup
Cheerios	250 mL	1 cup
Oatmeal, cooked	250 mL	1 cup
Shredded wheat	(10 mg Ca each biscuit)	2 to 5 pieces
Shreddies	250 mL	1 cup
Bread		
Cracked wheat	(22 mg Ca per slice)	slice
Mixed grain	(27 mg Ca per slice)	1 slice
Rye, light	(19 mg Ca per slice)	1 slice
White	(24 mg Ca per slice)	1 slice
Whole wheat 100%	(25 mg Ca per slice)	1 slice
Whole wheat 60%	(23 mg Ca per slice)	1 slice

FOOD	PORTION	
Table 8-4 (continued) **NONDAIRY SOURCES OF CALCIUM**		
	Metric	**Imperial**
Bread (continued)		
White bun, hamburger or hot dog	(07 to 44 mg Ca)	1
Pita, whole wheat, 16.5 cm diameter	(49 mg Ca)	1
Tortilla, corn	(42 mg Ca)	1
Vegetables		
Cabbage, raw, shredded	250 mL	1 cup
Carrot, raw, medium		1
Cauliflower, raw, cooked	250 mL	1 cup
Celery, diced, raw	250 mL	1 cup
Turnip, cooked	250 mL	1 cup
Spinach, raw, chopped	125 mL	½ cup
Olives, black		5 large
Olives, green		5 medium
Parsley, raw, chopped	25 mL	2 Tbsp
Peas, boiled	250 mL	1 cup
15 to 50 mg Ca		
Fruit		
Grapefruit, raw	1 medium	1 medium
Kiwi	1 large	1 large
Fig, dried, uncooked	1 medium	1 medium
Pear, raw	1 medium	1 medium
Raisins	125 mL	½ cup
Other		
Chocolate	30 g	1 square
Egg, whole, cooked	1 large	1 large
Maple syrup	15 mL	1 tbsp
Peanuts, oil roasted	50 mL	¼ cup
Sunflower seeds, kernel	50 mL	4 tbsp
Soy milk, liquid	250 mL	1 cup

* Contains oxalic acid, which impairs calcium absorption. Although the calcium is present in the food at the given level, the actual amount absorbed is significantly less.

Calcium Supplements

If all milk and dairy products are removed from the diet, it is often difficult to obtain sufficient calcium from these alternative sources on a regular basis. A supplement is then necessary. Calcium gluconate, calcium citrate malate, and the Kreb's cycle derivatives (citrate, fumarate, malate, succinate, glutamate) are the most well absorbed and utilized forms of calcium, and they are superior to calcium carbonate as a source of the mineral. These terms will appear on the

---

CALCIUM SUPPLEMENTS

◆ Calcium carbonate provides 625 to 750 milligrams of elemental calcium per 2.5 millileters (½ teaspoon).

◆ However, calcium citrate malate and calcium gluconate appear to be more effective supplements than calcium carbonate. In addition, some research studies indicate that they may interfere less with the absorption of iron than calcium carbonate.

---

label of the supplement, so you should become familiar with them when selecting an appropriate calcium supplement.

The use of calcium-based antacids is *not* recommended. Antacids are designed to neutralize stomach acid, which is necessary for the first stage of protein digestion (acid hydrolysis). In addition, the antacid produces an alkaline environment that may reduce the absorption of a variety of minerals, such as iron, zinc, copper, and calcium itself, which require an acidic environment for efficient absorption.

Heating and Processing of Milk

Heating or boiling milk will *not* make it non-allergenic, although a few of the proteins may be decomposed, reducing their allergenicity to some extent. Only those persons who are allergic to heat-labile proteins (see earlier discussion) will tolerate boiled milk and will also be able to tolerate canned milk (evaporated milk) that has been extensively heated. Milk as an ingredient in cooked products is sometimes tolerated when unheated milk is not. However, some allergenic milk proteins that are heat-stable will cause allergy in sensitive people, even after cooking. The cow's milk in infant formulas remains allergenic and will induce an allergic reaction in milk-allergic infants.

Milk from Other Animals

Goat's milk may be tolerated by a small number of people who are allergic to cow's milk. However, the incidence of allergy to goat's milk in these people is quite high: In two separate studies, 25 out of 44, and 22 out of 28, children allergic to cow's milk reacted to goat's milk. Also, immunological studies have indicated that cow's milk and goat's milk proteins are antigenically very similar. The chances of developing an allergy to goat's milk if a person is allergic to cow's milk is obviously quite high.

GOAT'S MILK

◆ Goat's milk proteins closely resemble those in cow's milk.

◆ Most people who are allergic to cow's milk proteins demonstrate, or soon develop, similar sensitivity to goat's milk proteins.

◆ Many goat's milk proteins cross-react with cow's milk proteins.

◆ The majority of children allergic to cow's milk are or will become allergic to goat's milk.

◆ Goat's milk is deficient in folate.

MARE'S MILK

◆ Fewer proteins are similar to cow's milk proteins.

◆ In a recent research study, only 1 of 25 cow's-milk-allergic children were allergic to mare's milk.

Substitutes for Milk in Meals and Recipes

The following products can substitute for milk in appearance, flavor and texture, *but they are not nutritionally equivalent to milk.* Some of these products contain potentially allergenic ingredients, such as soy or nuts, so care must be taken to ensure that the consumer is not allergic to these alternatives.

Soy Milk

Soy milk is an acceptable substitute for milk on breakfast cereals and in many recipes. However, some people who have a tendency to develop allergies may be allergic to, or become allergic to, soybeans and their products, so soy milk should be taken with caution initially.

Liquid soy milk can be substituted directly for milk, diluting it 1:1 with water (1 cup soy milk added to 1 cup water). Use soy milk undiluted in recipes calling for evaporated milk. If the taste of soy milk is unpalatable, the addition of lime juice will often make it more acceptable.

There are several soy-based beverages on the market that are designed as milk substitutes and are enriched with calcium. These require no dilution. Such products include SoGood, SoNice, EdenSoy, among others.

RICE "MILKS"

Rice "milks" are made from brown rice and safflower oil. They make an acceptable alternative to milk on cereals and in baking. The calcium-enriched type is recommended for people following a diet that is completely milk-free.

OTHER LIQUIDS

Meat stock, vegetable boullion, fruit juice, vegetable oil mixed with water, or just plain water may be added to recipes when only a small amount of milk (less than one cup) is needed. When making rice, tapioca, or semolina puddings, you can use fruit instead of milk. Use potato water instead of milk in making breads.

NUT MILKS

You can use protein-rich nuts and seeds in place of milk, as long as you are not allergic to them. Grind the nuts or seeds into the consistency of a fine flour in a blender or coffee grinder, and add water to make a smooth mixture. One cup of nut meal plus two cups of water makes a good mix for most purposes. You can add it to recipes in the same quantity as milk.

WHEY-FREE MARGARINES

Most margarines are fortified with whey, a fraction of milk that contains unimportant proteins (see Table 8-1). A few brands, in particular diet spreads, do not contain whey. All of the major ingredients are listed on the product label; read the labels carefully to determine which margarine is whey-free. Parkay Diet Spread, Fleischmann's low sodium, no salt margarine, and Canoleo margarine are examples. Use these in place of butter.

NONDAIRY CREAMERS AND CREAM SUBSTITUTES

There are several milk-free products on the market made from oils that are designed for use in tea and coffee; an example is Coffee Rich. "Nondairy" toppings (such as Dreamwhip) can replace whipped cream in desserts.

CHEESE SUBSTITUTES

Soybean cake (tofu) can be substituted for cheese in many recipes, and fresh soybean curd may be an acceptable substitute for cottage cheese. Make sure the tofu does not contain milk solids. Some products called "tofu cheese" do contain milk.

Feeding the Milk-Allergic Infant

MOTHER'S MILK

Without question, the best nutrition for the newborn baby and young infant is its own mother's breast milk. A baby will never be allergic to its mother's milk, but may react to allergenic proteins that get into to her milk from her diet. If the baby is showing signs of allergy, and is being exclusively breast-fed, then the mother's diet must be checked for the presence of allergenic foods to which her baby is reacting. Eggs and milk are the most common allergenic foods that seem to cause symptoms at this early life stage. The mother should avoid these, and any other foods suspected to be causing a reaction in her infant, for at least four weeks to determine if these foods are the cause of the baby's symptoms. Reintroducing the foods into the mother's diet and monitoring the baby's response is a good way to identify the foods that are causing the baby's problems.

If the breast-fed baby is lactose-intolerant (usually a temporary condition following intestinal infection at this age), the mother can continue to breast-feed, or pump her milk and treat it with lactase enzyme, until the baby's symptoms go away. Details concerning feeding the lactose-intolerant infant are provided in the section "Lactose Intolerance," later in this chapter. There is no point in the mother eliminating milk and milk products from her diet to treat lactose intolerance in her baby, because her milk will contain 6% lactose (6 milliliters lactose in 100 milliliters liquid) regardless of whether or not she consumes milk and milk products.

MILK-FREE FORMULAS

Soy-based formulas may be tolerated by milk-allergic infants. However, about 50% of babies with milk allergy seem to develop an allergy to soy also. In these cases, protein hydrolysate formulas are the best alternative. Protein hydrolysate formulas including the extensively hydrolyzed casein formulas (such as Alimentum, Enfalac Nutramigen, Enfalac Pregestimil) or extensively hydrolyzed whey formulas (such as Profylac), in which the proteins have been broken down into their constituent amino acids and peptides too small to be allergenic, are usually tolerated by the milk-allergic infant. The biggest disadvantage of these formulas is their high cost.

Partially hydrolyzed milk-based formulas such as partially hydrolyzed whey (for example, GoodStart) are not suitable for an infant with suspected or diagnosed hypersensitivity to cow's milk protein. Babies whose symptoms don't go away when they're on the extensively hydrolyzed casein formulas might tolerate an "elemental" amino acid formula such as Neocate. Children should be encouraged to continue on hydrolysate or amino acid formula (or soy-based formula if a soy protein allergy or intolerance has been ruled out) as long as it is acceptable. After the age of 12 months, when they are eating a good range of solid foods, milk-allergic children may do well on milk substitutes (e.g., fortified soy or rice milks) and other calcium-fortified foods, if allergy to these foods is not suspected.

Table 8-5 lists the foods allowed and foods restricted in a milk-free diet.

◆ About 50% of babies with IgE-mediated cow's milk allergy develop an allergy to soy.

◆ In addition, soy can cause a non-IgE-mediated response (intolerance) that is separate and distinct from allergy. The effects are localized in the digestive tract, with symptoms such as colicky pain, abdominal bloating, gas, and diarrhea. This is sometimes referred to as soy enteropathy.

LACTOSE INTOLERANCE

What Is Lactose?

Lactose is actually two sugar molecules joined together: it is known as a **disaccharide** (di = two; saccharide = sugar). The digestive enzyme **lactase** splits lactose into its two constituent sugars: glucose and galactose. These are single sugars, called **monosaccharides** (mono = one; saccharide = sugar). Monosaccharides are small enough to be transported across the cells that line the digestive tract and into circulation, where they are an important source of energy for many body functions. The lactose molecule is too large to pass through the cells lining the digestive tract; lactase breaks it down into smaller pieces so that it can reach the circulation and be used as a source of energy for the body.

◆ Lactose is milk sugar.

◆ Lactose intolerance is caused by a lack of the enzyme required to digest lactose in the digestive tract.

◆ Lactose intolerance is not an allergy.

◆ Milk allergy is caused by an immunological reaction against the proteins in milk.

Table 8-5
THE MILK-FREE DIET: FOODS ALLOWED AND FOODS RESTRICTED

Type of Food	Foods Allowed	Foods Restricted
Milk and Milk Products	<ul><li>Soy beverages</li><li>Soy-based infant formula</li><li>Casein hydrolysate formula</li><li>Rice Dream®</li><li>Coconut milk</li><li>Nut milks</li><li>Seed milks</li><li>* Non-dairy creamers:</li><li>e.g., Coffee Rich® Potato-starch-based drinks</li><li>(e.g., Darifree™) Clarified butter</li><li>Milk-free margarine</li><li>Whey-free margarine</li><li>Milk-free soybean cake</li></ul>	<ul><li>All cow's milk (whole, 2%, 1%, skim; Lactaid™, Lacteeze™, or other lactose-free or lactose-reduced milk; acidophilus milk)</li><li>Milk from all animals (goat, sheep, other)</li><li>All milk derivatives (cream, half-and-half, whipping cream, light cream, sour cream, ice cream)</li><li>All milk products (buttermilk, yogurt, quark, kefir, cheese of all types)</li><li>Any manufactured product containing ingredients indicating milk (see Table 8-2) such as<ul><li>Casein</li><li>Caseinates</li><li>Whey</li><li>Lactose</li><li>Lactalbumin</li><li>Lactoglobulin</li><li>Milk solids</li></ul></li></ul>
Breads and Cereals	<ul><li>Breads and baked goods made without milk or milk products</li><li>French or Italian bread</li><li>Some whole-wheat bread</li><li>Some rye bread</li><li>Soda crackers</li><li>Bagels</li><li>Pasta without cheese or milk-containing sauce</li><li>Plain cooked or ready-to-eat cereals</li><li>All plain grains, flours, and starches</li></ul>	<ul><li>Baked products made with milk or milk products such as breads, crackers, biscuits, muffins, pancakes</li><li>Cereals containing milk or milk solids</li><li>Commercial baking mixes</li><li>Any manufactured food containing ingredients indicating that they were derived from milk</li></ul>
Legumes	<ul><li>All plain legumes such as dried beans, dried peas; lentils; dals</li><li>Milk-free; casein-free tofu</li><li>Peanut butter</li><li>Soybeans</li><li>Any soybean product free from milk components</li></ul>	<ul><li>Any legume prepared with milk such as<ul><li>Milk</li><li>Cream</li><li>Cheese</li></ul></li></ul>

Note: This list is not exhaustive. Other foods may contain milk and not be listed here. It is up to the reader to read all ingredient labels carefully and to contact the manufacturer if there is any doubt.

Table 8-5 (continued)
THE MILK-FREE DIET: FOODS ALLOWED AND FOODS RESTRICTED

Type of Food	Foods Allowed	Foods Restricted
Fruit	• All pure fruits and pure fruit juices	• Any fruit with cream, milk, or butter as additional ingredients, toppings, or sauces
Meat, Poultry, and Fish	• All fresh or frozen meat, poultry, or fish • Processed meats made without milk or milk products	• Commercially prepared meat, poultry, or fish that is: – Breaded – Battered – Creamed • Commercially produced meat products containing milk ingredients such as meat loaf, hot dogs, cold cuts, sausages
Eggs	• Plain, boiled, fried, or poached • Omelette or scrambled made without milk or cheese • Milk-free mayonnaise	• Any egg dish containing milk ingredients such as – Milk – Cream – Cheese – Commercial mayonnaise
Nuts and Seeds	• All plain nuts and seeds	• Nuts, seeds, and nut and seed mixtures with coatings containing milk or lactose • Any nut or seed candies or confectioneries containing milk ingredients
Spices and Herbs	• All pure spices and herbs	• None
Sweeteners	• All pure sugar, syrup, honey • Sugar Twin®	• Sugar substitutes containing lactose
Fats and Oils	• Clarified butter • Pure vegetable oils • Milk-free margarines such as – Fleischmann's® low sodium, no salt – Parkay Diet Spread® – Canoleo® margarine – Real mayonnaise – Nondairy dessert topping – Shortening – Lard – Meat dripping – Gravy made without milk	• Cream • Sour cream • Cream cheese • Whipped topping • Butter • Margarine containing whey or milk • Salad dressings with milk or milk products

What Is Lactase?

Lactase, the enzyme that digests lactose, is made within the epithelial cells lining the digestive tract. If these cells are damaged, they cannot produce enough lactase. As a result, lactose is incompletely broken down into glucose and galactose and some lactose remains intact. The undigested lactose remains in the intestines and eventually finds its way into the large bowel. Here millions of bacteria use any undigested food for their own nourishment, multiplying rapidly and producing a large number of by-products. Usually a variety of gases, organic acids, and other irritating chemicals result from the activity of these microorgansims. We feel the effects as excessive flatus, abdominal bloating, pain, loose stool, or diarrhea, and general distress in the lower intestines.

*Lactose intolerance does **not** involve the immune system, and no antibodies are produced. Therefore, lactose intolerance is **not** an allergy.*

Incidence of Lactase Deficiency

IN BABIES AND YOUNG CHILDREN
Virtually every baby has enough lactase to digest the lactose in its mother's milk at birth. Lactase deficiency in infants is uncommon because lactose is the principal sugar in human milk and the baby needs lactase in order to digest lactose. Because lactose is so important to babies' nutritional needs, they are usually born with enough of the enzyme to digest it. There is a medical condition known as congenital alactasia, or primary lactase deficiency, in which the baby is born without the ability to produce the enzyme, but this is *an extremely rare event*.

A *temporary* lactase deficiency can develop in babies when the inflammation associated with a bacterial or viral infection in the digestive tract damages the cells that produce the enzyme. This is known as secondary lactase deficiency, to distinguish it from primary congenital alactasia. Happily, in secondary lactose intolerance the cells rapidly return to normal when the infection clears up, and the usual level of lactase production is quickly reestablished.

IN OLDER CHILDREN AND ADULTS
Most adults lose *some* degree of lactase activity after puberty. In certain ethnic groups, such as the Oriental races, African blacks, persons of Middle Eastern origin, aboriginal peoples of North and South America and the Arctic, and people from the Mediterranean region, lactose intolerance may be as high as 80% of the population. In contrast, only about 20% of people of northern European ori-

gin lose the ability to produce lactase. In most cases, complete loss of lactase does not occur, but these people produce the enzyme at such a low level that consumption of large quantities of milk and milk products with normal levels of lactose leads to the uncomfortable symptoms of lactose intolerance.

Secondary lactase deficiency can occur in adults as well as children. Bacterial and viral infections, and sometimes the use of strong drugs and medications taken by mouth, such as antibiotics, may damage the fragile epithelial cells in the digestive tract. If lactose was tolerated prior to the epithelial damage, regular lactase activity will resume as soon as the cells return to normal.

Distinguishing Between Milk Allergy and Lactose Intolerance

It is frequently very difficult to distinguish milk allergy from lactose intolerance on the basis of clinical symptoms alone, because some of the symptoms, such as abdominal pain, diarrhea, nausea, vomiting, gas, and bloating, are common to both conditions. However, milk allergy often results in symptoms in other organs, such as the upper respiratory tract (for example, a stuffy, runny nose), pain, itching, fluid drainage from the ears, or skin reactions (such as eczema or hives), and lactose intolerance does not.

Because secondary lactase deficiency is a consequence of inflammation in the digestive tract, the intestinal inflammation caused by milk allergy can sometimes result in lactase deficiency. Thus, both milk allergy and lactose intolerance can exist together. Because milk is the only source of lactose in the normal diet, eliminating milk from the diet will cure both conditions, but it will not distinguish which condition caused the symptoms. It is important to determine which condition is causing the problem: Milk and milk products are a significant source of nutrients, especially for infants and young children, and they should not be eliminated from the diet unless it is absolutely necessary to do so. Furthermore, eliminating milk entirely is not easy, because so many different foods, such as baked goods, soups, salad dressings, gravies, desserts, and so on, contain milk. Not being able to eat these foods can make meal planning very difficult.

Laboratory Tests for Lactose Intolerance

There are a number of laboratory tests that can identify lactose intolerance:

The *fecal reducing sugar test* is considered by many clinicians as very reliable. After the patient takes a drink containing lactose, the feces are collected and Fehling's solution is added. The presence of lactose is indicated by a change in color, from blue to red. The lactose "reduces" the chemical in the solution. Thus, a change in color indicates that a deficiency of lactase has led to undigested lactose being excreted in the feces.

The *hydrogen breath test* is a common test for lactose intolerance. In this test the patient drinks a given quantity of lactose and after a prescribed interval, a breath sample is analyzed for the presence of hydrogen. If hydrogen is detected, it indicates that bacteria in the digestive tract have acted on undigested lactose and produced hydrogen as one of their metabolic by-products. Unfortunately, this test is not specific for lactase deficiency, because any sugar remaining in the digestive tract will be metabolized by bacteria with the production of hydrogen. Undigested sucrose, maltose, or a starch will give a similar result.

The *blood glucose test* involves measuring the level of glucose in the blood after the patient takes a drink containing 50 grams of lactose. An increase in blood glucose indicates that lactose has been broken down to glucose and galactose, the levels of which rise in the blood when the body is producing enough lactase. Measuring the level of galactose would be equally informative. If there is no increase in the level of glucose in the blood, lactose intolerance is confirmed.

If the feces collected after the above lactose drink are acidic, with a pH of 6 or lower (the *fecal pH test*), it indicates that microorganisms in the large bowel have fermented the undigested lactose. The microbial activity results in the production of acids, which lower the pH of the stool. Thus, the diagnosis of lactose intolerance is further reinforced.

Management of Lactose Intolerance

Lactase deficiency is easier to manage than cow's milk protein allergy, because any milk or milk product free from lactose can be consumed without gastrointestinal symptoms. Lactose-free milk is available as products such as Lacteeze or Lactaid. Alternatively, a commercial form of lactase (sold as Lactaid liquid) can be added to any milk before consumption. After 24 hours in the fridge, the lactose is split into its two component sugars, glucose and galactose, which the body can absorb and use without harm. All of the nutrients and proteins in milk are thus available to the body, and there will be no risk of nutritional deficiency as a result of long-time avoidance of milk.

It is more difficult to avoid lactose in prepared foods; anything containing milk or milk solids is likely to contain lactose also. Some people find that they can consume lactose-containing foods without a problem if they take Lactaid in the form of a tablet before eating those foods.

Lactose intolerance is dose-related. Usually the epithelial cells of the digestive tract are producing a limited amount of the enzyme lactase, and the body can process small doses of foods containing lactose. Problems occur when the amount of lactose in the food *exceeds* the capacity of the enzyme to digest it. The important thing is to determine tolerance levels. By remaining within one's own limits, a person should not have symptoms. Most people who are lactose-intolerant can drink a 6-ounce glass of milk without symptoms, but will experience abdominal discomfort if they exceed this amount.

When lactose intolerance has been diagnosed, the degree of lactase deficiency can be assessed by having the patient take increasing quantities of lactose in a variety of dairy products (Table 8-6). Most lactase-deficient people can process the lactose in one glass of milk, which is about 11 grams of lactose. But taking several types of milk and dairy products in a 24-hour period would exceed their enzyme's capacity to break down lactose and digestive tract symptoms would result.

Table 8-6
LEVELS OF LACTOSE IN NORMAL SERVING SIZES OF COMMON FOODS AND BEVERAGES

Product	Serving Size	Lactose (grams)
Sweetened condensed milk	125 mL (½ cup)	15
Evaporated milk	125 mL (½ cup)	12
Whole milk	250 mL (1 cup)	11
2% milk	250 mL (1 cup)	11
1% milk	250 mL (1 cup)	11
Skim milk	250 mL (1 cup)	11
Buttermilk	250 mL (1 cup)	10
Ice milk	125 mL (½ cup)	9
Ice cream	125 mL (½ cup)	6
Half-and-half light cream	125 mL (½ cup)	5
Yogurt, low-fat	250 mL (1 cup)	5
Sour cream	125 mL (½ cup)	4
Cottage cheese, creamed	125 mL (½ cup)	3
Whipping cream	125 mL (½ cup)	3
Cottage cheese, uncreamed	125 mL (½ cup)	2
Sherbet, orange	125 mL (½ cup)	2
American (jack) cheese	30 g (1 oz)	2
Swiss cheese	30 g (1 oz)	1
Blue cheese	30 g (1 oz)	1
Cheddar cheese	30 g (1 oz)	1
Parmesan cheese 3	g (1 oz)	1
Cream cheese (e.g., Philadelphia)	30 g (1 oz)	1
Lactaid milk	125 mL (½ cup)	0.025
Butter	5 mL (1 tsp)	trace

Feeding the lactose-intolerant baby

The Breast-Fed Baby

A breast-fed baby will ingest significant quantities of lactose in mother's milk. *The lactose composition of her milk will remain constant regardless of whether or not the mother consumes milk and dairy products.*

- If the lactose intolerance is secondary to a gastrointestinal tract infection or other condition that is expected to be temporary, some authorities advise continuing breast feeding and expect the diarrhea to gradually go away as the underlying inflammation disappears.

- Some authorities recommend placing a few drops of Lactaid directly into the baby's mouth before each feeding. This may provide enough of the enzyme to break down the lactose in mother's milk, and so reduce or eliminate the baby's digestive tract symptoms.

- Alternatively, the mother can pump her breast milk and treat the milk with Lactaid drops (4 drops per 250 millimeters of milk) and allow the enzyme to act for 24 hours in the fridge. The baby is fed the lactose-free milk the next day. This is continued until the diarrhea stops, when the baby can be gradually put back to the breast.

The Formula-Fed Baby

Infant formulas that are lactose-free can be given to a lactose-intolerant infant. If the baby is *not* allergic to milk, the milk-based formula Lacto-Free (Mead Johnson) or Similac LF (Ross), which are free from lactose, are suitable. If the infant is allergic to cow's milk proteins, but tolerates soy, soy-based formulas such as Prosobee (Mead Johnson), Alsoy (Nestle), or Isomil (Ross) may be suitable. Infants who are allergic to both cow's milk and soy proteins may tolerate a casein hydrolysate formula such as Alimentum (Ross), Nutramigen (Mead Johnson), or Pregestimil (Mead Johnson). All of these formulas are free from lactose.

Managing Lactose Intolerance

Lactose Restrictions

- Assume that foods, medications, and beverages containing milk and milk solids contain lactose, unless they are labelled "lactose-free."

- Avoid products labelled as containing lactose, milk, milk solids, milk powder, cheese and cheese flavor, curd, whey, cream, butter, and margarine containing milk solids.

◆ Products containing lactic acid, lactalbumin, lactate, and casein **do not** contain lactose and can be consumed.

Acidophilus milk has had a bacterium called *Lactobacillus acidophilus* added to it. These bacteria do not break down lactose to any great extent, so lactose-intolerant people would not be able to tolerate this milk.

Milk and Milk Products Suitable for a Lactose-Restricted Diet

◆ Adding the enzyme lactase (commercially available as Lactaid) to liquid milk, and allowing the enzyme to act for a minimum of 24 hours in the refrigerator, will make it digestible. No milk substitutes are then necessary. The amount of the enzyme that needs to be added will depend on the degree of lactase deficiency. Follow the instructions that are provided with the product.

    15 drops in 1 liter of milk will render it 99% lactose free.

    10 drops reduces the lactose to 90%.

     5 drops will provide a milk that is 70% lactose-free.

◆ Lactaid tablets may be taken before eating or drinking lactose-containing products and may be sufficient to break down the amount of lactose consumed in the following meal.

◆ Lactaid milk and Lacteeze milk, which are 99% lactose-free, are available in the dairy section of grocery stores. These are tolerated by lactose-deficient people, but they are more expensive than regular milk.

◆ Hard, fermented cheeses may be tolerated because most of the lactose is removed with the whey during their manufacture.

◆ Although butter and regular margarines contain a small amount of lactose (in whey), they are usually tolerated because the level of lactose is so low and these products are eaten in small quantities.

◆ Fermented milks such as yogurt and buttermilk may be tolerated because the level of lactose in these products is reduced (but not completely eliminated) by bacterial enzymes. Mixing Lactaid drops in the yogurt in the doses indicated above, and refrigerating the product for 24 hours, may make it acceptable for someone who is severely lactose-intolerant.

The Lactose-Free Diet

Phase I: Avoidance of Lactose

Restriction of all lactose will be required initially. The patient should follow Phase I (Table 8-7) until the digestive tract symptoms improve. Then, by gradually introducing increasing amounts of lactose-containing foods, the person's limit of tolerance for lactose will be determined (Phase II).

Table 8-7 PHASE I: AVOIDANCE OF LACTOSE		
Type of Food	**Foods Allowed**	**Foods Restricted**
Milk and Milk Products	• Milk treated with Lactaid™ drops according to manufacturer's instructions • Lactaid milk • Lacteeze milk • Other lactose-free milks • Milk-free substitutes, such as • Rice Dream™, Darifree™ • Coffe-Rich™ • Soy beverages such as SoGood™, SoNice™, EdenSoy™,	• Avoid all except those on the "Allowed" list.
Breads and Cereals	• Breads and baked goods without milk or milk derivatives • *Read labels carefully* to ensure no milk is included in the list of ingredients because some of the manufactured products below may contain milk. – French bread – Italian bread – Whole-wheat bread – Rye bread – Soda crackers – Bagels – Pasta • Plain cooked cereals • Some ready-to-eat cereals • Plain grains	• Baked goods made with milk or derivatives of milk
Vegetables	• All pure fresh or frozen vegetables and their juices, without added ingredients	• Prepared as – Creamed – Scalloped • Mashed with milk • Breaded or battered • Instant potatoes and similar manufactured foods
Fruit	• All pure fresh or frozen fruits and their juices, without added ingredients	• Fruit dishes with milk-containing ingredients or toppings, such as – Custard – Cream – Ice cream • Any manufactured, packaged, or frozen fruit dishes with added milk solids

Table 8-7 (continued)
PHASE I: AVOIDANCE OF LACTOSE

Type of Food	Foods Allowed	Foods Restricted
Meat, Poultry, and Fish	• All fresh or frozen without added ingredients • Any processed meats without milk ingredients • Meat, poultry, or fish canned without milk ingredients	• Any with added ingredients containing milk, such as – Sauces – Creamed – Breaded – Battered
Eggs	• Plain, without added milk or milk products: – Boiled – Fried – Scrambled – Poached – Omelette	• Prepared with – Milk – Cheese – Butter – Margarine – Any other milk derivative
Legumes	• All plain legumes, such as – Beans – Peas – Dried peas and beans – Lentils – Peanuts and peanut butter	• Any prepared with milk or milk derivatives, such as – Butter – Margarine – Milk or cheese sauces
Nuts and Seeds	• All plain nuts and seeds	• Any with added milk-derived ingredients
Fats and Oils	• Pure vegetable oils • Milk-free margarines such as – Fleischmann's low-sodium, no salt – Parkay diet spread – Canoleo margarine – Some other diet spreads (read labels carefully) • Real mayonnaise • Shortening • Lard • Meat drippings • Gravy made with allowed ingredients	• Salad dressings with milk or milk derivatives • Butter • Margarines containing whey (read labels)
Spices and Herbs	• All fresh, or dried	• None
Sweeteners	• All except those with added lactose or other milk-derived ingredients – Sugar – Pure syrups – Honey	• Sugar substitutes containing lactose (read labels carefully)

PHASE II: DETERMINING LACTOSE-TOLERANCE LEVELS

In Phase II, lactose tolerance is determined by introducing milk and milk products in gradually increasing portions. Lactose intolerance is dose-related. Usually, a certain amount of the lactase enzyme is being produced, and some lactose can be processed. It is important to establish how much lactose can be broken down at one time (Step 1) and how much lactose can be processed over the day (Step 2).

Step 1

Day 1: Morning (Breakfast)

◆ Eat a portion of food containing 1 gram lactose, for example, 1 oz or 2 tbsp of cream cheese.

◆ If there are no symptoms of intolerance, double the amount of lactose on day 2.

Day 2: Morning (Breakfast)

◆ Eat a portion of food containing 2 grams of lactose, for example, 2 ounces or ¼ cup of cream cheese *or* ½ cup of uncreamed cottage cheese.

◆ If there are no symptoms of intolerance, increase the amount of lactose on day 3.

Day 3: Morning (Breakfast)

◆ Eat a portion of food containing 5 grams of lactose, for example, 1 cup of yogurt (regular or low-fat).

◆ If there are no symptoms of intolerance, increase the amount of lactose on day 4.

Day 4: Morning (Breakfast)

◆ Eat a portion of food containing 10 grams lactose, for example, 1 cup (250 mL) of milk (homogenized; fat-reduced 2%; 1% or skim).

Step 2

To establish how much lactose may be tolerated over the day, go back to the amount last tolerated. (For example, on day 2, 2 grams of lactose were tolerated, but on day 3, there was bloating, cramping, and diarrhea following 1 cup of yogurt.)

Day 1: Morning (Breakfast)

◆ Eat a portion of food containing the amount of lactose tolerated in step 1 (for example, 2 grams of lactose).

Day 1: Evening (Dinner)

◆ Repeat the morning procedure.

◆ If there are no symptoms of intolerance, increase the number of servings on day 2.

Day 2: Morning (Breakfast)
- ◆ Eat a portion of food containing the amount of lactose tolerated in step 1.
- ◆ Repeat the process at lunch and dinner.

Ideas for Milk Substitutes on a Lactose-Reduced Diet

BEVERAGES

Lactaid Milk and Lactaid Hot Chocolate
>   Combine 1 tbsp (15 mL) of pure cocoa with 1 tbsp sugar.
>   Mix in 1 tbsp cold water until smooth.
>   Stir in 1 cup of hot Lactaid milk.

Fruit and Vegetable Juices
>   All pure vegetable and fruit juices without added ingredients

Coffee and Tea
>   Clear coffee, tea, and herbal tea
>   In place of milk, add
>>   Lactaid milk
>>   Rich's Coffee Rich
>>   Soy beverages (SoGood, SoNice) without milk-derived additives
>>   (*read labels*)

Others
>   Soft drinks and mineral water
>   Alcoholic beverages except cream-based liqueurs

Liquid Meal Replacers
>   Liquid nutritional supplements containing casein, but free from whey, such as Boost, Enercal, Ensure, Resource

SOUP

For a soup base:
>   Clear stock
>   Clear broth or bouillon
>   Defatted meat drippings
>   Tomato or vegetable juice

Read labels on canned stock based soups, and *avoid* milk or cream-based soups.

DESSERTS

All desserts and baked goods made without milk or milk products, for example:
   Angel food cakes
   Gelatin fruit desserts (Jello)
   Rice Dream dessert
   Milk-free soy ice desserts
   Fruit ices
   Popsicles
   Fresh, frozen, or canned fruit

Sorbet made in a food processor
   1 banana
   A dash of lemon juice
   1 to 1¼ cups of frozen berries
   Add sugar or Sugar Twin to taste

CONDIMENTS AND SNACKS
   Salt and pepper
   Tabasco, Worcestershire sauce, soy sauce
   Ketchup, mustard, relish, pickles
   Air-popped popcorn
   Potato chips
   Tortilla or nacho chips and salsa
   Hard and gelatin candy in moderation

Avoid milk chocolate and candies made with restricted ingredients, such as
   Toffee
   Caramels
   Chocolates

DINING IN RESTAURANTS
- Dining in regular restaurants should pose no difficulty as many milk-free foods are included on all restaurant menus
- Check with the server to ensure that the dish is milk-free
- Most fast-food restaurants will have lists of the ingredients in all their menu items; avoid those that contain milk or its derivative.
- Avoid all cream-based sauces and dressings; request dishes without added sauces.

— CHAPTER 9 —

EGG ALLERGY

Eggs contain many different proteins that can lead to allergy. Each egg-allergic person is likely to be sensitized to more than one such protein. Someone who has a proven allergy to eggs is usually advised to avoid egg in any form. This is wise in the case of children under the age of 7, because there is a higher risk of a severe or anaphylactic reaction to eggs in this age group. However, for adults, such a risk is much less, and if they have not experienced anything resembling an anaphylactic reaction, it is often useful for them to determine to what degree they need to restrict their intake of eggs. Because there is a great deal of difference between the proteins in egg yolk and the proteins in egg white (the latter tend to be more allergenic than the former), it is sometimes useful to find out which of these egg components is the cause of the allergy so that the diet need not be so restricted. In addition, some egg proteins are destroyed by heat, which means that a person sensitized to heat-labile proteins can consume eggs that are well-cooked, especially in small quantities in baked goods, without any harmful effects. However, a person allergic to heat-stable proteins, which are unaffected by heat, must avoid eggs in any form. So, a discussion of egg allergy should start with a brief description of the different proteins in eggs. Then we can discuss the diet suitable for a person with allergy to any of these components.

EGG PROTEINS

The white of an egg contains about 10% protein and 80% water. The yolk is made up of 50% water, 34% fat, and 16% protein. Egg white is considered to be the source of the major egg allergens, which include *ovalbumin, conalbumin (ovotransferrin)*, and *ovomucoid*. Some egg yolk proteins, especially *alpha-livetin*, may also induce the production of IgE antibodies, and there may be some degree of antigenic cross-reactivity between egg yolk and egg white proteins. Table 9-1 lists the major egg white and egg yolk proteins that are known to cause allergic reactions in sensitive people.

Table 9-1
EGG PROTEINS

Antigenic Egg White Proteins:

Major Proteins
Ovalbumin
Conalbumin (Ovotransferrin)
Ovomucoid
Ovomucin
Lysozyme

Trace Amounts* of
Catalase
Ovoflavoprotein
Ficin inhibitor
Ovoglycoprotein
G2 and G3 globulins
Ovomacroglobulin
Ribonuclease
Ovoinhibitor
Avidin

Antigenic Egg Yolk Proteins:

Major Proteins
Lipovitellin
Phosvitin
Low-density lipoproteins
Livetins

* Trace amount means that the component is present in such small quantities that it is almost undetectable.

COMPOSITION OF THE AVERAGE CHICKEN EGG

Egg white: 56 – 61%
Yolk: 27 – 32%
Shell: 8 – 11%

Proteins in eggs from different bird species sometimes cross-react antigenically. However, evidence from a single study indicates that people allergic to duck and goose eggs were not allergic to hen's eggs. The subject of cross-reactivity between eggs from different bird species needs to be investigated further.

In most cases of egg allergy, IgE antibodies are produced specifically to egg proteins, which differ from the proteins in chicken flesh. However, some *livetins* are derived from the blood of the hen. IgE antibodies to these proteins might result in allergy to both egg and chicken because blood is sometimes found in the chicken egg.

Although cooking may decompose many of the egg proteins so that cooked eggs may be tolerated in cases where raw egg causes an allergic reaction, some egg proteins, especially ovomucoid, are heat-stable and people who are allergic to this component will react to cooked as well as raw egg.

Avoidance of egg as an *individual ingredient* in a meal (such as omelette, scrambled, boiled, fried, and so on) is relatively easy. However, eggs are frequently included as an ingredient in prepared foods. As such they may not be so easily recognized unless you take care in reading food labels, becoming familiar with terms that indicate the presence of egg protein, and being aware of the foods traditionally made with eggs.

The Egg-Free Diet (Table 9-2)

The egg-free diet omits eggs and products containing eggs.

Because it is almost impossible to separate the white and yolk of the egg, a person with an egg white allergy or an egg yolk allergy, especially if it results in anaphylaxis, *should avoid **all** egg proteins* until it has been clearly demonstrated that only one part of the egg is responsible for the allergic reaction. If there is any risk of an anaphylactic reaction, all forms of egg should be carefully avoided, even if it is known that only the white or the yolk is responsible: Both can be contaminated with proteins from the other.

There is evidence that eggs from a variety of different bird species have common allergens, so a person allergic to eggs from one species should avoid eggs from all species unless it is certain that allergy to specific species does not exist.

Important Nutrients in Eggs

Eggs contribute vitamin D, vitamin B12, pantothenic acid, selenium, folacin, riboflavin, biotin, and iron, and in smaller amounts, vitamin A, vitamin E, vitamin B6, and zinc. These nutrients can easily be supplied in meat, fish and poultry products, legumes, whole grains, and vegetables, so an egg-free diet should not pose any risk of deficiency of any of these nutrients.

Table 9-2
THE EGG-FREE DIET: FOODS ALLOWED AND FOODS RESTRICTED

Type of Food	Foods Allowed	Foods Restricted
Milk and Milk Products	* Milk (whole, 2%, 1%, skim) • Cream • Sour cream • Sour cream • Yogurt • Buttermilk • Ice cream without egg • Frozen yogurt without egg • Cheese	* Eggnog * Any milk drinks made with egg • Desserts containing egg such as custard, cream pies, puddings, some gelatin desserts • Commercial ice creams containing egg
Breads and Cereals	• Bread, buns, and baked goods made without egg • French or Italian bread • Soda crackers • Plain cooked grains • Plain oatmeal • Regular Cream of Wheat® • Cream of Rice® and other cooked cereals • Ready-to-eat cereals made without egg • Egg-free pasta • Egg-free baking mixes • Homemade baked goods without egg or made with egg-free substitutes (see page 156)	• Commercial or homemade baked goods made with egg such as cakes, muffins, pancakes, waffles, fritters, doughnuts; toaster pastries • Quick breads • Cakes, breads, and other baked products with egg glaze • All baking mixes containing egg • Instant oatmeal and flavored oatmeal • Instant Cream of Wheat • Commercial pasta (spaghetti, macaroni, egg noodles, etc.) • Confectioneries containing egg such as divinity, fondants, marshmallows, nougat, meringue, pavlova, mousse, soufflé
Vegetables	• All pure vegetables and their juices	• Vegetable dishes made with egg • Salads containing egg • Salad dressings containing egg such as traditional Caesar salad • Mayonnaise • Sandwich spreads containing egg
Fruit	• All pure fruits and fruit juices	• Any fruit dish containing egg such as meringue, mousse, soufflé, fruit whips
Meat, Poultry, and Fish	• All pure fresh, frozen, or canned meat, poultry, and fish	• Meat, poultry, and fish dishes made with egg as a binder or glaze, such as meat loaf and meatballs • Sausages, loaves, croquettes made with egg • Some processed meats (check labels) • Soups such as egg drop soup • Consommé cleared with egg white

Note: This list is not exhaustive. Other foods may contain egg and not be listed here. It is up to the reader to read all ingredient labels carefully and to contact the manufacturer if there is any doubt.

Table 9-2 (continued)
THE EGG-FREE DIET: FOODS ALLOWED AND FOODS RESTRICTED

Type of Food	Foods Allowed	Foods Restricted
Eggs	• None	• Eggs from all bird species including • Chicken • Duck • Ostrich • Turkey • Quail • Goose • Plover • Other • Manufactured foods with ingredients indicating the presence of egg such as: • Albumin • Globulin • Livetin • Ovalbumin • Ovomucin • Ovomucoid • Ovovitellin • Ingredients made from derivatives of eggs, for example • Lysozyme • Simplesse
Legumes	• All pure legumes such as dried peas, beans, lentils, dals • Plain tofu • Plain peanut butter	• Legume dishes containing egg or derivatives of egg (see list under "Eggs")
Nuts and Seeds	• All plain nuts and seeds	• Glazed or coated nuts (read label) • Nuts or seeds in baked goods made or glazed with egg
Fats and Oils	• Butter, cream, sour cream • Margarine • Vegetable shortening • Pure vegetable oils • Lard • Meat drippings • Gravy	• Salad dressings that list egg in any form as an ingredient • Caesar salad dressing • Real mayonnaise • Sauces made with egg such as hollandaise, béarnaise, Newburg
Spices and Herbs	• All	• None
Sweeteners	• All	• None

General Guidelines for the Egg-Free Diet

◆ *Avoid all obvious sources of eggs* (omelette, scrambled, boiled, fried) and foods made principally with eggs (eggnog, custard, souffle, quiche, timbale, egg noodles, angel food cake).

◆ *Avoid packaged foods containing eggs*, even as a minor ingredient. Foods with the ingredients egg, egg powder, egg white, egg yolk, or egg protein obviously should be avoided. Become familiar with the terms on food labels indicating the presence of egg (see Table 9-3).

◆ In a restaurant, or when eating a meal with unknown ingredients, avoid foods traditionally made with eggs, including: mayonnaise; Caesar salad; some salad dressings; sauces such as hollandaise, bearnaise, Newburg, Foyot; meat, fish, or vegetables coated with a batter (such as fritters and tempura); pancakes; waffles. In Chinese restaurants, egg swirl soup, wonton soup, and any dish with noodles traditionally contain egg.

◆ Some soft drinks (root beer), wine, and beer may contain egg, which is used as a "clarifier."

◆ Many baked goods contain egg, and egg may be present in baking powder.

◆ Some candies are made with egg, such as nougat and divinity. Check labels carefully.

◆ Ice creams usually contain eggs.

◆ Many desserts, such as cream pies, pavlova, and packaged dessert mixes containing custards, may have egg in them.

◆ Egg may be present as a garnish on some dishes and may be used as a "binding agent" in meat loaf and dumplings.

EGG SUBSTITUTES

Eggs serve three purposes in recipes:

1. Act as a leavening agent
2. Act as a binder
3. Provide a source of liquid

Substitutes are designed to perform these functions as far as possible, but the finished product may not be exactly the same as when an egg is used.

Substitutes for Egg as a Leavening Agent

1 tbsp egg-free baking powder plus 2 tbsp liquid = 1 egg

Table 9-3
TERMS ON LABELS THAT INDICATE THE PRESENCE OF EGG

Albumin	Eggs of all bird species	Mayonnaise
Ovalbumin	chicken	Simplesse
Globulin	duck	Egg powder
Ovoglobulin	goose	Egg white
Ovomucin	turkey	Egg yolk
Ovomucoid	ostrich	Egg protein
Ovovitellin	quail	Frozen egg
Livetin	plover	Dried egg solids
Lysozyme	other	Powdered egg
		Pasteurized egg
		Egg Beaters™

Nonfood Items That May Contain Egg
Photographic film
Printed natural fabrics
Some fur garments
Some vaccines are produced from viruses grown in eggs. The risk of injecting such a vaccine in a highly egg-allergic person should be discussed with his or her physician.

2 tbsp flour plus ½ Tbsp shortening
plus ½ tsp egg-free baking powder   ] = 1 egg
plus 2 tbsp liquid

("Liquid" can be water, vinegar, fruit juice, broth, or any liquid that would be appropriate for the recipe.)

Some recipes call for only 1 egg and a large proportion of baking powder (2 tsp) or baking soda (1½ tsp). Try these recipes without egg and add 1 tbsp of vinegar instead of the egg with the baking powder or baking soda.

Substitutes for Egg as a Binder

RECIPE 1

Combine ⅓ cup water and 3 – 4 tsp brown flax seeds. Bring to a boil on high heat, then simmer on low heat for 5 –7 minutes until a slightly thickened gel begins to form. Strain the flax seed out of the liquid and use the gel in the recipes.

This recipe makes enough substitute for one egg. Increase the amounts as needed to substitute for 2, 3, or more eggs.

Some people prefer to leave the flax seeds in the mixture after thickening or to blend them into the gel before using. This may alter the recipe's taste a little.

RECIPE 2
⅓ cup ground flax seed plus 1 cup water
Bring mixture to a boil. Simmer 3 minutes. Refrigerate.
One tablespoon of the mixture replaces one egg.

RECIPE 3
⅓ cup extra water plus 1 tbsp arrowroot powder plus 2 tsp guar gum

RECIPE 4
2 ounces tofu = 1 egg

Substitutes for Egg as a Liquid

⅓ cup apple juice = 1 egg
OR: 4 tbsp pureed apricot = 1 egg
OR: 1 tbsp vinegar = 1 egg

Commercial egg substitutes can be used (for example, Jolly Joan egg replacer or Egg Replacer marketed by Ener-G-Foods).

DO NOT use Egg Beaters, which is made from egg white.

If egg yolk is tolerated, but egg white causes a adverse reaction, egg yolks separated from the whites can be used, *as long as the egg white does not cause an anaphylactic reaction*. If the egg white has caused anaphylaxis in the past, **do not** use egg yolk, because the small amount of albumin that will adhere to the yolk might be enough to cause a reaction.

Egg-Free Baking Powder Recipes

GLUTEN-FREE BAKING POWDER
Baking soda	1 part (⅓ cup)
Cream of tartar	2 parts (⅔ cup)
Cornstarch	1 part (⅓ cup)

Mix and sift all ingredients together. Use in same quantities as baking powder in recipes.

CORN-FREE (ARROWROOT) BAKING POWDER

Baking soda	part (⅓ cup)
Cream of tartar	2 parts (⅔ cup)
Arrowroot starch	2 parts (⅔ cup)

Mix well and store in an airtight container.
1 tsp regular baking powder = 1½ tsp arrowroot baking powder

HYPOALLERGENIC BAKING POWDER

Baking soda	1 part (⅓ cup)
Cream of tartar	2 parts (⅔ cup)
Ground rice (or brown rice flour)	1 part (⅓ cup)

Sift all ingredients together thoroughly. Use in same quantities as baking powder in recipes.

— CHAPTER 10 —

WHEAT AND GRAIN ALLERGY

Perhaps the most difficult foods to eliminate from your diet are the grains and the flours made from them. Most people eat bread, pasta, baked goods, breakfast cereals, and many snack foods, daily. Just think of your usual routine: for breakfast, cereal, toast, pancakes, or perhaps a toaster pastry; a mid-morning snack that may be a muffin or Danish pastry; for lunch, a sandwich made with bread, perhaps with a bowl of noodle soup; a cookie at mid-afternoon "to keep up your energy" until supper, which may consist of lasagna, spaghetti, or some other pasta dish, or possibly pizza whose crust is, of course, bread. And then before bed, perhaps another cookie. . . . It is difficult to imagine a day without products made from flours and grains.

When you suspect that you may be reacting to wheat or another staple grain, or perhaps have been to the allergist and have been told that your skin or blood test for wheat or other grains is positive, you are going to have to eliminate grains and flours from your diet, at least for a short time. The task at first seems almost impossible especially if you have a hectic lifestyle and rely heavily on convenience foods that need little preparation. It is hard indeed to find prepared foods that do not contain grains and flours. But don't despair, this chapter is designed to help you through this process.

The first thing we need to do is discuss why grains can cause allergies and how you can best avoid the ones that cause problems. Understanding which part of the grain needs to be avoided will help you have a clearer idea of what to substitute for it. And this is what we want to achieve–not to deprive you of grains and baked goods entirely, but to give you the information that will help you to find acceptable substitutes. This will be especially important if you discover, after the process of elimination and reintroduction, that you are going to have to continue to avoid perhaps wheat and its related grains for the long-term.

COMPOSITION OF GRAINS

Although the carbohydrate content of grains is much higher than their protein content, it is the protein that causes the immune system response in an allergic reaction. Wheat is the grain most commonly reported to cause allergic reactions; it is also the grain most common in the Western diet. Allergy to other grains (e.g., oats, rye, barley, corn, rice) is experienced less frequently.

Proteins in Wheat

Protein makes up about 12% of the dry wheat kernel. There are four classes of wheat proteins:
Gliadins
Glutenins
Albumins
Globulins

Gliadins and glutenins form the **gluten** complex. Gliadins contain as many as 40 to 60 distinct components; glutenins contain at least 15. The molecular size of the protein components in wheat is 10 to 40 kilodaltons, the size considered optimal for triggering a Type I hypersensitivity reaction. Other cereal grains contain similar mixtures of proteins which theoretically could trigger a hypersensitivity reaction.

Allergy to Wheat Proteins

No single protein or class of proteins seems to be responsible for wheat allergy. People who are allergic to wheat tend to react to the albumins and globulins, rather than to the gliadins and glutenins. However, some researchers disagree with this generalization and believe there is more evidence for immune responses to gliadins and globulins than to albumins and glutenins. Interestingly, despite this demonstrable immune reactivity (IgE positivity in RAST [radio-allergo sorbent test] in most cases), some people show no clinical evidence of wheat allergy when they consume wheat. On the other hand, many people with demonstrable symptoms after consuming wheat are RAST-negative. (See Chapter 5, page 86, for more information on RAST.) These findings simply emphasize the importance of elimination and challenge in identifying of a sensitivity to wheat or any other grain before it is excluded from a person's diet for a prolonged period of time.

The most common symptoms of wheat allergy are asthma (in asthmatics), rhinitis, and conjunctivitis, resulting from flour or grain dust in work environments.

Grains and Celiac Disease

Individuals with gluten-sensitive enteropathy (celiac disease, also called sprue) react to the alpha-gliadin component of gluten. Although researchers have proposed a variety of mechanisms involving immune reactions as the primary trigger of celiac disease, there is no definitive evidence that it is due to an allergy.

Symptoms of celiac disease are diarrhea, weight loss, malabsorption (especially of fat), signs of iron or folate deficiency, sometimes rickets, and indications of other vitamin and mineral deficiencies. Occasionally the condition is accompanied by an itchy rash (dermatitis herpetiformis).

Celiac disease is most definitively diagnosed by a jejunal biopsy (removal and examination of tissues from a specific area of the small intestine) that reveals villous atrophy (flattened, short, or absent villi) and other abnormal changes of the lining of the jejunum. A number of blood tests are available for detecting the presence of a variety of specific antibodies whose presence is indicative of celiac disease. A suspicion that celiac disease is the cause of a person's symptoms should always be confirmed by laboratory data so that treatment is not undertaken inappropriately. Treatment is lifelong and consists of the strict avoidance of all grains that contain gluten, namely, wheat, rye, oats, and barley. However, it is important to realize that *not all wheat intolerance, grain intolerance, or even gluten intolerance is due to celiac disease.*

Symptoms of Wheat Allergy

Wheat has been reported to be the provoking allergen in a number of different allergic conditions. Abdominal pain and loose stools beginning within 12 to 72 hours after eating wheat are the most frequently reported symptoms of wheat allergy. In children this pattern often accompanies an allergy to cow's milk proteins.

Ingested and inhaled wheat flour has been demonstrated to cause asthma in both adults and children and is one of numerous food and environmental allergens implicated in causing eczema. Wheat allergy also may provoke hives and angioedema (tissue swelling, especially of the face). An anaphylactic reaction to wheat has been reported in young infants, but is a very rare occurrence. Exercise-induced anaphylaxis after eating wheat has been reported several times (see Chapter 2, page 19).

Allergy to Other Cereal Grains

The incidence of allergy to other cereal grains and the degree of cross-reactivity among cereal grains is unknown. Allergy to oats, rye, or barley is uncommon, and therefore restricting these grains is rarely necessary except for the treatment of celiac disease. Corn allergy is rare but has been documented in a number of reports, mainly in children. Allergy to rice appears to be equally uncommon. If allergy to any grain is suspected, elimination and challenge should be carried out to confirm the suspicion and determine the specific grain causing the adverse reaction.

Allergy to cereal grains other than wheat is discussed later in this chapter, on page171.

THE WHEAT-FREE DIET

In Western countries, it is difficult to avoid wheat because wheat is a principal ingredient in many commonly eaten foods. Breads, breakfast cereals, crackers, cookies, muffins, pasta, snack foods, luncheon meats, sausages, candies, desserts, cakes, pies, pancakes, waffles, and many other wheat-containing products are the basis of the "convenience foods" associated with the fast-paced Western lifestyle. These products supply the nutrients occurring naturally in wheat, as well as those added in the fortification of wheat flour, namely, thiamin, riboflavin, niacin, and iron. However, they can be obtained from other sources, so a wheat-free diet need not result in the loss of any important nutrients.

Important Nutrients in Wheat

Wheat and wheat products are a significant source of thiamin, riboflavin, niacin, iron, selenium, chromium, and in smaller amounts, magnesium, folate, phophorous, and molybdenum. Many of these micronutrients are added to wheat cereals and flours as fortifiers. Alternative choices of foods to replace these include oats, rice, rye, barley, corn, buckwheat, amatanth, and quinoa, some of which are fortified with micronutrients similar to those found in wheat products. Flours that are suitable as replacements for wheat flour include flours and starches from rice, potato, rye, oats, barley, buckwheat, tapioca, millet, corn, quinoa, and amaranth.

Spelt, kamut, triticale, and flours derived from these grains are too closely related to wheat to be considered safe on a wheat-free diet, unless specifically demonstrated to be tolerated by elimination and challenge.

If you can tolerate rye, oats, barley, corn, and rice, then you can consume baked products, cereals, and pastas using these grains instead of those using wheat. In addition, unusual grains and flours such as millet, quinoa, amaranth, buckwheat, tapioca, sago, arrowroot, soy, lentil, pea, and bean, as well as nuts and seeds, may be used in interesting combinations to make baked products and cereals.

Label-Reading Guidelines for a Wheat-Free Diet

When restricting any food from the diet, you need to become familiar with terms that may appear on product labels indicating that the food is present. Wheat may appear in food products under the terms listed in Table 10-1.

Table 10-1
FOOD PRODUCTS THAT CONTAIN WHEAT

Terms That Indicate the Presence of Wheat

Bread crumbs	Cracked wheat	Semolina
Bran	Cracker meal	Spelt
Bulgur	Durum	Triticale
Gluten	Durum flour	Kamut
High-gluten flour	Enriched flour	Couscous
Vital gluten	Self-rising flour	Anything with "wheat" in the
Protein flour	Pastry flour	name, for example:
High-protein flour	Bread flour	—Wheat berries
Graham flour	Unbleached flour	—Wheat germ
Graham crackers	All-purpose flour	—Wheat bran
Crackers	Phosphated flour	—Wheat starch
Matzoh	White bread	—Sprouted wheat
Cereal extract	Sourdough bread	—Wheatena
Fanina	Multigrain flour	—Wheat gluten
Flour	Multigrain bread	—Whole-wheat bread and flour
	Seitan	—60% wheat bread

Products That May Contain Wheat
(unless source is declared to be other than wheat)

Gelatinized starch	Vegetable starch Soy sauce
Hydrolyzed vegetable protein (HVP)	Malt
Hydrolyzed plant protein (HPP)	Grain coffee substitute
Malt	Postum
Starch (unless origin is specified, e.g., "corn starch")	Granola
Modified starch (unless origin is specified)	Granola bar
Vegetable gum	

Hydrolysed plant protein (HPP), hydrolysed vegetable protein (HVP), and monosodium glutamate (MSG) may be made from wheat. However, because the hydrolysis process breaks down the protein to a form that is unlikely to be allergenic, avoiding these products is not considered necessary.

Wheat-Free Diet

The wheat-free diet on the next four pages omits wheat and foods containing wheat products. (Table 10-2). *This diet is not suitable for the treatment of celiac disease because it is* not *gluten-free.*

Table 10-2
THE WHEAT-FREE DIET: FOODS ALLOWED AND FOODS RESTRICTED

Type of Food	Foods Allowed	Foods Restricted
Milk and Milk Products	• Milk (whole milk; 2%, 1%; skim; lactose-reduced (Lactaid®, Lacteeze®); acidophilus) • Cream • Sour cream • Buttermilk • Yogurt • Cheese of all types • Cottage cheese • Ricotta • Feta • Quark • Any other food made from pure milk	• Any milk product containing wheat (usually as a thickener), such as – Instant cocoa – Hot chocolate mixes – Malted milk – Ovaltine – Coffee substitutes (e.g., Postum) • Cheese sauces, spreads, and other dairy foods containing wheat
Grains, Cereals, Flours, and Starches	Grains, cereals, flours, and starches made with or derived from • Amaranth • Arrowroot • Barley • Buckwheat • Corn • Kasha • Lentil or pea flour • Nut meal and flour (all types) • Oats • Quinoa • Rice (all types) • Rye • Sago • Seed meal and flour • Soy flour • Tapioca	Grains, cereals, flours, and starches made with or derived from • Bulgur • Couscous • Cracked wheat • Durum • Farina • "Gluten enriched" flour • Graham • Kamut • Malt* • Matzoh • Semolina • Spelt • Starch* • Triticale • Wheat • Wheaten • Wheat bran and germ • Wheat berries
	Breads and baked goods: Any made from allowed flours and starches such as • Rice bread • Rice and soy bread • Rye bread	*Breads and baked goods:* Any item made from restricted flours or starches • Any regular white or whole-wheat bread, buns, croissants, or bagels

Note: This list is not exhaustive. Other foods may contain wheat and not be listed here. It is up to the reader to read all ingredient labels carefully and to contact the manufacturer if there is any doubt.

Table 10-2 (continued)
THE WHEAT-FREE DIET: FOODS ALLOWED AND FOODS RESTRICTED

Type of Food	Foods Allowed	Foods Restricted
Grains, Cereals, Flours, and Starches (continued)	• Cornmeal bread made without wheat flour • Breads, muffins, cookies, pancakes, waffles, and cakes made with allowed grains	• Cakes, muffins, pancakes, cookies, waffles, etc., made with wheat or white flour • Bread crumbs • Cracker meal
	Crackers and snacks Any made from allowed grains such as • Corn chips • Corn nachos • Corn taco chips • Potato chips • Rice cakes, plain, with seeds or with other allowed grains • Rice crackers	*Crackers and snacks* Any containing wheat, such as • Graham crackers • Cheese crackers • Ritz™ crackers • Saltines™ • Champagne™ crackers • Vegetable Thins™ • Matzoh
	Breakfast cereals Any made from any grain on allowed list, e.g., oats, barley, rye, millet, and corn, such as • Oatmeal • Corn flakes • Cream of Rice® • Rice Krispies® • Puffed rice • Puffed millet • Kenmei Rice Bran® • Puffed amaranth	*Breakfast cereals* Any breakfast cereal containing wheat, such as • Shredded wheat • Puffed wheat • Weetabix • Wheaties • Wheatena • Cream of Wheat • Red River Cereal • Miniwheats • Others (read labels carefully)
Pasta	Pasta made from any grain on allowed list, such as • Soy pasta • Buckwheat pasta • Mung bean pasta • Bean vermicelli • Rice noodles and pasta • Brown rice pasta • Wild rice pasta • Corn pasta • Potato pasta • Quinoa pasta	Any pasta made with wheat flour including • Spinach • Carrot • Egg noodles • Vermicelli • Others (read labels carefully)

Table 10-2 (continued) THE WHEAT-FREE DIET: FOODS ALLOWED AND FOODS RESTRICTED		
Type of Food	**Foods Allowed**	**Foods Restricted**
Vegetables	• All prepared with allowed ingredients • All vegetable juices • All pure fresh, frozen, or canned vegetables	• Vegetables prepared with a dressing or garnish containing wheat • Salad dressings containing wheat (starch) as a thickener • Sprouted wheat
Fruit	• All pure fruits and fruit juices	• Commercial pie fillings • All fruit dishes containing wheat • Fruit pies with a crust made from wheat flour • Fruit pies with Graham cracker crust
Meat, Poultry, and Fish	• All plain, fresh, frozen, or canned meat, poultry, or fish • Those prepared without wheat, wheat batters, or bread crumbs	Meat dishes that may contain wheat, such as • Battered • Breaded • Croquettes • Luncheon meats • Meat loaves • Meat balls • Patties • Pâté • Sausages • Spreads • Stuffing • Weiners • Processed meats
Eggs	• All eggs and egg dishes prepared without wheat	• Egg dishes containing wheat • Scotch eggs (wheat is in the sausage)
Legumes	• All prepared without wheat • Plain tofu • Peanut butter • Tamari sauce	• Legume dishes containing wheat, usually as a thickener • Soya sauce
Nuts and Seeds	• All plain seeds and nuts	• Snack nuts and seeds with HVP, HPP, or MSG
Fats and Oils	• Butter • Cream	• Wheat germ oil • Salad dressings containing wheat

Table 10-2 (continued)
THE WHEAT-FREE DIET: FOODS ALLOWED AND FOODS RESTRICTED

Type of Food	Foods Allowed	Foods Restricted
Fats and Oils (continued)	• Margarine • Shortening • All pure vegetable, nut, and seed oils • Fish oils • Lard • Meat drippings • Peanut and other pure nut and seed butters • Homemade gravy thickened with nonwheat starch (e.g., corn, tapioca, arrowroot) • Nut and seed butters	• Sauces containing wheat (usually as a thickener) • Gravy thickened with wheat flour or starch

Spices and Herbs	• All plain spices and herbs	• Seasoning mixes containing wheat, HVP*, HPP*, or MSG*, such as
		  – Packaged soup seasoning mixes
		  – Bouillon cubes

Sweets and Sweeteners	• Sugar • Honey • Molasses • Jams • Jellies • Preserves • Baking chocolate and pure cocoa powder	All sweets containing wheat, such as • Icing sugar* • Candy* • Marshmallows*

*Avoid these products unless the source is known **not** to be wheat.

GRAIN ALLERGY

Symptoms of Grain Allergy

People who are grain-allergic may experience symptoms similar to those of wheat allergy. Symptoms occur in three major organ systems:

- Gastrointestinal tract: diarrhea, nausea, vomiting, gas, bloating, pain
- Respiratory tract: nasal congestion, sneezing, runny nose, itchy/watery eyes
- Skin: hives; angioedema; eczema

A Type I hypersensitivity reaction (immediate-type allergy) can occur within a few minutes to a few hours after ingesting the grain. A delayed reaction may occur up to 72 hours after eating the grain (more commonly within 24 to 48 hours). People showing this type of reaction must avoid the grains that cause it. The following information provides you with guidelines for avoiding all major cereal grains. Reintroducing each grain separately in a controlled "challenge" should enable you to identify the specific grain that is responsible for your symptoms.

Corn Allergy

Corn is a difficult allergen to avoid in the Western diet because so many prepared foods contain corn in the form of corn starch, corn syrup, or their derivatives. There are likely to be corn products in cereals, baked goods, snack foods, syrups, canned fruits, beverages, jams, jellies, cookies, luncheon meats, candies, other convenience foods, and infant formulas.

Corn oil is not usually allergenic, unless the product is contaminated during its manufacture by protein from the grain. Because corn protein is an extremely rare cause of anaphylaxis and because the quantity likely to be present is very small, it is not usually necessary to restrict corn oil as an ingredient in foods.

Elimination of corn does **not** lead to nutritional deficiencies as long as the usual intake of corn itself is small. However, if the usual diet contains many convenience foods, alternative corn-free products will be needed for adequate nutrition.

Corn is likely to be present in foods containing

Corn	Corn flour
Cornmeal	Corn starch
Cornflakes	Popcorn
Cornmeal	Caramel corn
Corn sweetener	Maize
Corn syrup solids	Corn alcohol

Baking powder	Food starch
Hominy	Modified starch
Grits	Vegetable starch
Vegetable gum	Vegetable protein
Vegetable paste	Starch

Hydrolyzed plant protein (HPP), hydrolyzed vegetable protein (HVP), and textured vegetable protein (TVP) may be made from corn. However, as with similar products derived from wheat, the hydrolysis process breaks down the protein to the point where it is unlikely to be allergenic. As a result, it is usually unnecessary to exclude these from a corn-restricted diet.

The Grain-Restricted Diet

This diet is designed to eliminate a variety of grains *in addition to wheat* to determine their possible role in causing symptoms of allergy or intolerance. The grains most likely to be involved as causative factors in grain-associated allergy include

◆ Wheat and grains derived from wheat, such as triticale, kamut, and spelt
◆ Rye
◆ Oats
◆ Barley
◆ Corn

More information on restricted foods can be found in Table 10-3 on the next page.

Table 10-3
THE GRAIN-RESTRICTED DIET

The following are restricted:

Wheat	Corn
Semolina	Cornstarch
Spelt	Oatmeal
Triticale	Barley
Bulgur	Kamut
Couscous	Farina
Durum	Cornmeal
Rye	Oats

Flours, breads, and crackers made from any of the above grains are restricted:

White bread	Rye bread
Whole-wheat bread	Oat bread
Sourdough bread	Barley bread
All-purpose flour	Bread crumbs
Gluten flour	Cracker meal
Graham flour	Graham crackers
Phosphated flour	Matzos
Protein flour	Starch
Cracked wheat flour	Cream of Wheat
Durum flour	Wheat germ
Pastry flour	Bran
Self-rising flour	

These corn and corn products are restricted:

Corn sugar*
Corn dextrose*
Corn syrup*
Sorbitol*

The following Mexican foods are frequently made with corn:

Tamales	Nachos
Tortillas	Tacos
Masa harina	

* Sugar, syrup, and sugar alcohols derived from grains are usually non-allergenic. However, if they are contaminated with a small amount of protein, they may cause an allergic reaction in extremely sensitive individuals. It is wise to avoid them until the limit of tolerance is known.

The following products *may* contain grains as a "hidden ingredient" and should be avoided by people who are grain-allergic *unless it is certain that they do not contain the grain responsible for the allergy:*

Weiners	Meat loaf
Sausages	Breaded meat or fish
Luncheon meats	Meat or fish in batter
Stuffing	Some canned soups (*read labels*)
Spreads	"Thickened" soups or gravies
Pate	Bouillon cubes
Pies	Ice cream cone
Pie fillings	Some salad dressings
Croquettes	Icing sugar
Patties	Cereal coffee substitutes (Postum)
Root beer	Commercial baking powder
Mustard pickles	Some soy sauces

Grain-derived alcoholic beverages (see below)
Any product containing bread or bread crumbs
Any product labeled "gluten-enriched"
Malted milk
Some cheese spreads or "cheese foods"

These products *may* contain corn (*read labels*):

Commercial baking powder
Breads, cookies, cereals, desserts (may contain cornstarch; *read labels*)
Commercial gravies and sauces (may be thickened with cornstarch)
Luncheon meats

Miscellaneous products that are derived from grains, especially hydrolyzed proteins and MSG, are unlikely to cause an adverse reaction, because the protein is broken down to a form that is usually *not* allergenic. They need to be avoided only in the rare case where there is any risk of an anaphylactic reaction to grains.

Malt	Malt flavoring
Malt vinegar	Sprouted wheat
Monosodium glutamate	Sprouts from any restricted grain
Hydrolyzed vegetable protein (HVP)	Beer, lager, ale, porter
Hydrolyzed plant protein (HPP)	Bourbon, vodka, and gin (may contain corn)

Table 10-4		
THE GRAIN-RESTRICTED DIET: FOODS ALLOWED AND FOODS RESTRICTED		
Type of Food	**Foods Allowed**	**Foods Restricted**
Breads, Cereals, and Substitutes	Breads, baked goods, cereals, pancakes, pasta, and snack foods made from any restricted grain: • Rice flour and starch • Potato flour and starch • Millet flour • Buckwheat groats and flour • Kasha • Amaranth flour • Quinoa flour • Tapioca starch • Sago starch and flour • Soy flour • Lentil flour • Pea and bean flours • Chickpea flour • Arrowroot starch and flour • Nut meal and flour • Seed meal and flour from allowed grains	Breads, baked goods, cereals, pancakes, pasta, and snack foods made from any restricted grain: • Wheat • Kamut • Spelt • Triticale • Semolina • Durum • Bulgur • Farina • Couscous • Matzoh • "Gluten enriched" flour • Malt • Rye • Oats • Barley • Corn
Milk and Milk Products	All milk and milk products without restricted ingredients, including: • Milk • Yogurt • Buttermilk • Cheeses • Cream cheese • Cottage cheese • Butter • Ice cream (check composition for presence of restricted ingredients)	Any containing restricted ingredients, especially • Cocoa powders • Chocolate mixes • Hot chocolate • Cheese sauces • Cheese spreads • Malted milk
Meat, Fish and Poultry	• All plain, fresh, frozen or canned without restricted ingredients • Battered with allowed grains, flours, or crumbs • Plain deli products without restricted ingredients	Meats that might contain restricted ingredients (check labels): • Luncheon meats • Weiners • Sausages • Pâtés • Spreads • Stuffing

Note: This list is not exhaustive. Other foods may contain grain and not be listed here. It is up to the reader to read all ingredient labels carefully and to contact the manufacturer if there is any doubt.

Table 10-4 (continued)
THE GRAIN-FREE DIET: FOODS ALLOWED AND FOODS RESTRICTED

Type of Food	Foods Allowed	Foods Restricted

Meat, Fish and Poultry (continued)		• Meat loaf
		• Croquettes
		• Battered meats
		• Breaded meats
		• Manufactured products containing
		  – HVP
		  – HPP
		  – MSG

Eggs	All plain or prepared without restricted ingredients	Egg dishes containing restricted grains such as • Quiche • Mousse • Pavlova • Soufflé
Nuts and Seeds	• All plain, uncoated nuts and allowed seeds • Raw or roasted with allowed oils	Snack nuts and seeds coated with restricted ingredients or coated with flavoring agents such as • HPP • HVP • MSG
Vegetables	• All fresh, frozen, or canned plain vegetables • Prepared with allowed ingredients • Sprouted grains and seeds on allowed list • All plain vegetable juices	Any vegetable prepared with any restricted grain as • Coating • Breading • Marinade • Garnish • Sprouted
Legumes	All plain peas, beans, and lentils prepared with allowed ingredients • Dals prepared without added restricted flours and grains • Plain tofu • Soy products • Peanut butter	All legume dishes containing restricted grains and flours, such as • Dals with added wheat • Tofu patties coated with wheat flour or bread crumbs

Table 10-4 (continued)
THE GRAIN-FREE DIET: FOODS ALLOWED AND FOODS RESTRICTED

Type of Food	Foods Allowed	Foods Restricted
Fruits	All pure fruit and fruit juices, fresh, frozen, or canned	All fruit dishes containing restricted ingredients, such as • Pie fillings • Fruit sauces • Dessert fillings and toppings

Fats and Oils	• Butter
	• Margarines made from allowed oils
	• All pure vegetable, nut, seed, and fish oils, such as
	  – Olive
	  – Sunflower
	  – Safflower
	  – Canola
	  – Avocado
	  – Grapeseed
	  – Soy
	  – Peanut
	  – Sesame
	  – Mustard
	  – Walnut
	• Lard
	• Meat drippings
		• Margarine made with oil from restricted grains such as corn
		• Wheat germ oil
		• Corn oil
		• Salad dressings made from restricted ingredients
		• Gravy thickened with any restricted flour or starch

Herbs and Spices	All plain herbs and spices	Seasoning mixes with restricted ingredients • HPP • HVP • MSG
Sweeteners	• Sugar • Honey • Molasses • Maple syrup • Jams • Jellies • Preserves • Date sugar	Sweets containing restricted ingredients, such as • Icing sugar • Corn sugar and syrup • Corn dextrose • Sorbitol • Marshmallows

Oils from Restricted Grains

Pure oils are nonallergenic, however, if the oil is not completely pure, it may contain a small amount of the grain protein as a contaminant. It is wise to avoid corn oil and wheat germ oils until the limit of tolerance is known.

Ideas for Substituting Grains in Selected Meals

BREAKFAST FOODS
Cooked grains make enjoyable breakfast cereals when fruit, honey, nuts, or seeds are added.

Cook amaranth, millet, quinoa, and buckwheat grain like brown rice:
Combine a cup of grain with 2¼ or 2½ cups of water.
Bring to boil, lower heat, and simmer for 45 to 60 minutes depending on the degree of "doneness" desired.

You can cook the grains in large batches (for example, 4 cups of grain), freeze it in 1-cup quantities, can reheat it in the microwave. Cooked grain provides the basis for an instant breakfast cereal.

SOUP
Commercial soups are frequently thickened with restricted grains or contain restricted noodles or pasta. Bouillon cubes may contain grains. Homemade meat, poultry, or vegetable soup stocks are safe. Meat drippings can be chilled, the fat lifted off, and the meat juices used for a soup base. They may be thickened with tapioca, arrowroot, or starch if desired.

Easy Vegetable Stock
Use any combination of washed and trimmed onion skins, potato and carrot peelings, celery strings and leaves, parsley stems, green bean and tomato ends, outer lettuce leaves. Save trimmings in a plastic bag in the fridge or freezer. Cover with water in a saucepan. Add a bay leaf and pepper and bring to a boil. Simmer for 30 minutes. Strain and add salt to taste. Use instead of consommé or soup base. Freeze leftovers in ice cube trays.

DESSERTS
The following desserts are allowed:

◆   All desserts and baked goods made with allowed ingredients
◆   Plain gelatin desserts

- Fruit ices
- Popsicles
- Ice cream made with allowed ingredients but **not** ice cream cones
- Sherbet

BREADS AND BAKED GOODS

No single flour will replace wheat flour in a recipe. The texture will be different when you use a non-wheat flour, but more importantly, any baked product that is risen as an important part of its production will not retain its risen shape as it cools unless gluten is part of its structure. Non-gluten grains will drop noticeably as they cool. You can substitute alternative grains for wheat in a combination that provides an acceptable texture to the product, but you must adjust for the dense nature of the finished product.

EXAMPLES OF ALLOWED FLOURS AND STARCHES

Amaranth flour	Potato flour	Arrowroot starch or flour
Quinoa flour	Buckwheat flour	Rice flour (brown and white)
Channa flour	Rye flour	Chickpea flour (Besan)
Sago flour	Lentil flour	Soy flour
Millet flour (Bajri)	Tapioca starch or flour	Nut meal or flour (any type)
T'eff		

Substitutes for Restricted Flours in Recipes

In place of restricted flours in recipes, combinations of alternative flours make better cakes, cookies, breads, pancakes, and waffles than a single flour alone. A combination of rice, soy, potato, and arrowroot (or tapioca,) starch makes an acceptable bread mix. Use 1 cup of the mix in place of 1 cup of wheat flour in recipes.

Combining "light," "intermediate," and "heavy" flours in the ratio on the next page will give a better baked product than using any single flour.

Light Flours	Intermediate Flours	Heavy Flours
White rice	Potato	Soy
Tapioca	T'eff	Buckwheat
Arrowroot	Brown rice	Millet
Sago		Amaranth
		Chickpea
		Any nut
		Quinoa

Combine in a ratio:
   ½ cup heavy flour
   ¼ cup light flour
   ¼ cup intermediate flour

1 cup of the combined flours will substitute for 1 cup of any restricted flour in recipes, but some adjustments in liquid levels or cooking times may be required to obtain an equivalent texture, especially in breads.

— CHAPTER 11 —

SOY
ALLERGY

Soy beans are legumes. Soy and peanut (peanut belongs in the same botanic family as soy) are the most allergenic of the *Leguminosae* family, which has over 30 species including fresh and dried peas, fresh and dried beans, all types of lentils, carob, and licorice. Research studies indicate that developing symptoms to more than one member of the legume family is rare. A person who is allergic to peanut and/or soy will not necessarily be allergic to both or other members of the family. Each type of legume must be investigated individually to determine sensitivity to it; avoiding all legumes when only one causes allergy will place unnecessary restrictions on a person's diet. This can be especially detrimental to the nutritional health of vegetarians, and even more so to that of vegans.

If you have been diagnosed with an allergy to soy, or if you suspect that you may have soy allergy, it is important that you follow a completely soy-free diet, at least for a short period of time. At first glance, this may seem fairly straightforward–avoid tofu, soy-based beverages (soy milks), and soy sauce, and don't eat in Oriental restaurants. No big deal! But wait; let us look at the subject of soy a little more carefully. It may not be as simple as you think!

Traditionally, soy is an important part of the Oriental diet, being consumed as tofu in many Chinese and Japanese dishes and, in its fermented form, as soy sauce, miso soup, and similar foods. Tofu and other soy products are an important and necessary part of the vegetarian diet, providing essential protein and other nutrients to replace those found in foods from animal sources. Although soy itself is not a common part of the traditional Western diet, it may surprise some people to realize that all of us have been consuming an increasing amount of soy as an ingredient in many manufactured foods. In fact, it is very difficult to avoid soy entirely. Because it increases the nutrient value of any manufactured food, and adds flavor and texture to the product, it is a very popular addition to many processed and convenience foods. Take a look at the ingredient labels on the packaged foods you have on your shelf–you may be surprised at how many of them list soy. Many breads, pancake mixes, baking mixes of all types, breakfast cereals, packaged soups, and packaged entrees contain soy. Luncheon meats, "cold cuts," frozen dinners, hamburger patties, meat pies, and sausages contain soy. Soy is often used as a "meat extender," making the product less expensive (an important selling point in some markets). It is often disguised as "vegetable protein" and other terms in which soy is not immediately apparent. You need to be aware of all of these terms. (A table is provided later for you in this chapter.)

In some areas, soy-based infant formulas have become very important as alternatives to cow's milk based formulas when a child has been diagnosed as allergic or suspected to be allergic, to cow's milk protein. Such formulas are inexpensive, and with the addition of certain essential micronutrients (vitamins and minerals) may provide an acceptable substitute to cow's milk formulas for feeding in infancy, as long as the child is not allergic to soy, of course.

As you can see, we need to look a little more closely at this food which is becoming so important in our daily lives.

WHY IS SOY IMPORTANT AS AN ALLERGEN?

Unlike its relative, peanut, soy is a rare cause of anaphylaxis, but it can cause symptoms such as asthma, rhinitis (stuffy nosy), urticaria (hives), angioedema (tissue swelling), and gastrointestinal disturbances. An estimated 43% of babies who are allergic to cow's milk develop an allergy to soy when given soy-based infant formulas. Allergy to soy protein has many features similar to those of allergy to cow's milk protein. Like cow's milk, soy is a frequent contributor to atopic dermatitis (eczema) in atopic children. In infants, soy allergy can cause loose stool and diarrhea, vomiting, abdominal discomfort, irritability, crying, intestinal blood loss, anemia, and slow or nonexistent weight gain (failure to thrive). Respiratory tract symptoms include cough, wheeze, asthma, and rhinitis. Symptoms in the skin include hives and angioedema, as well as eczema.

How Can I Know When Soy is Present in a Food?

Most manufactured foods that contain soy will indicate the presence of soy protein on the label. However, sometimes, the word "soy" may not appear on the label, so persons who are soy-allergic need to become familiar with terms that indicate the likely presence of soy.

On a food label, soy may be indicated by terms such as "textured vegetable protein" or "hydrolyzed plant protein." Lecithin is often derived from soy, and oriental foods such as tempeh, tofu, miso, and bean curd are made from soy, which may not be obvious to the consumer who is unfamiliar with oriental foods.

Unlabeled products such as bulk foods, unwrapped breads, and baked goods may contain soy, especially if flour is an ingredient. Persons who are allergic to soy are advised not to purchase these products unless they can find out the specific ingredients.

Table 11-1 lists the terms most commonly used to indicate the presence of soy.

Table 11-1
terms indicating the presence of soy in food products

Terms That Indicate the Presence of Soy Protein

Tofu	Kyodofu (freeze-dried tofu)	Miso
Okara (soy pulp)	Shoyu	Sobee
Supro	Tamari	Tempeh
Yuba	Soy milk	Soy beverage
Soy nuts	Soy sauce	Soy sprouts
Soybean	Soybean paste	Soy flour
Soy grits	Soy albumin	Soy protein
Soy protein isolate	Soy lecithin	Textured vegetable protein* (TVP)

Ingredients That May Contain Soy

Emulsifiers*	Sprouts (source unspecified)	Vegetable broth*
Stabilizers*	Bean sprouts	Vegetable gum*
Lecithin*	Hydrolyzed plant protein (HPP)*	Vegetable paste*
	Hydrolyzed vegetable protein (HVP)*	Vegetable protein*
	Monosodium glutamate (MSG)*	Vegetable shortening*
		Vegetable starch*

* Unless the source is specified and is not soy

THE SOY-FREE DIET (TABLE 11-2)

The soy-free diet omits soybeans and all soy products. Soy is widely used in commercial food preparation. People who are soy-allergic need to examine labels carefully as certain brands of the foods listed may not be soy-free.

	Table 11-2	
	THE SOY-FREE DIET: FOODS ALLOWED AND FOODS RESTRICTED	
Type of Food	**Foods Allowed**	**Foods Restricted**
Milk and Milk Products	• All except those on the restricted list	• Cheese substitutes • Soy cheese • Tofu cheese • Ice cream, frozen desserts, and dessert mixes unless labeled soy free • Milk or cream replacers • Soy-based infant formula • Soy milk • Soy beverage • Soy yogurt
Breads and Cereals	• All except those on the restricted list	• Homemade and commercial breads and baked goods containing soy • Pancake mixes • Soy grits • Soy flour • Baking mixes • Cereals containing soy • Mixed grain cereals • Multigrain breads • Granola and granola bars • Infant cereals containing soy • High-protein flour and bread • English muffins • Stuffings
Vegetables	• All pure, fresh, frozen, or canned vegetables and their juices	• All vegetable dishes made with soy or unknown ingredients • Soy sprouts • Mixed sprouts • Salads with sprouts • Salad dressings containing soy • Some frozen french fries • Commercial vegetable products • Some commercial soups • Commercial dry soup mixes • Some bouillon cubes
Fruit	• All pure fresh, frozen, or canned fruits and their juices	• Fruit dishes made with soy products • Some commercial canned fruit products

Note: This list is not exhaustive. Other foods may contain soy and not be listed here. It is up to the reader to read all ingredient labels carefully and to contact the manufacturer if there is any doubt.

Table 11-2 (continued) THE SOY-FREE DIET: FOODS ALLOWED AND FOODS RESTRICTED		
Type of Food	**Foods Allowed**	**Foods Restricted**

Meat, Poultry, and Fish	• All fresh or frozen meat, poultry, or fish
	• Fish canned in water
		• Meat, poultry, or fish dishes with soy
		• Tuna and other fish canned in oil
		• Tofu (soybean curd)
		• Miso
		• Meat extenders
		• Textured vegetable protein
		• Vegetarian meat replacers (analogs)
		• Veggie burger
		• Meat products that may contain soy include
		  – Cold cuts
		  – Luncheon meat
		  – Frozen dinners
		  – Hamburger patties
		  – Meat paste
		  – Meat pate
		  – Meat pies
		  – Minced beef
		  – Sausages
		  – Imitation bacon bits

Eggs	• All plain eggs	• Egg dishes prepared with soy products
Legumes	• All plain legumes except soy and tofu • Dried peas and beans • All green beans and peas • Lentils • Split peas • Peanuts	• All legume dishes containing soy or tofu • Any soy products • Mixed beans • Bean mixtures (e.g., 12-bean soup) • Mixed bean salads
Nuts and Seeds	• All packaged plain, pure nuts and seeds • All pure nut and seed oils and their butters, e.g., tahini, almond butter • Peanuts • Peanut butter	• Soy nuts • Soy butter • Nuts or mixes containing soy derivative • Any oils or nuts of undisclosed origin
Fats and Oils	• Butter • Cream	• Salad dressings that list "oil" without revealing the source

Table 11-2 (continued)
THE SOY-FREE DIET: FOODS ALLOWED AND FOODS RESTRICTED

Type of Food	Foods Allowed	Foods Restricted
Fats and Oils (continued)	• Pure vegetable, nut, or seed oil with source specified • Lard and meat drippings • Gravy made with meat drippings • Pure olive oil spray • Peanut oil	• Soy oil • Margarine unless sources of all oils are revealed and margarine is soy-free • Vegetable oil • Vegetable oil sprays • Shortening

Spices, Herbs, and Seasonings	• All pure herbs and spices
	• Blends of herbs and spices, without added oils
		• Seasoning packets with undisclosed ingredients
		• Sauces containing soy, such as
		  – Barbecue
		  – Oriental
		  – Soy
		  – Tamari
		  – Worcestershire
		• Hydrolyzed vegetable protein (HVP)
		• Hydrolyzed plant protein (HPP)
		• Texturized vegetable protein (TVP)

Sweets and Sweeteners	• Plain sugar, honey, molasses, maple syrup • Corn syrup • Pure chocolate • Pure cocoa • Cocoa butter • Artificial sweeteners • Pure jams and jellies • Homemade cookies and candies with allowed ingredients	• Chocolate • Chocolate bars • Marzipan (almond paste) • Cookies and candies • Cake icing, unless sources are revealed and are soy-free

Soybeans are legumes; however, **cross-reactivity** with other legumes, including peanuts, is rare and should not be assumed without careful investigation. Food-specific diagnosis is necessary to avoid overly restricting the diet.

Soy Oil

Pure soy oil is not considered to be allergenic, unless contaminated by soy protein in its manufacture. This latter source of soy allergen is difficult to detect in a manufactured product. Therefore, people who are very allergic to soy are advised to avoid soy oil also, although most will tolerate a small amount of the oil in manufactured foods (perhaps up to a teaspoon) without any difficulty.

Soy oil and soy lecithin do not contain detectable soy protein and therefore are not usually antigenic. However, sometimes the refining process does not exclude all soy proteins, so a person who is highly sensitive to soy is advised to avoid soy oil and soy lecithin also. Cold-pressed soy oils (also referred to as "pure-pressed," "expeller-pressed," or "unrefined") are very likely to contain soy proteins.

People who are highly sensitive to soy, or who are in the process of identifying soy allergy, should avoid **all** products containing soy oil, especially when it is the main ingredient (e.g., soy oil, soy-based margarines, cooking sprays).

Nutrients in Soybeans

Soybeans contribute thiamin, riboflavin, vitamin B6, phosphorus, magnesium, iron, folacin, calcium, and zinc to the diet. However, soy is typically used in commercial products in amounts that are too small to be considered a significant source for these nutrients. Therefore, elimination of soy from the diet does not compromise the nutritional quality of most diets.

— CHAPTER 12 —

PEANUT ALLERGY

Peanuts are one of the most frequently cited causes of life-threatening ana-phylactic reactions. Because of the intense fear among sufferers, parents, and doctors about the risks associated with anaphylactic reactions, peanuts have become the *bete noire* of food allergy practice. In reality, peanuts have caused very few deaths; deaths from anaphylactic reactions to antibiotics and other medications, injected radio-contrast dyes used in X-ray diagnostic tests, and insect venom from wasp and bee stings vastly outnumber deaths from peanuts. Even when we consider the number of deaths from anaphylactic reactions to foods, tree nuts and shellfish seem to be more frequent culprits than peanuts. However, because of their bad reputation, peanuts have been banned by many airlines, in classrooms from kindergarten onward, and from most places where young children congregate. It is indisputable that whenever that is a risk for ana-phylaxis, all possible precautions need to be taken, especially when the victim may be a young child. So, it is probably safer to err on the side of caution, and whenever there is even a slight risk of anaphylaxis, careful avoidance of expo-sure to even a minute quantity of peanuts is justified. The first thing we need to do, therefore, is to understand the nature of peanut allergy and to be informed about where we can expect to encounter peanuts in the normal diet. That's what this chapter is all about.

ALLERGIC REACTIONS TO PEANUTS

The most important, and most severe reaction to peanuts is **anaphylaxis.** An **anaphylactic reaction** involves all systems of the body (is systemic) and, in its severest form, can rapidly progress to anaphylactic shock and death. (For details of the anaphylactic reaction, refer to Chapter 2, page 18.)

Other symptoms of peanut allergy include hives, angioedema (tissue swelling), wheezing, asthma, nausea, vomiting, nasal congestion, itching, and allergic conjunctivitis (itchy/watery eyes). An allergy to peanuts is often life-long.

*People who have been diagnosed as anaphylactic to peanuts must avoid **all** sources of peanuts.* Even when the reaction has been mild on previous occasions, if you have had any reaction at all to peanuts, the potential for a severe allergy exists. Therefore, most doctors advise treating *all* peanut allergies as if they were life-threatening.

Peanut Allergens

Peanuts are unrelated botanically to nuts that grow on trees, and most people are able to eat a variety of tree nuts, such as walnuts, pecans, Brazil nuts, almonds, cashew nuts, hazelnuts, macadamia nuts, and so on, without difficulty. However, because tree nuts are highly allergenic foods, they are also frequent causes of strong allergic reactions and anaphylaxis. An allergy to nuts should be distinguished from an allergy to peanut and other legumes, otherwise the diet can become stressful and cumbersome if the allergic person avoids all traces of peanuts and all other nuts.

In order to be sure that all sources of peanuts have been identified, especially in manufactured foods, the peanut-allergic person must become familiar with terms on ingredient labels that indicate the presence of peanuts and must be aware of the foods most likely to contain peanuts or peanut protein (Table 12-1).

A cautionary note here is that sometimes no differentiation is made in the marketing of peanuts and nuts, and the two are often found together in "nut mixtures." When nuts and peanuts are sold in bulk, a utensil used to handle nuts has often been previously used with peanuts without cleaning in between. In the manufacture of candies, confectioneries, and ice cream, there is frequent cross-contamination between nuts of different species and peanuts, so a person with severe peanut allergy is advised to avoid any product containing "nuts" because of the danger of encountering peanuts inadvertently.

"Mandalona" nut is one of the names given to a manufactured product made from deflavored, decolored peanut meal that is pressed into molds, reflavored and colored and sold as a cheaper substitute for tree nuts such as almonds, pecans, and walnuts. *People with peanut allergy must be cautious when consuming any food that may contain such a product.*

Table 12-1
TERMS ON FOOD LABELS THAT INDICATE
THE PRESENCE OF PEANUT PROTEIN

Ingredients That Indicate the Presence of Peanut

Peanut protein	Peanut flour	Beer nuts
Hydrolyzed peanut protein	Mandalona nuts	Mixed nuts
Peanut oil	Artificial nuts	Goober nuts
Cold-pressed peanut oil	Nu-nuts flavored nuts	Goober peas
Peanut butter		

Products That May Contain Peanut

Marzipan (almond paste)	Chinese dishes	Prepared and frozen desserts
Prepared soups	Satay sauces	Ice cream with nuts
Dried soup mixes	Baked goods	Chocolate ice cream
Chili	Cookies	Vegetable oil
Egg rolls	Candies	Hydrogenated vegetable oil
Thai dishes	Chocolate bars	Vegetable shortening

Peanut Oil

Research studies have indicated that peanut-allergic adults can tolerate pure peanut oil without any clinical reactions. This is true of oils from any source, including soy. The allergic reactivity occurs to the protein that may contaminate the oil, not to the oil itself. However, people who are anaphylactic to peanut, nuts, or a grain are usually cautioned to avoid the oil derived from the allergenic plant because there may be traces of plant protein in the oil.

Research indicates that refined peanut oil is safe for peanut-hypersensitive people. However, there is no guarantee that any peanut oil is completely free from peanut protein. A person who is anaphylactic to peanut is strongly advised to avoid peanut oil entirely. Cold-pressed oils (also labeled "pure-pressed," "expeller pressed," or "unrefined") in particular should be avoided.

THE PEANUT-FREE DIET (TABLE 12-2)

The peanut-free diet omits peanuts and foods containing peanuts. It is important that peanut-sensitive people avoid **all** sources of if there is even a moderate risk of an anaphylactic reaction to it. However, there is no evidence that even a severe allergy to peanut requires avoidance of all other *legumes*. Avoidance of legumes such as soy, lentils, dried peas, and beans is necessary only when allergy to the individual foods has been identified. It is also unnecessary to avoid tree nuts, which are botanically unrelated to peanuts. However, because of the risk of contamination of tree nuts, especially nut mixtures, to contain, or to be contaminated, by peanuts, a person who has demonstrated allergy to peanuts is usually advised to avoid nuts of all types in the interests of safety.

Nutrients in Peanut

Peanuts supply niacin, magnesium, vitamin E, manganese, pantothenic acid, chromium, and in smaller amounts vitamin B6, folacin, copper, and biotin. These nutrients are easily replaced by including meat, whole grains, legumes, and vegetable oils in the diet.

The Peanut-Allergic Baby

Protein from peanuts in the mother's diet can pass into her breast milk and cause allergic symptoms in the breast-fed baby. If the breast-fed infant is allergic to peanut protein, the elimination of all peanut and peanut-containing products from the mother's diet should be beneficial. If peanut elimination only partially eases the infant's distress, carefully kept exposure diaries by the mother may isolate other possible dietary or medication irritants.

Table 12-2
THE PEANUT-FREE DIET: FOODS ALLOWED AND FOODS RESTRICTED

Type of Food	Foods Allowed	Foods Restricted
Milk and Milk Products	• Milk • Cream • Plain yogurt • Ice cream made with allowed ingredients • Plain cheese • Sour cream • Quark® • Dips made with allowed ingredients	• Milk based desserts and confectioneries (e.g., ice cream) containing peanuts or nuts • Chocolate ice cream or other milk-based confectioneries unless labeled "peanut-free" • Cheese foods (e.g., slices, dips, spreads, cheese balls) containing nuts or undisclosed ingredients
Breads and Cereals	• Any breads, buns, or baked goods that are known to be free from peanut and peanut oil • Plain cooked grains • Plain oatmeal • Regular Cream of Wheat® • Ready-to-eat cereals without added oil or nuts • Homemade granola without peanut • Dried pasta	• Commercial or homemade baked goods made with peanut oil or peanuts • Baked goods made with undisclosed sources of "nuts," oil, or shortening • Baking mixes • Ready-to-eat cereals with added oils and nuts, such as granola
Vegetables	• All pure vegetables and their juices	• Vegetable dishes with sauces containing peanuts, peanut oil, or unknown nuts or oils • Salads with dressings containing unknown oil or nuts • Vegetables canned in undisclosed oils
Fruit	• All pure fruit and fruit juices	• Fruit dishes containing peanuts or nuts • Fruit dishes made with oil or shortening of unknown origin
Meat, Poultry, and Fish	• All pure fresh or frozen meat, poultry, or fish • Fish canned in broth, water, or non-peanut oils	• Meat, poultry, or fish dishes made with peanut or undisclosed nuts or oils • Fish canned in undisclosed oils • Chinese dishes • Thai dishes • Egg rolls • Commercial chili • Vegetarian burgers unless labeled "peanut-free" • Peanut protein

Note: This list is not exhaustive. Other foods may contain peanut and not be listed here. It is up to the reader to read all ingredient labels carefully and to contact the manufacturer if there is any doubt.

Table 12-2 (continued)
THE PEANUT-FREE DIET: FOODS ALLOWED AND FOODS RESTRICTED

Type of Food	Foods Allowed	Foods Restricted
Eggs	• All without restricted ingredients	• Egg dishes prepared with oils or nuts of unknown sources • Egg rolls

Legumes	• All pure legumes except peanut
	• Tofu
		• Peanut and peanut products including
		  – Artificial nuts
		  – Goober nuts
		  – Goober peas
		  – Hydrolyzed peanut protein
		  – Mandalona nuts
		  – Mixed nuts
		  – Peanut butter
		  – Peanut flour
		  – Peanut oil
		  – Peanut protein
		• Legume dishes containing peanut or oils or nuts of undisclosed source

Nuts and Seeds	• All packaged plain, pure nuts and seeds
	• All pure nut and seed oils and their butters, such as
	  – sesame tahini
	  – almond butter
	  – almond paste
	  – cashew butter
		• Mixed nuts
		• Mandalona nuts
		• Artificial nuts
		• Nuts or oils of undisclosed origin
		• Goober nuts
		• Goober peas

Fats and Oils	• Butter • Cream • Pure vegetable, nut, or seed oil with source specified (except peanut) • Lard • Meat drippings • Gravy made with meat drippings	• Peanut oil • Salad dressings that list "oil" without revealing source • Margarine, unless source of all oils is revealed and is peanut-free
Spices and Herbs	• All pure herbs and spices • Blends of herbs and spices, without added oils	• Seasoning packets with undisclosed ingredients • Vegetables such as garlic or sun-dried tomatoes packed in oil, unless source of oil is disclosed and is peanut-free
Sweets and Sweeteners	• Plain sugar, honey, molasses, maple syrup • Corn syrup • Pure chocolate • Pure cocoa • Artificial sweeteners • Homemade cookies and candies with allowed ingredients	• Chocolates with unknown ingredients • Chocolate bars • Marzipan (almond paste) • Cookies and candies • Any confectionery containing nuts unless specified to be peanut-free

— CHAPTER 13 —

NUT AND SEED ALLERGY

THE ALLERGENS

Nuts represent the reproductive part of the plant. In the majority of cases, the most highly allergenic molecules of plants are associated with the storage proteins in the seed. Nuts, grains, legumes (peas, beans, lentils), as well as the foods we call "seeds," all contain similar types of storage **albumins,** which tend to be highly allergenic. The seed-storage albumins are used by the growing plant during germination. They may have a defensive role against pathogens, because many of these types of albumins have antifungal properties. It is possible that many of the huge number of dicot seeds contain cross-reacting albumins. However, the *degree* of clinical **cross-reactivity,** in which a person allergic to one nut, seed, grain, or legume is allergic to another from a different plant species, has not yet been determined. It appears that each storage albumin is unique to the species of plant that produces it.

Nuts

Nuts are produced by trees of diverse and unrelated botanical genera, so it is usually only necessary to avoid the specific species of nut that has been identified as the culprit allergen. However, allergy to certain tree nuts is frequently associated with anaphylactic reactions. Therefore, in the interests of safety, *a person who is known to be allergic to one species of nut should avoid all nuts*, because it is almost impossible to identify individual nuts in nut mixtures. Additionally, the risk of cross-contamination of one type of nut with another is high.

Seeds

Some edible seeds are also highly allergenic, and it is important that the specific seed responsible for a person's allergic reaction be correctly identified. Sesame seed in particular is a frequent cause of allergy. However, as with nuts, a seed-allergic person who has experienced an anaphylactic reaction in response to eating seeds should avoid **all** seeds in the interest of safety.

SYMPTOMS OF NUT AND SEED ALLERGY

Symptoms that have been reported in response to nuts and seeds include:

◆ Contact dermatitis, especially of oral tissues
◆ Oral allergy syndrome
◆ Tingling of lips
◆ Itching of mouth, ears, and eyes
◆ Conjunctivitis (often from transfer of the allergen to the eye by contaminated hands)
◆ Throat tightening
◆ Hives
◆ Angioedema (tissue swelling)
◆ Asthma (in asthmatics)
◆ Anaphylaxis
◆ Gastrointestinal symptoms such as abdominal pain, diarrhea, vomiting

These symptoms occur immediately on contact with or consumption of the culprit nut or seed.

DIET FREE FROM TREE NUTS

Tree nuts are not a common constituent of foods, and they are included in recipes and manufactured foods selectively. Therefore, a specific "nut-free diet" is not required. It is necessary only to recognize the terms that would indicate the presence of nuts on manufacturers' labels or in recipes. Table 13-1 lists the most commonly used terms.

Nut antigens from different types of trees are usually unrelated. Therefore, if a person is allergic to a nut, its identity should be established, and he or she should learn all of the names and terms indicating the presence of that species.

People who are at risk for an anaphylactic reaction to a nut should avoid **all** types of nuts because of the danger of cross-contamination of one nut species by another.

Table 13-1
TERMS ON LABELS THAT INDICATE THE PRESENCE OF NUTS

Terms That Indicate the Presence of Nuts

Almond	Pecan	Nut butters
Brazil nut	Pine nut	Almond butter
Cashew	– Pinon	– Cashew butter
Chestnut	– Indian nut	– Chestnut spread
Filbert (Hazelnut)	– Pignoli	– Other
Hickory nut	Pistachio	Nut paste
Macadamia nut	Walnut	– Almond paste
Mashuga nuts		– Marzipan
		Nut oils
		Nut meal

Foods That May Contain Nuts

Artificial nuts	Flavored ice creams such as
Nougat	– Maple walnut
Nutella® (chocolate/hazelnut spread)	– Pecan
Gianduja (mixture of chocolate and chopped nuts)	– Pistachio
Candy bars	– Other nut flavors
Chocolate bars	– Chocolate
Boxed chocolates	Dessert toppings
	Cheese balls
	"Gourmet" cheese spreads

ALLERGENIC SEEDS

Some seeds are eaten "as is"; others are used as seasoning; and some are pressed for their oil. A person who is allergic to a specific seed should avoid **all** sources of the seed.

Table 13-2 on the next page lists the seeds known to have caused allergy in susceptible individuals. *It is not a complete list of all potentially allergenic seeds.*

Table 13-2 ALLERGENIC SEEDS		
Usually Consumed as a Distinct Food	**Usually Consumed as a Seasoning**	**Usually Used as the Oil**
Cotton seed (often added to "multigrain" products such as breads) Flax Melon Pomegranate Psyllium Pumpkin Sunflower Sesame	Yellow mustard White mustard Black mustard Celery Pomegranate (anardana) Poppy	Flax (linseed)

— CHAPTER 14 —

FISH AND SHELLFISH ALLERGY

ALLERGY TO FISH

Fish species are abundant and exist in many edible forms in most countries of the world. The allergenic part of the fish is usually in the meat (muscle) of the fish. However, there is evidence that fish gelatin made from skin and bones may also be allergenic. Fish gelatin contains a high level of collagens. **Collagen** is an important protein in all connective tissue; it converts to gelatin when it is boiled. Consequently, there is concern that certain collagens made from fish might be a cause of allergy. Collagens are used in a variety of cosmetics and may be a cause of allergy in fish-allergic users of these products, as well as people who consume collagen protein in fish. This subject needs to be investigated further.

It is not yet known whether antigens in different types and species of fish cross-react, making it necessary for fish-allergic people to avoid all species of fish if they are allergic to one species. In most cases, it is usually necessary for allergic people to avoid the *specific type of fish* to which they are allergic. However, there is increasing evidence that certain fish allergens may be common to several species. Not a great deal is known about individual fish allergens except for the antigen in cod named gad c 1, which was one of the first food allergens to be studied. The antigen is a type of protein called parvalbumin, and it can be found in a variety of fish species unrelated to cod, for example, carp, tuna, and salmon. It is still unclear whether a person allergic to one of these species should avoid all fish. At the present time, the advice is this: If there is *no* risk of an anaphylactic reaction, avoid only the fish species that have caused a reaction when consumed. If there *is* a risk of an anaphylactic reaction, avoid **all** fish and their derivatives in the interests of safety.

Fish and shellfish are quite distinct antigenically, so a person who is allergic to shellfish rarely needs to avoid free-swimming fish. To avoid unnecessary dietary restrictions, it is important to clearly identify the species of fish to which a person reacts adversely.

It is usually easy to avoid fish because its presence in a recipe is obvious, and its inclusion in a manufactured food is almost always indicated on the label. Table 14-1 lists terms that indicate the presence of fish or fish product in manufactured foods and recipes.

Nutrients in Fish

Fish is a significant source of niacin, vitamin B6, vitamin B12, vitamin E, phosphorus, selenium, and in smaller amounts vitamin A, magnesium, iron, and zinc. These nutrients are also present in meats, grains, legumes, and oils, which can be eaten on a fish-free diet.

Table 14-1
TERMS ON LABELS THAT INDICATE THE PRESENCE OF FISH

Terms That Indicate the Presence of Fish Protein

Fish (all species)
Roe
Caviar
Surimi

Fish oils, such as
– Cod liver oil
– Halibut liver oil
– Salmon oil
– Menhaden oil
– Efamol Marine®

Foods That May Contain Fish Protein

Asian dishes such as
– Egg rolls
– Sushi
– Sashimi
– Tempura
– Thai recipes
– Chinese recipes
– Satay sauces

Caesar salad (with anchovy)
Chili

Baked goods
Cookies
Candy bars
Prepared and frozen desserts
Any food containing gelatin,
    unless the source of the
    gelatin is given

Note on Fish Oils

Although pure oils are nonallergenic, it is very likely that any fish oil is contaminated with protein of the fish from which it was extracted. Fish-allergic people should avoid oil from the species of fish to which they are sensitive. If they don't know which fish species they are allergic to, then they should avoid all fish oil, especially if there is a risk of anaphylaxis.

SHELLFISH-FREE DIET

A person who is allergic to shellfish is usually advised to avoid shellfish of **all** types because even unrelated species tend to cause an adverse reaction when eaten by a sensitized individual. Therefore, a shellfish-restricted diet eliminates all species of crustaceans, such as crab, lobster, shrimp, prawn, and all species of mollusks (bivalves), such as clams, mussels, scallops. However, a person who reacts to shellfish does not need to avoid fish, since there is no evidence to suggest a relationship between the two types of seafood.

Table 14-2 lists names and terms that indicate the presence of shellfish. Kosher food products do not contain shellfish and therefore are safe for a person with shellfish allergy.

Table 14-2
TERMS ON LABELS THAT INDICATE THE PRESENCE OF SHELLFISH

Terms That Indicate the Presence of Shellfish

Crustaceans	Mollusks	Octopus
Crab	Abalone	Squid
Lobster	Oyster	Calamari
Shrimp	Clam	Escargot (snail)
Prawn	Cockle	Quahog
Scampi	Mussel	
Crawfish (crayfish)	Scallop	
	Whelk	
	Winkle	

Food That May Contain Shellfish Protein

Asian dishes	Shrimp noodles	Taro cake
Japanese dishes	Shrimp balls	Daikon cake
Vietnamese dishes	Shrimp chips	Flavoring in imitation fish
Thai dishes	Shrimp salad roll	products
Chinese dishes:	Prawn chips	Stuffing
– Congee	Haw Gow	
– Oyster sauce	Sui My	
– Satay sauce	Sashimi	
– XO sauce	Sushi	
– Fish sauce		
– Fish soup		
– Fish balls		

Note: This list is not exhaustive. The shellfish-allergic person should inquire about the source of ingredients whenever a new food is eaten, especially in an Oriental restaurant.

— CHAPTER 15 —

THE "TOP TEN" ALLERGENS

In each of the preceding seven chapters, we have discussed elimination of one specific food or one type of food. In practice, people often need to avoid more than one food, especially while they are trying to determine exactly which ones they are allergic to. If you need to avoid only one, two, or three foods, the previous chapters will give you enough information to do so without risking nutritional deficiencies. By consuming the "foods allowed" for each food restriction, it should not be a problem for you to ensure that you obtain adequate nutrition while on the exclusion diet. However, in some cases, more than two or three foods need to be avoided. This chapter will provide you with the information that will allow you to avoid the ten most allergenic foods and still not risk nutritional deficiency.

THE ALLERGENIC "TOP TEN" FOODS

Milk and milk products, egg, wheat, corn, soy, peanut, tree nuts, chocolate, fish, and shellfish are the most frequent causes of food allergy. The more foods a person needs to avoid, the greater is the risk for nutritional deficiency. When many foods are removed from the diet at the same time, it is important to find substitute foods that will replace the important nutrients that are restricted. Table 15-1 lists substitute foods to ensure adequate nutritional intake when a person is avoiding these ten most highly allergenic foods at the same time.

How Long Should I Stay on a Restricted Diet?

A very restricted diet should not be followed initially for longer than four weeks, after which time each food should be retested to confirm that it really needs to be avoided. If one or more of the specified foods do not cause symptoms when they are consumed after elimination, they can be included in the diet, which will then become more nutritionally complete and easier to manage.

Each of the ten foods restricted on the diet in Table 15-1 can be found in many products and has many derivatives. It would require extensive lists of foods and their products to cover all possible dietary sources. Reading of food labels is essential to detect the allergen as an ingredient in processed and prepared foods. Because so many foods are restricted on this diet, information is provided only for the *foods allowed*. Most of the information for individual restrictions has already been included in Chapters 8 to 14.

If enough of the foods allowed in the "top ten allergens" elimination diet in Table 15-1 are consumed, and the diet is limited to four weeks, nutritional deficiency should not be a problem. Possibly the only supplements required are calcium and vitamin D. However, a person following this diet for longer than four weeks is strongly advised to check with a physician and a dietitian for guidance in choosing appropriate supplements.

Table 15-1
DIET FREE FROM MILK, EGG, WHEAT, CORN, SOY, PEANUT, TREE NUTS, FISH, SHELLFISH, AND CHOCOLATE

Type of Food	Foods Allowed

Milk and Milk Products	• Milk and soy-free products such as
	  – Rice Dream® (made from brown rice and safflower oil)
	  – Darifree® (made from potato starch)
	• In recipes, substitute
	  – fruit or vegetable juice
	  – homemade soup stock
	  – water used to cook vegetables or potatoes
	• Instead of butter use
	  – whey-free, soy-free, corn-free margarine (e.g., Canoleo®)
	  – pure jelly
	  – jam
	  – honey
	  – herb-flavored olive oil
	• Dressings on vegetables and salad:
	  – olive oil with herbs
	  – homemade salad dressings made with allowed ingredients

Grains, Cereals, and Bakery Products	*Grains and flours:*
	• Amaranth and amaranth flour
	• Barley and barley flour
	• Buckwheat and buckwheat flour
	• Chickpea or garbanzo bean flour (besan)
	• Millet and millet flour (bajri)
	• T'eff
	• Oats and oat flour
	• Potato starch and flour
	• Quinoa and quinoa flour
	• Rice and rice flour
	• Wild rice and wild rice flour
	• Rye and rye flour
	• Sago and sago flour
	• Tapioca; tapioca starch and flour
	• Cassava flour and starch
	
	Breads and baked goods:
	• Baked goods and specialty baking mixes containing allowed ingredients such as:
	  – Ener-G® rice, brown rice, or tapioca bread
	  – Celimix® rice or flaxmeal bread
	• Homemade baked goods made with allowed flours and grains

Note: This list is not exhaustive. Other foods may contain the substances listed in the title of this table and not be listed here. It is up to the reader to read all ingredient labels carefully and to contact the manufacturer if there is any doubt.

Table 15-1 (continued)
DIET FREE FROM MILK, EGG, WHEAT, CORN, SOY,
PEANUT, TREE NUTS, FISH, SHELLFISH, AND CHOCOLATE

Type of Food	Foods Allowed

Grains, Cereals, and Bakery Products (continued)	*Crackers and snacks:*
	• Potato chips made with allowed oil, such as Nalley 100% Golden Light Chips®
	• Pure rye crisp crackers
	• Rice cakes
	• Rice crackers
	
	Cereals:
	• Made from any of the allowed grains such as
	  – Cream of Rice®
	  – Kenmei Rice Bran,
	  – Puffed rice
	  – Rice flakes
	  – Oatmeal
	  – Rolled oats
	  – Oat bran
	  – Rye flakes
	  – Granola made with allowed ingredients only
	  – Puffed amaranth
	  – Puffed millet
	  – Quinoa flakes
	
	Pasta:
	• Made from any allowed grains and free from wheat and other restricted ingredients, such as
	  – Brown rice pasta
	  – Wild rice pasta
	  – Mung bean pasta
	  – Green bean pasta
	  – Buckwheat pasta (soba noodles)
	  – Rice pasta
	  – Rice noodles
	  – Potato pasta
	  – Quinoa pasta

Vegetables	• All plain fresh and frozen vegetables and their juices *except*
	  – Corn
	  – Soybeans
	  – Soybean sprouts
	  – Mixed sprouts

Table 15-1 (continued)
DIET FREE FROM MILK, EGG, WHEAT, CORN, SOY,
PEANUT, TREE NUTS, FISH, SHELLFISH, AND CHOCOLATE

Type of Food	Foods Allowed
Fruit	• All plain fresh and frozen fruits and their juices
Meat and Poultry	• All fresh or frozen pure meat or poultry *Avoid* any meat mixed with additional ingredients, such as processed meats, sausages, and all deli meats.
Fish and Shellfish	• None
Eggs	• None • Use egg-free egg replacer products such as Ener-G® Egg Replacer
Legumes	• All plain legumes and legume dishes prepared with allowed foods, *except* soy and peanut
Nuts	• None

Seeds	• All seeds such as
	  – Anise
	  – Caraway
	  – Cumin
	  – Fennel
	  – Flax
	  – Melon
	  – Mustard
	  – Pepper
	  – Poppy
	  – Pumpkin
	  – Sesame
	  – Sunflower

Fats and Oils	• Vegetable oils such as
	  – Olive
	  – Canola
	  – Sunflower
	  – Safflower
	  – Flaxseed
	• Meat drippings
	• Lard
	• Poultry fat
	• Homemade gravy with allowed ingredients
	• Tahini (sesame seed butter)

Spices and Herbs	• All pure fresh or dried herbs and spices

— CHAPTER 16 —

YEAST AND MOLD ALLERGY

Yeasts and molds belong to the kingdom Fungi. Fungi are neither plants nor animals, but because they are made up of living cells, like all cells they contain proteins, and these proteins can be allergenic. We are constantly surrounded by fungi, in the air we breathe, and in the food we eat. Most people are familiar with the commonest forms of fungi–mushrooms, molds, and yeasts. Some people are allergic to inhaled fungi, especially to the spores that are their reproductive structures, in a similar way that seeds are the reproductive parts of plants. You will usually experience allergy to inhaled molds and mold spores as asthma or other respiratory-tract symptoms. Sometimes molds and their spores are inadvertently eaten in moldy foods.

We also consume fungi as food–all of the mushrooms are fungi–and some people may be allergic to mushrooms, although such allergy is rare. Illness (and occasionally death) caused by eating a poisonous mushroom is more common than an allergic reaction to a nonposionous one. We use yeasts in a variety of food manufacturing processes, such as in brewing beers, making wines and vinegars, and baking bread and other bakery products. A range of different fungi, especially molds, are used in making cheese and other fermented food products.

Just like plants, each fungus contains its own protein, which is responsible for a person's allergy. However, because it is extremely difficult to separate the different types of fungal proteins, when a person has a proven allergy to fungus, he or she is usually advised to avoid fungi of all types. This chapter will provide you with the information you need to avoid the most allergenic food fungi—the yeasts and molds. So, let us start with a discussion of these fungi in a little more detail, so you will know what you are dealing with.

209

Occurrence of Yeast and Mold

Yeasts and molds are tiny single-celled fungi. Mold colonies are often seen growing on the surface of moist foods such as bread, jam, and cheese. Yeasts (*Saccharomyces* species) are used in food production to ferment the nutrient source on which they grow. This property is used in the leavening of bread (by baker's yeast) and the manufacture of wine and vinegar (by brewer's yeast). Yeast is a source of B vitamins and is present in many multivitamin preparations containing B vitamins.

Sensitivity to Yeast and Mold

The spores of some mold fungi, such as species of the genera *Aspergillus* and *Cladosporium* (sometimes called *Hormodendrum*), are common causes of inhalant allergy, especially for people with asthma. Anyone who is sensitive to inhaled fungal spores must avoid all sources of the fungi such as the moist soil of house plants and damp rooms, especially basements where molds grow. Because mold spores are released from damp ground softened by the first thaw of spring, mold-sensitive persons with asthma may need to limit their time outdoors to avoid inhaling the spores in the air at this time of year.

A small percentage of asthmatic persons sensitive to inhaled fungal spores, and some people who are not asthmatic, develop urticaria (hives) when they eat or drink substances containing yeast or molds. Extremely sensitive persons can suffer an anaphylactic reaction, with breathing difficulty, hives, angioedema (tissue swelling) especially in the throat, and cardiac symptoms. These people must be particularly careful to avoid all sources of fungi in their diet.

Managing Yeast and Mold Sensitivity

Management of yeast and/or mold sensitivity requires the elimination of all foods that might contain yeast or mold (Table 16-1). Foods excluded as obvious possibilities are leavened (risen) baked products, most cheeses, certain fruits and vegetables, certain beverages, and moldy foods. Some lists of foods to avoid for yeast sensitivity cite milk because it could be a source of penicillin, an antibiotic derived from fungi belonging to the genus *Penicillium*. In the past, dairy cows were treated with penicillin to protect them from infection. However, this practice has been discontinued because of the danger to penicillin-sensitive people, so milk need not be avoided.

Some diets free of yeast and mold advocate avoiding wheat flour. However, because modern flour milling does not permit the use of moldy wheat, sensitive persons do not need to avoid flour. Nevertheless, they must avoid all baked goods containing flour leavened with yeast. Also, because enriched flours contain vitamins that may be derived from yeast, these products must also be avoided.

Malt is made by fermenting barley or other grains with yeast and is used to flavor foods such as cereals, candies, and beverages. All sources of malt should be avoided.

All obvious sources of mold such as moldy jams and jellies must be avoided. Leftover foods and leftover tea and coffee are potential media for the growth of molds; therefore, only fresh foods and freshly brewed tea and coffee should be consumed. Fruit may also be a source of mold, so fruit should be eaten only if it is fresh or freshly cooked.

Candida albicans

Candida albicans is a dimorphic fungus, which means that it grows as a yeast form in a carbohydrate-rich environment and forms hyphae (strands) when the growth environment is low in nutrients. Thus it is commonly referred to as a "pseudoyeast." Other species of *Candida* exist and have the same characteristics as *C. albicans*: that is, they are "pseudo yeasts."

The role of species of candida, especially *C. albicans*, as a cause of allergy has been much disputed. Positive skin reactions often occur in persons without clinical evidence of candida infection or allergic disease. Candida species are extremely common members of the body's resident microflora. Usually they are harmless, as they are kept in check by other resident microorganisms such as bacteria. This balance can be upset, however–for example, when antibiotics eliminate several species of bacteria or the immune system is not functioning efficiently. In these instances, candida multiply unchecked and soon cause infections such as oral thrush, vaginal candidiasis (sometimes called monoliasis), and skin eruptions.

Some practitioners believe that repeated imbalances of this sort can lead to chronic candida sensitivity, which in turn can lead to numerous food and chemical sensitivities. A "candida diet" is prescribed to treat this condition, usually excluding foods that contain sugars and other carbohydrates such as simple starches. In addition, the sensitive person should avoid dietary forms of other fungi, which are believed to cross-react with candida and produce similar reactions.

Although candida infection or sensitivity may contribute to mold and yeast sensitivity, this connection is not scientifically proven. The instructions in this chapter are for a yeast and mold allergy (Type I hypersensitivity) and should not be used to manage a suspected candida sensitivity.

Table 16-1 **THE YEAST- AND MOLD-FREE DIET:** **FOODS ALLOWED AND FOODS RESTRICTED**		
Type of Food	**Foods Allowed**	**Foods Restricted**
Milk and Milk Products	• Butter • Buttermilk • Cottage cheese • Cream • Ice cream • Panir • Plain milk • Quark® • Ricotta cheese • Sherbet • Yogurt	• Feta cheese • Malted milk • Sour cream • Fermented cheeses such as Danish Blue and Camembert, and all others with mold as the fermentation agent
Breads and Cereals	• Any flour or grain not enriched with vitamins • Any bread, bun, pita, or pizza dough not leavened with yeast or sourdough starter, or with malt, or with enriched flour	• Flour or grains enriched with vitamins • All others, including – Au gratin dishes – Bread coating – Bread crumbs – Bread stuffing – Bread pudding
Vegetables	• All pure fresh, frozen or canned vegetables and their juices except those listed at right	• Fungi such as mushrooms, truffles, and morels • Sauerkraut
Fruit	• All pure fresh, frozen, or canned fruits and their juices except those listed at right	• Grapes, raisins, and other dried fruit
Meat, Poultry, and Fish	• All fresh, frozen, or canned meat, poultry, or fish prepared without bread crumbs	• Meat, poultry, and fish dishes made with bread crumbs: – Breaded fish – Croquettes – Fish cakes – Hamburger patties not labeled as 100% meat – Luncheon meats – Sausages
Eggs	• All	• Any prepared with restricted foods, such as eggs Benedict with cheese sauce, quiche with cheese, cheese in omelettes, etc.

Note: This list is not exhaustive. Other foods may contain yeast and mold and not be listed here. It is up to the reader to read all ingredient labels carefully and to contact the manufacturer if there is any doubt.

Table 16-1 (continued)
THE YEAST- AND MOLD-FREE DIET:
FOODS ALLOWED AND FOODS RESTRICTED

Type of Food	Foods Allowed	Foods Restricted
Legumes	• All plain legumes	• Fermented legumes such as soy sauce
Nuts and Seeds	• All plain nuts and seeds	• Any nut products containing restricted ingredients (e.g., snacks)
Fats and Oils	• Butter, cream, margarine, shortening • Pure vegetable oils • Salad dressings made with oil and lemon • Lard and meat drippings • Gravy	• Salad dressings with vinegar or fermented products such as soy sauce
Spices and Herbs	• All fresh, frozen or dried herbs and spices	• Herb or spice mixes containing restricted foods
Sweeteners	• Sugar, honey, molasses • Jams, jellies, and sweet syrups (once opened, refrigerate and use quickly)	• Malted sweetener • Moldy jam, jelly, and syrups • Candies and candied fruits
Beverages	• Milk and milk drinks without malt • Fruit and vegetable juices • Carbonated beverages except root beer • Freshly brewed coffee • Tea made from fresh herbs such as mint • Mineral water • Distilled alcoholic beverages such as vodka, rum, gin, and whiskey	• Malted milk drinks and any beverage containing malt • Leftover coffee • Tea other than herbal teas • "Health" drinks made with nutritional yeast • Wine, beer, cider, and other fermented alcoholic beverages
Fermented Foods	• None	• Marmite® and other manufactured foods containing yeast extract • All types of vinegar and all foods containing vinegar, such as pickles, ketchup, relishes, and sauces for meat such as Worcestershire, HP Sauce®, barbecue sauce • Soy sauce and other fermented oriental sauces

Table 16-1 (continued)
THE YEAST- AND MOLD-FREE DIET:
FOODS ALLOWED AND FOODS RESTRICTED

Type of Food	Foods Allowed	Foods Restricted
Vitamins and Medications	• Check with your pharmacist for yeast-free vitamin supplements; these are permitted. • Check with your pharmacist for medications free of penicillin and its derivatives.	• B vitamins and multivitamin supplements with B vitamins derived from yeast • Penicillin and its derivatives • All other antibiotics derived from fungi
Miscellaneous		• Yeast such as brewer's yeast, baker's yeast, torula yeast, nutritional yeast

— CHAPTER 17 —

NICKEL ALLERGY

Nickel is a well-known cause of contact dermatitis in nickel-sensitive people, inducing a reaction wherever it is in close contact with the skin or mucous membrane. This response is known as a cell-mediated immune reaction (Type IV hypersensitivity reaction). The nickel induces **local T-cell lymphocytes** to produce cytotoxic **cytokines** that cause the itching, reddening, and scaling of contact dermatitis.

Food allergy caused by nickel was first suspected when dermatologists noticed that some people showed symptoms of dermatitis on skin surfaces that were *not* in contact with any known allergen. These dermatologists suspected that the allergenic source might be in something ingested and looked for sources of known contact allergens, such as nickel, in commonly eaten foods. They noticed that sometimes the nickel in food is not a natural component but instead is introduced during processing, for example, from metal containers or from cooking and processing utensils.

This chapter will provide you with the information you need to avoid the major sources of nickel in your diet if you, or your doctor, suspect that nickel allergy may be contributing to your skin rash or dermatitis.

MANAGEMENT OF NICKEL ALLERGY

Clinical studies suggest that some nickel-sensitive people benefit from avoiding food sources of nickel. However, opinions differ on what constitutes a nickel-restricted diet. In one research study, an oral dose of nickel (as nickel sulfate) as low as 0.6 mg produced a positive reaction in some nickel-sensitive persons.

However, another report indicated that 2.5 mg was required to induce a flare-up. Because the levels of nickel required to induce a reaction have varied widely in different studies, it is difficult to determine a "safe level" of dietary nickel for nickel-sensitive persons.

To further confuse the subject, the level of nickel in foods varies with the plant species and with the nickel content of the soil in which the plant was grown or, in the case of seafood, of the aquatic environment[1]. Processing of foods can increase the level of nickel in a food product as well. For example, minute traces of nickel from metal grinders used in milling flour can increase the level of nickel in flour considerably, and stainless steel cookware will increase the level of nickel in the food cooked in it.

Often dietary nickel is not the sole cause of the dermatitis, however. In these cases, nickel avoidance may improve the situation but does not make the symptoms disappear.

Human beings require a minute amount of dietary nickel for essential metabolic processes. For adults, the U.S. RDA (Recommended Dietary Allowance) for nickel is 50 µg daily. (The Canadian Dietary Standard does not include a recommendation for nickel.) The richest sources of dietary nickel are nuts, dried peas and beans, whole grains, and chocolate.

The Relationship Between Nickel and Iron

Most ingested nickel remains unabsorbed and is excreted in the feces. Usually less than 10% of the nickel in food is absorbed, but this amount *increases* in iron-deficient persons and lactating mothers. Nickel and iron use the same transport system to cross from the intestine into circulation, so, if iron is being transported, nickel is excluded. Accordingly, people who are sensitive to nickel should include iron-rich foods in their diet.

Nickel Contact Dermatitis and Oral Tolerance

The most common cause of nickel dermatitis is direct contact with nickel-containing objects. People who have tested positive for nickel using a patch test (on skin of the forearm or back) should avoid contact with *all* objects containing the metal.

A recent study indicated that the severity of contact dermatitis related to nickel can be reduced by oral exposure to nickel, for example, in the form of a

---

[1] J. M. V. Joneja, "Level of Nickel in Common Foods," *Dietary Management of Food Allergy and Intolerances,* 2nd ed. (Vancouver: J. A. Hall 1998), pp. 168-172.

dental appliance. According to other studies, oral exposure to nickel can worsen established nickel contact dermatitis initially, but prolonged exposure can reduce the clinical symptoms.

The subject of nickel contact dermatitis, nickel allergy, and achievement of tolerance is confusing from a practical point of view because of the extremely complex series of events that occur in the immune system. Nickel contact dermatitis is caused by a Type IV hypersensitivity reaction; nickel allergy is possibly a Type I hypersensitivity; and the precise mechanism that allows the immune system to achieve tolerance, especially to foods, is unclear at present.

CAUSES OF NICKEL CONTACT DERMATITIS

The most common cause of nickel dermatitis is direct contact with nickel-containing objects. Some frequent causes of nickel contact dermatitis include

Jewelry	Thimbles
Coins	Needles
Detergents	Pins
Keys	Wire supports in bras
Buckles	Hairpins, curlers, bobby pins
Clasps	Eyeglass frames
Zippers	Paper clips
Snap fasteners	Staples
Hook-and-eye fasteners	Metal pens and clips
Dental instruments	Stainless steel cutlery
Door handles	Metal objects held in mouth
Knitting needles	Medals
Metal shoe eyelets	Safety pins
Bullets	Screws, etc., in orthopedic devices
Metal pots and pans	

Nail polish with a metal mixing ball in the container should be avoided; the solvents in the polish can leach out the nickel.

The site of the reactions will be a good indicator of the source of the nickel.

THE NICKEL-RESTRICTED DIET

People suspected of having an allergy to nickel that is caused by eating foods that contain the metal often try a nickel-restricted diet for a limited period of time. Usually 4 to 6 weeks is sufficient to determine the effectiveness of the diet. Table 17-1 provides the nickel-restricted diet.

Table 17-1 THE NICKEL-RESTRICTED DIET		
Food Category	**Low Nickel Content (Foods Allowed)**	**High Nickel Content (Foods Restricted)**
Milk and Milk Products	All, including • Milk • Butter • Margarine • Yogurt • Cheese	• None
Breads and Cereals	All not on "high nickel" list, including • Rice • Corn • Popcorn • Rye • Wheat bread in moderation • Pasta in moderation	• Oats • Oatmeal • Buckwheat • Wheat germ • Wheat bran • Multigrain bread • Multigrain cereals
Vegetables	All not on "high nickel" list	• Beans (fresh and frozen) • Spinach • Green peas • Kale • Asparagus • Broccoli
Legumes, Dried Peas, and Beans	• None	All, including • Lentils • Yellow split peas • Chickpeas • Beans—brown, white, and green • Soybeans • Soybean products • Soy flour • Bean sprouts
Fruit	All not on "high nickel" list	• Pear • Banana • Pineapple • Plum • Prune • Raspberry • Fig
Meat, Poultry, Egg	• Egg • Chicken • Turkey • Other poultry • Meat from all species	• None

Note: This list is not exhaustive. Other foods may contain nickel and not be listed here. It is up to the reader to read all ingredient labels carefully and to contact the manufacturer if there is any doubt.

Table 17-1 (continued) THE NICKEL-RESTRICTED DIET		
Food Category	**Low Nickel Content (Foods Allowed)**	**High Nickel Content (Foods Restricted)**
Fish	Fish, including • All fin fish	All shellfish, including • Shrimp • Prawn • Oysters • Mussels
Nuts and Seeds	• None	All nuts, including • Peanut • Walnut • Almond • Hazelnut • Alfalfa seed • Flaxseed • Poppy seed • Sunflower seed
Beverages	• Coffee • Soft drinks • All fruit juices except those on "high nickel" list • Alcoholic beverages	• Tea • Cocoa • Chocolate drinks • Pineapple juice • Prune juice • Raspberry juice • Pear Juice • (All other juices are low in nickel)
Sweets and Confectioneries	All not on "high nickel" list, including • White sugar • Brown sugar • Honey	• Chocolate • Licorice • Almond paste (marzipan) • Any candy bars containing nuts or seeds
Herbs and Spices	• All in moderation	• None
Flavorings	• All in moderation including yeast-containing breads and mustard	• None
Other	• Vitamin and mineral supplements without nickel	• Vitamin and mineral supplements with nickel • Commercial baking powder

The table is based on a compilation of data from several different sources. It is not possible to provide a reliable scale of the level of nickel in foods, because levels of the metal vary in foods for a number of reasons, including

◆ The species or variety of plant from which the food was derived.
◆ The amount of nickel in the soil in which the plant was grown.
◆ In the case of fish, the amount of nickel in the water from which the fish was harvested.
◆ In the case of flours, how much nickel was introduced into the flour during the process of milling with metal grinders. Stone-grinding of flours avoids this source of the metal, but nickel is present to varying levels in the grain itself, depending on the species and the content of nickel in the soil in which it was grown.

Nutrients

The nickel-free diet offers a good variety of foods in all food groups, and basic nutrient needs should be easily met. However, two nutrients worthy of special consideration are iron and fiber.

IRON

Excellent sources of easily absorbed iron (heme iron from animal sources) are liver, beef, turkey (dark meat), eggs, lamb, pork, and baked salmon. Good sources of nonheme (from plant sources) iron are blackstrap molasses, dried apricots, cooked beet greens, green peas, and dates.

Foods rich in vitamin C such as citrus fruit, tomatoes, and peppers help increase iron absorption. Iron absorption is also increased if you avoid coffee with meals and for one hour after meals.

FIBER

With the restriction of wheat bran, oats, some vegetables and fruits, legumes, nuts, and seeds, many of the commonly used high-fiber foods are restricted. Some alternative choices include:

◆ **Grains**: brown and wild rice, corn and popcorn, corn bran, cereal, rye bread, crackers
◆ **Vegetables**: Brussels sprouts, corn, parsnips, carrot, eggplant, winter squash, sweet potato, yams
◆ **Fruits**: blackberries, dates, raisins, blueberries, boysenberries, crabapple, cranberries, currants (red and white), kiwi fruit, lemon, lime, orange, rhubarb

Substitutes for Other Nickel-Containing Foods

SOUPS
Some dried, packaged soup powders appear to be high in nickel. Better choices include homemade stocks from allowed vegetables plus meat; stocks from defatted meat drippings with tomato or vegetable juice or milk.

DESSERTS
All desserts and baked goods made without chocolate, oats, nuts, seeds, and fruits on the "high nickel" list are allowed. Also, try angel food cake instead of chocolate cake and gingersnaps or tea biscuits instead of chocolate chip cookies. Vanilla, butterscotch, and caramel ice cream (check ingredients) are allowed.

CONDIMENTS AND SNACKS
- Salt and pepper, and all herbs and spices, are allowed.
- Tabasco and Worcestershire sauce are fine, but avoid any soy-based sauces.
- Ketchup, mustard, relish, pickles, and salsa are allowed.
- Popcorn, potato, corn, and tortilla chips are good choices for snacks.
- Eat hard (mints) and gelatin candies instead of chocolates.

Cooking

Enamel-coated pans, pans with nonstick coating, or glass or microwave-safe plastic containers should be used. Stainless steel cookware and contact with chromium-plated utensils should be avoided.

— CHAPTER 18 —

DISACCHARIDE INTOLERANCE

Intolerance of disaccharides almost always leads to digestive-tract symptoms, such as abdominal bloating, pressure, and pain, often accompanied by diarrhea, sometimes alternating with constipation, and occasionally nausea and vomiting. The reason for the problem is an inability to digest disaccharide sugars. The most well-known and the commonest disaccharide intolerance is lactose (milk sugar) intolerance, which is discussed separately and in more detail in Chapter 8, page 136. But intolerance of other disaccharides such as sucrose (table sugar, syrup, and fruit sugar), and less frequently maltose (the sugar usually derived from grains), is experienced by some people, often as an inherited condition. This chapter will discuss the symptoms and causes of intolerance of all the disaccharides you are likely to encounter in your diet. More importantly, it will tell you how to avoid your particular "problem sugar" and give you the information you need to obtain complete, well-balanced nutrition despite your dietary restrictions.

Disaccharide intolerance may occur in a variety of conditions that damage the tissues and cells lining the digestive tract. These conditions include deficiency in digestive enzymes, for example, lactase deficiency and sucrase-isomaltase deficiency; cow's milk and soy protein-sensitive allergy or enteropathy; gluten-sensitive enteropathy (celiac disease); infections in the digestive tract caused by parasites such as amoebae, helminths, nematodes, and microorganisms such as *Giardia lamblia* and viruses such as the rotavirus group. In infants, additional causes include immaturity of the digestive tract and congenital absence of enzymes or components of the transport systems needed to digest sugars. In all cases, symptoms are confined to the digestive tract.

THE CAUSE OF DISACCHARIDE INTOLERANCE

Sugars, starches, and complex carbohydrates in foods are broken down (digested) by **enzymes** produced in the body. In order to be transported across the lining of the digestive tract and into circulation to be used in body processes, carbohydrates must be broken down to **monosaccharides** ("single sugars"). The carbohydrate composition of the normal diet is about 60% starch, 30% sucrose, and 10% lactose. Each carbohydrate is treated slightly differently in the process of digestion.

When carbohydrates reach the small intestine, they have been largely broken down to **disaccharides**—sugars made up of two sugar molecules. However, these still have to be broken down to monosaccharides before they can be transported into circulation. This final degradation is carried out by **disaccharidase** enzymes. These enzymes are produced in cells lining the small intestine, called brush border cells. This is in contrast to other types of digestive enzymes that are produced in organs at a distance from the digestive tract, such as the pancreas, and are brought to the intestines after they are formed. However, if the cells lining the small intestine are damaged, adequate amounts of the disaccharidase enzymes cannot be produced, and the disaccharide sugars remain intact and undigested. The undigested sugars then pass into the large bowel (the colon) where bacteria act on them in a process of fermentation. The products of microbial fermentation cause the symptoms of disaccharide intolerance.

SYMPTOMS

Fluid is drawn into the large intestine to normalize the increased osmotic pressure produced by excess sugar. Gases are produced as a result of an increase in microbial growth and fermentation in the bowel. This results in abdominal bloating, pain, and flatulence. Organic acids are produced by microbial fermentation in the bowel, which also causes a change in osmotic pressure, leading to more water being retained in the bowel. Watery diarrhea or loose stool results from the increase in fluid in the bowel.

CONDITIONS LEADING TO DISACCHARIDASE DEFICIENCIES

There are several reasons why the cells lining the small intestine stop producing disaccharidases:

1. In many cases the cells are damaged by inflammation resulting from an intestinal infection (enteritis). The infection is often due to a virus or bacterium, or sometimes to intestinal parasites such as amoebae, *Giardia lamblia*, helminths, or nematode worms.
2. Inflammation may also be caused by a food allergy. The intolerance is secondary to (follows) the allergy, but will persist as long as the food allergy continues.
3. Use of strong drugs and medications taken by mouth, such as antibiotics, may cause damage to the fragile cells.
4. It may be the result of an inherited tendency. This is most commonly seen in lactose intolerance: loss of the ability to produce **lactase**, the disaccharidase that breaks down lactose, the sugar in milk. This usually occurs after the age of five years.
5. In rare cases, an infant inherits the condition and is disaccharidase-deficient from birth.

Duration of the Condition

If the disaccharidase deficiency is a result of damage to the intestinal cells, caused by infection, food allergy, or strong drugs, it is called a *secondary deficiency* and is usually temporary. When the primary cause is removed, the cells will start to heal and gradually resume production of disaccharidase enzymes. Over time, you will be able to tolerate many foods to which you are presently intolerant.

If the deficiency is a result of an inherited tendency, it is likely that the disaccharide intolerance will be lifelong: This is called a *primary deficiency*. The foods that cause the most problems must always be avoided. In some cases, the deficient disaccharidase enzyme can be provided in the form of medication (liquid or tablets) to be eaten with the food, or drops can be added to foods (for example, lactase in the form of Lactaid) and you will be able to tolerate a certain amount of the treated food.

In most cases, a disaccharide intolerance is dose-related. Usually the cells are producing a limited amount of disaccharidase enzyme, and small doses of foods containing disaccharides can be processed. Problems occur when the amount of disaccharide in the food exceeds the capacity of the enzymes to digest it. The important thing is to determine your own body's capacity to handle disaccharide. As long as you remain within your personal limits, you should remain symptom-free.

The Problem Disaccharides

Lactose

This is the sugar in milk. It occurs mostly in the whey (liquid) fraction of milk, although foods made mainly of casein (such as cheeses) may still contain a small amount of lactose. The enzyme that breaks down lactose is called lactase. It splits lactose into two monosaccharides: glucose and galactose. A person whose intestinal cells are producing very little lactase will not be able to break down much lactose. Lactose intolerance is quite different from milk allergy, in which a person's immune system fights the protein in milk.

Sucrose

Table sugar and syrups are examples of sucrose. Table sugar usually comes from sugar beet or sugar cane, but is also present in many plants, especially fruits, grains, and vegetables. Syrup may be made from many types of grains, or from plants such as the maple tree from which maple syrup is extracted. The enzyme that breaks down sucrose is called sucrase. It splits sucrose into two monosaccharides: glucose and fructose.

Maltose

Maltose is found mostly in grains and starchy vegetables. The enzymes that break down maltose include maltase and isomaltase: They split maltose and starches into molecules of the monosaccharide, or "single sugar," glucose.

Starches

Starches are made up of long chains of glucose molecules. The linkages between the glucose molecules all have to be split to release the free glucose before it can be absorbed. If there is a deficiency in the enzymes that split these linkages, free glucose molecules will not be released, and the remaining undigested starch or sugar will be passed to the large bowel where bacteria will ferment it, resulting in the symptoms discussed earlier.

IDENTIFYING THE DISACCHARIDE THAT IS DEFICIENT

Except in the case of a lactase deficiency, which improves dramatically when lactose is removed from the diet, it is often difficult to separate specific disaccharide intolerances from each other.

If the deficiency is due to damage to intestinal cells, loss or reduction in activity of all the disaccharidases often results. In such a case it is usually advisable to follow a diet restricting all disaccharides at first. Because this is usually a temporary situation, avoidance will lead to healing and the foods may be tolerated in increasingly large amounts the longer the diet is followed.

If the deficiency is permanent, it is often due to loss, or lack, of the ability to produce one specific disaccharidase; in this case, efforts should be made to identify the specific deficiency. In the majority of cases, it will be a lactase deficiency as this is usually an inherited tendency, often associated with certain racial groups. Eighty percent of the world's adult population tend to lose the ability to produce lactase. Only people of northern European descent tend to retain the ability to produce lactase throughout life; 80% of this group usually can digest lactose.

Requirement for Nutritional Supplements

In general, if you are eating a wide range of the allowed foods and the disaccharide intolerance is a secondary (temporary) deficiency, you should not need a supplement. The amount of supplement that may be required will depend on individual tolerances to the disaccharide-containing food; some people will be able to tolerate a small amount of the food, so any deficiencies will be minimal.

For people with primary (permanent) deficiencies, or those who need to follow the diet for an extended period of time, the following supplements may be necessary:

Lactose restricted: calcium and possibly vitamin D
Sucrose restricted: vitamin C
Maltose restricted: vitamin B complex

Feeding the Disaccharide-Intolerant Baby

Infant formulas that are lactose-free and sucrose-free can be given to a disaccharidase-deficient infant. If the baby is *not* allergic to cow's milk proteins the milk-based formulas Enfalac (Enfamil), LactoFree (Mead Johnson), and Similac LF (Ross), which are free from lactose and sucrose are suitable. If the infant *is* allergic to cow's milk proteins, but tolerates soy, the soy-based formulas Enfalac (Enfamil) and ProSobee (Mead Johnson), which are sucrose-free, are suitable. The infant who is allergic to *both* cow's milk and soy proteins may tolerate a casein hydrolysate formula such as Enfalac (Enfamil), Nutramigen (Mead Johnson), or Pregestimil (Mead Johnson), which are free from lactose and sucrose.

A breast-fed baby will ingest significant quantities of lactose in mother's milk. The lactose composition of her milk will remain constant, regardless of whether or not the mother consumes milk and dairy products. If the baby's lactose intolerance is secondary to a gastrointestinal tract infection or other condition that is expected to be temporary, some authorities advise continuing breast-feeding and expect the diarrhea to gradually diminish as the underlying inflammation disappears.

Alternatively, the mother can pump her breast milk, treat it with Lactaid drops (4 drops per 250 milliliters of milk), and allow the enzyme to act for 24 hours in the fridge. The baby will be fed the lactose-free milk the next day. This is continued until the diarrhea stops, when the baby can be gradually put back to the breast.

THE DISACCHARIDE-FREE DIET (TABLE 18-1)

Restriction of **all** disaccharides is required initially.

Phase I should be followed for a minimum of four weeks to find out if disaccharidase deficiency is the cause of the gastrointestinal symptoms, specifically diarrhea. When the diarrhea improves, loosening of these restrictions will determine each individual's tolerance for each disaccharide.

Phase II involves introduction of one food from the "restricted" lists every other day until diarrhea recurs. Maltose tolerance is determined by introducing grains, especially "white" grains and flours. Sucrose tolerance is determined by introducing vegetables, fruits, nuts and seeds, and finally sugars. Lactose tolerance is determined by introducing dairy products and milk. Specific details of lactose intolerance are provided in Chapter 8, page 136.

Table 18-1
THE DISACCHARIDE-FREE DIET: FOODS ALLOWED AND FOODS RESTRICTED

Type of Food	Foods Allowed	Foods Restricted

Milk and Milk Products	• Cheeses (not processed):
	  Brie
	  – Camembert
	  – Cheddar
	  – Gruyère
	  – Limburger
	  – Monterey Jack
	  – Mozzarella
	  – Port du Salut
	• Non-dairy creamers, e.g.,
	  Coffee Rich®
		• All except those listed at left

Grains, Breads, and Cereals	• None	All, including: • Flours made from grains • Amaranth • Barley • Buckwheat • Bulgur • Corn • Millet • Oats • Quinoa • Rice • Rye • Spelt • Triticale • Wheat
Vegetables	Fresh, frozen, canned, without added sugar or starch: • Celery • Chives • Cucumber • Endive • Garlic • Green onion • Kale • Lettuce • Mushrooms • Parsley • Parsnips • Peppers, green and red • Potatoes, french fried or hash browns	• Canned with additives • Added sauces • Added butter or margarine • Asparagus • Artichokes • Broccoli • Cabbage, green and red • Carrots * Cauliflower • Corn • Kohlrabi • Leeks • Okra • Onion (mature, cooking) • Potatoes (boiled) • Pumpkin

Note: This list is not exhaustive. Other foods may contain disaccharides and not be listed here. It is up to the reader to read all ingredient labels carefully and to contact the manufacturer if there is any doubt.

Table 18-1 (continued)
THE DISACCHARIDE-FREE DIET: FOODS ALLOWED AND FOODS RESTRICTED

Type of Food	Foods Allowed	Foods Restricted
Vegetables (continued)	• Radishes • Spinach • Swiss chard • Tomatoes • Tomato juice • Turnip • Watercress • Avocado	• Squash, all types • Sweet potatoes • Yams • V-8 Vegetable Juice®

Fruit	Fresh, frozen, canned in own juice
	• Berries:
	  – Blackberry
	  – Blueberry
	  – Cranberry
	  – Gooseberry
	  – Loganberry
	• Cherry
	• Currants, red and black
	• Damson plums
	• Figs, raw
	• Guava
	• Grapes
	• Grape juice
	• Kiwi fruit
	• Lemon
	• Lime
	• Passion fruit (granádilla)
		• Added sugar or syrup
		• Apple
		• Apricot
		• Banana
		• Date
		• Grapefruit
		• Mango
		• Melon, all types
		• Nectarine
		• Orange
		• Papaya (pawpaw)
		• Peach
		• Pear
		• Pineapple, raw
		• Plum, prune type
		• Raspberry
		• Strawberry
		• Tangerine
		• Watermelon

Meat, Poultry, and Fish	All fresh or frozen: • Lamb • Beef • Pork • Wild game • Chicken • Duck • Turkey • Game birds • Fin fish • Shellfish	• Processed • Breaded • Smoked • Cured • Canned • Corned Beef
Eggs	• Cooked, plain (e.g., fried, boiled, scrambled)	• With added milk, flour, or sugar

Table 18-1 (continued)
THE DISACCHARIDE-FREE DIET: FOODS ALLOWED AND FOODS RESTRICTED

Type of Food	Foods Allowed	Foods Restricted
Legumes	• Tofu	• Bean sprouts • Black eyed peas • Broad beans (fava beans) • Chickpeas (garbanzos) • Green and wax beans • Kidney beans • Lentils • Navy beans • Peanut • Peas • Soybeans • Split peas
Nuts and Seeds	• None	All, including • Almond • Beechnut • Brazil nut • Butternut • Cashew • Hazelnut (filbert) • Hickory • Macadamia • Peanut • Pecan • Pistachio • Pumpkin seed • Sesame seed • Soybean (roasted) • Sunflower seed • Walnut

Fats and Oils	• Pure vegetable oil:
	  – Canola
	  – Corn
	  – Flaxseed
	  – Olive
	  – Safflower
	  – Soy
	  – Sunflower
	• Margarine without milk solids, e.g., Fleischmann's Low Sodium, No Salt Margarine®
	• Parkay Diet Spread®
	• Some other diet spreads
	• Lard and meat drippings
		• Butter
		• Margarine containing whey or milk solids

Table 18-1 (continued)
THE DISACCHARIDE-FREE DIET: FOODS ALLOWED AND FOODS RESTRICTED

Type of Food	Foods Allowed	Foods Restricted
Sugars and Sweeteners	• Glucose • Dextrose • Fructose (fruit sugar) • Levulose • Honey • Sugar substitutes (lactose-free and in moderation) • Aspartame • Cyclamate • Saccharine • Sugar Twin® • Equal® • Sweet 'n' Low®	• Sucrose (table sugar) • Lactose (milk sugar) • Maltose (grain sugar) • Foods containing sugars • Syrups
Spices and Herbs	• Allspice • Anise seed • Basil • Bay leaf • Caraway • Cayenne • Celery • Chervil • Chili powder • Cinnamon • Cloves • Coriander, leaf or seed • Cumin seed • Dill, seed or weed • Fennel seed • Fenugreek seed • Garlic powder • Ginger • Mace • Marjoram • Mustard • Nutmeg • Onion powder • Oregano • Paprika • Parsley • Pepper, black and white • Poppy seed • Poultry seasoning • Rosemary • Sage • Savory • Tarragon • Thyme • Turmeric	• Herb or spice mixes or seasoning packets • Curry

— CHAPTER 19 —

BIOGENIC AMINES INTOLERANCE:

HISTAMINE AND TYRAMINE SENSITIVITY

Biogenic amines, including **histamine** and **tyramine**, are products of certain amino acids that make up specific proteins. They may be present in both plants and animals consumed as food. In fact, small quantities of biogenic amines are present in almost all foods and usually cause no problems. Large quantities result from microbial activities during rotting of foods and during manufacture of fermented foods such as cheese, wine, vinegar, fermented sausages, soy sauce, and sauerkraut. Large quantities, especially of histamine in foods, cause symptoms of food poisoning in most people; individuals who are considered "intolerant" to biogenic amines experience symptoms when they consume levels that cause no problems in nonsensitive people.

Varying opinions exist on the significance of biogenic amines in non-immunologically-mediated reactions to foods. Because histamine is the most important mediator responsible for the symptoms of "classical allergy" in the Type I (IgE-mediated) hypersensitivity reaction (see Chapter 3, page 41), it is difficult for clinicians to distinguish between reactions due to allergy and those resulting from too much histamine, since the symptoms are the same in both cases. The "classical" symptoms of food allergy, such as urticaria (hives), angioedema (tissue swelling), nasal congestion, asthma (in asthmatics), headaches, oral allergy symptoms, and digestive-tract complaints such as nausea, flatulence, abdominal cramps, and diarrhea, are also typical of histamine intolerance and, to some extent, tyramine intolerance.

HISTAMINE

Histamine is an important physiological fluid in the body. It is always present in **plasma**, the fluid portion of blood in which blood cells are suspended. The level of histamine in blood goes up and down throughout the day in a specific type of rhythmic variation. Histamine plays important regulatory roles in gastric acid secretion in the stomach, in determining how easily substances pass through blood vessels, in muscle contraction, and in the immune response. It is a key mediator in inflammation, which is the way the immune system protects the body from invasion by infective microorganisms and other events, such as trauma (tissue injury), that are a threat to health.

Histamine is manufactured and stored in a number of cells in the body, particularly **mast cells** (see Chapter 3, page 32), which occur throughout body tissues, especially mucous tissue. In an allergic reaction (IgE-mediated Type I hypersensitivity), histamine is released from mast cells in vast quantities and is one of the most important inflammatory mediators of the swelling, itching, reddening, and increased movement of blood cells and fluid from inside blood vessels into tissues that are characteristic of symptoms of allergy.

Events other than Type I hypersensitivity can cause the release of histamine from mast cells. Some foods and food additives have shown this ability in the absence of allergy.

Histamine Intolerance

High doses of histamine are toxic for all humans, but individual tolerance determines reactivity to small quantities. Just about everyone who ingests histamine from a contaminated food at a level of more than 2.7 milligrams per kilogram of body weight will show symptoms of "histamine poisoning," but at lower concentrations only a few sensitive individuals will have a reaction. It is likely that differences in levels of tolerance are of genetic origin, but tolerance can be reduced by disease, especially allergy and autoimmune diseases and medications, such as some antidepressants, some asthma medications, and some antihypertensive drugs.

CAUSE OF HISTAMINE INTOLERANCE

The cause of histamine intolerance is thought to be a defect in the breakdown of histamine. In humans, breakdown of histamine is done by two **enzymes**, diamine oxidase (DAO) and histamine methyltransferase (HMT), that have different characteristics. DAO occurs predominantly in the lining of the intestine as well as the placenta, kidney, and the **thymus** gland. HMT has a wider distribution, occurring in the stomach, lung, spleen, kidney, thymus, and particularly the brain. Both enzymes can be slowed or stopped by a variety of compounds, many of which are used as medications. Reduced DAO activity has been the subject of several investigations of conditions such as "idiopathic" (of unknown cause) urticaria and angioedema in which an allergic response has been ruled out. Laboratory findings of increased plasma levels (greater than 2 nanograms per milliliter) of histamine and reduced DAO activity have been suggested as indicators of reduced histamine breakdown and possible enzyme deficiency.

SYMPTOMS OF HISTAMINE INTOLERANCE

Symptoms occur when the enzyme system that breaks down histamines cannot keep the histamines at a "normal" level.

Urticaria (hives) and angioedema (tissue swelling) are symptoms that occur in response to excessively high levels of histamine in the body. Rhinitis (nasal congestion) is another symptom of too much histamine. Histamine has also been implicated as an important mediator in some types of headaches that are thought to differ from migraine.

Histamine is the only proven inflammatory mediator to cause itching. Histamine can also cause blood vessels to become more permeable, thus allowing fluid to move from the blood vessels into tissue, causing swelling. It can also cause blood vessels to widen. Sensitive people may experience symptoms such as hypotension (drop in blood pressure) and tachycardia (increased pulse rate) as a result.

DIETARY MANAGEMENT OF HISTAMINE INTOLERANCE

A histamine-restricted diet has often proved beneficial in reducing total body histamine levels when the cause of the condition is unknown but the symptoms indicate that histamine is the principal mediator. Conditions such as idiopathic urticaria (chronic hives of unknown cause), angioedema ("giant hives"), chronic itching, and some headaches have responded well to a histamine-restricted diet. It is worthwhile to restrict these foods for four weeks in cases where all other treatments have not helped relieve symptoms.

SYMPTOMS INDICATING TOO MUCH HISTAMINE IN THE BODY

◆ rhinitis and rhinorrhea (stuffy, runny nose)
◆ conjunctivitis (irritated, watery, reddened eyes)
◆ urticaria (hives)
◆ angioedema (swelling, especially of facial tissues)
◆ itchiness (especially of eyes, nose, ears, skin)
◆ headache

Food Sources of Histamine

Histamine is present in most fermented foods. Microbial enzymes convert the amino acid histidine (present as a part of all proteins) to histamine. Any foods that have been subjected to microbial fermentation in the manufacture of the food, such as cheeses, fermented soy products, fermented foods (sauerkraut), alcoholic beverages, and vinegars, contain histamine.

Foods that have been exposed to microbial contamination will contain histamine; the level is determined by how fast the microbial metabolism takes place. Histamine levels will rise to a reactive level long before any signs of spoilage occur in the food. This is particularly important in fish. Bacteria in the gut will start to convert histidine to histamine as soon as the fish dies. The longer the fish remains ungutted, the higher the level of histamine in the flesh.

Some foods, such as tomato, eggplant, and spinach, contain high levels of histamine naturally. In addition, a number of food additives such as azo dyes, particularly tartrazine, and preservatives are known to cause histamine to be released. Some of these (such as benzoates) occur naturally in foods, especially fruits, and may have the same effect as the food additive in releasing histamine. (Sensitivity to azo dyes is discussed in more detail in Chapter 21; sensitivity to berzoates, in Chapter 22.) The histamine-restricted diet excludes all the foods that are known to contain high levels of histamine. It also excludes chemicals that can release histamine when they enter the body.

Histamine excess is dose-related. Each function and food adds its own level of histamine up to the person's limit of tolerance. Once the limit is reached, histamine "overflows" and symptoms result (Figure 19-1). The severity of the symptoms depends on the amount of excess histamine in the system.

General Instructions for Avoiding Histamine-Rich Foods

MEAT, POULTRY, FISH, EGG

Avoid the following:

- ◆ Fish and shellfish whether fresh, frozen, smoked, or canned, if processing is unknown. If the fish is freshly caught, gutted, and cooked within ½ hour, it may be eaten.
- ◆ Egg. A small quantity of cooked egg in a baked product such as pancakes, muffins, and cakes is allowed.
- ◆ Processed, smoked, and fermented meats such as luncheon meat, sausage, weiner, bologna, salami, pepperoni, smoked ham, cured bacon.

◆ Left-overs. Freeze any uneaten protein-based food. Bacteria will quickly act on protein at room and refrigerator temperatures, resulting in histamine production.

MILK AND MILK PRODUCTS
Avoid all *fermented* milk products, including

◆ Cheese of any kind such as cheddar, Colby, blue cheese, Brie, Camembert, feta, Romano
◆ Cheese products such as processed cheese, cheese slices, cheese spreads
◆ Cottage cheese
◆ Ricotta cheese
◆ Yogurt
◆ Buttermilk
◆ Kefir

FRUITS
Avoid

◆ Orange, grapefruit, lemon, lime
◆ Cherries
◆ Grapes
◆ Strawberries
◆ Apricots
◆ Avocado
◆ Raspberries
◆ Pineapple
◆ Cranberries
◆ Prunes
◆ Loganberries
◆ Dates
◆ Raisins
◆ Currants (fresh or dried)

VEGETABLES
Avoid

◆ Tomatoes, tomato sauces, ketchup
◆ Soy and soy products
◆ Spinach
◆ Red beans
◆ Eggplant
◆ Olives in vinegar or brine

- Pumpkin
- Pickles, relishes, and other foods containing vinegar

FOOD ADDITIVES
Avoid
- Tartrazine and other artificial food colors
- Preservatives, especially benzoates and sulphites

SEASONINGS
Avoid
- Cinnamon
- Cloves
- Vinegar
- Chilli powder
- Anise
- Curry powder
- Nutmeg

MISCELLANEOUS
Avoid
- Fermented soy products (such as soy sauce, miso)
- Fermented foods (such as sauerkraut)
- Tea (regular or green)
- Chocolate, cocoa, and cola drinks
- Alcoholic beverages of all types
- "De-alcoholized" beverages (e.g., beer, ale, wine)

MEDICATIONS AND VITAMIN SUPPLEMENTS
- Tartrazine is in some medications (both prescription and nonprescription) and some vitamin supplements. Essential medications should be tartrazine-free.
- Pharmacies keep a list of manufacturers who produce tartrazine-free products.

CONTACT ALLERGY
- Some toiletries and cosmetics containing histamine-releasing substances may cause contact dermatitis. Avoid any that contain cinnamaldehyde, Balsam of Peru, benzoates of any type, sulfites, and dyes.

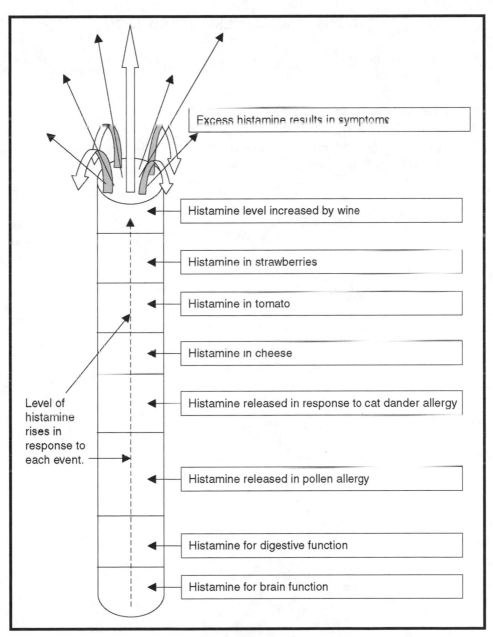

Excess histamine results in symptoms

Histamine level increased by wine

Histamine in strawberries

Histamine in tomato

Histamine in cheese

Histamine released in response to cat dander allergy

Histamine released in pollen allergy

Histamine for digestive function

Histamine for brain function

Level of histamine rises in response to each event.

Figure 19-1
Diagram Representing a Person with Allergies to Pollen and Cat Dander
Who Has Eaten a Meal Containing Histamine-Rich Foods
(Cheese, Tomato, Strawberries) with Wine

The Histamine-Restricted Diet

Table 19-1 lists the foods allowed and the foods not allowed in the histamine-restricted diet. This diet excludes **all:**

◆ Foods with naturally high levels of histamine
◆ Fermented foods
◆ Artificial food colors, especially tartrazine
◆ Preservatives, particularly benzoates and sulphites

Table 19-1
THE HISTAMINE-RESTRICTED DIET

Type of Food	Foods Allowed	Foods Restricted
Milk and Milk Products	• Plain milk • Cream • Ice cream without artificial additives • Curdled milk products	• Any manufactured dairy products made with restricted ingredients • Cheese of all types • Yogurt • Buttermilk • Any milk products produced by fermentation
Breads Cakes and Cookies Breakfast Cereals Crackers Pasta and Noodles	• Any unbleached flour or grain • Corn; cornstarch and plain popcorn • Plain rice and wild rice • Parboiled rice • General Foods Minute Rice® • Any plain fresh whole-grain bread, buns, biscuits, pizza dough with allowed ingredients. • Homemade or purchased baked cookies, pies, etc., made with allowed ingredients • Breakfast cereals with allowed ingredients, including: – All plain grains – Corn flakes – Shredded wheat – Rice Krispies – Plain oats and oatmeal – Cream of Wheat – Puffed wheat – Puffed rice – Cream of rice • Plain crackers with allowed ingredients: – Grissol Melba Toast® – RyVita® – Rye Krisp® – Wassa® Crisp bread – Rice cakes – Rice crackers • Plain pasta • Pasta dishes with allowed ingredients	• Bleached flour (benzoyl peroxide is the bleaching agent) • Popcorn with artificial flavors • Manufactured rice entrées • Any baked product with restricted ingredients • Breakfast cereals with restricted additional ingredients such as artificial colors, flavors, and preservatives • Flavored instant oatmeal • All manufactured pasta meals in packages or cans

Note: This list is not exhaustive. Other foods may contain histaminet and not be listed here. It is up to the reader to read all ingredient labels carefully and to contact the manufacturer if there is any doubt.

Table 19-1 (continued)
THE HISTAMINE-RESTRICTED DIET

Type of Food	Foods Allowed	Foods Restricted
Vegetables	• All pure fresh and frozen vegetables and their juices *except* those on the restricted list • Homemade salad dressings containing allowed ingredients, e.g., oil, garlic, and herbs	• Eggplant (aubergine) • Pumpkin • Sauerkraut • Spinach • Tomato • Avocado • Olives in vinegar or brine • Vegetable dishes with restricted ingredients • Most commercial salad dressings, including mayonnaise
Fruit	• Apple • Banana • Figs • Guava • Kiwi • Longans • Lychees • Mango • Melons of all types, such as: 　– Cantaloupe (rock melon) 　– Honeydew 　– Watermelon • Passion fruit • Pear • Rhubarb • Starfruit • Fruit dishes, juices, jams, jellies, and conserves made with allowed fruits and ingredients	• Apricot • Blueberry • Cherry • Cranberry • Currant • Dates • Grapes • Loganberry • Nectarine • Orange • Grapefruit • Lemon • Lime • Mulberry • Papaya (pawpaw) • Peach • Pineapple • Prunes • Plums • Raisins • Raspberries • Strawberries • Fruit dishes, juices, jams, jellies and conserves made with restricted fruit and other ingredients
Meat, Poultry, and Fish	• All pure, freshly cooked meat or poultry without restricted ingredients • Fresh fish if it has been caught, gutted, and cooked or frozen without delay	• All fermented processed meats such as 　– Salami 　– Bologna 　– Pepperoni 　– Weiners

Table 19-1 (continued)
THE HISTAMINE-RESTRICTED DIET

Type of Food	Foods Allowed	Foods Restricted
Meat, Poultry, and Fish (continued)		– Smoked or pickled meats – All leftover cooked meat • All shellfish • All fish, whether fresh, frozen, or canned, unless it has been freshly caught, gutted, and cooked without delay • Pickled fish • Smoked fish • Any meat, poultry, or fish made with restricted ingredients
Eggs	• Egg as a minor ingredient in any allowed products (e.g., cakes, muffins, breads, and other baked goods)	• Dishes in which egg is the main ingredient, such as: – Soufflé – Mousse – Quiche – Omelet • Scrambled, boiled, fried eggs • Egg dishes prepared with restricted foods • Raw egg white (as in eggnog, Hollandaise sauce, traditional Caesar salad dressing, mayonnaise, some milk shakes)
Legumes	• All plain legumes except those on the restricted list • Pure peanut butter	• Soy beans • Red beans
Nuts and Seeds	• All plain nuts and seeds *except pumpkin seeds*	• Pumpkin seeds • Any nut or seed mixtures with restricted ingredients (e.g., artificial barbecue flavor)
Spices and Herbs	• All fresh, frozen, or dried herbs and spices except those on the restricted list	• Anise • Cinnamon • Cloves • Curry powder • Nutmeg • Seasoning packets with restricted ingredients • Foods labeled "with spices"

Table 19-1 (continued)
THE HISTAMINE-RESTRICTED DIET

Type of Food	Foods Allowed	Foods Restricted
Fats and Oils	• Pure butter • Pure vegetable oils • Homemade salad dressing with allowed ingredients • Lard and meat drippings • Homemade gravy	• All fats and oils with color and/or preservatives • Hydrolyzed lecithin • Margarine • Prepared salad dressings with restricted ingredients • Gravy made from mixes or in cans
Sweeteners	• Sugar, icing sugar • Maple syrup, corn syrup • Honey • Jams, jellies, marmalade, and conserves made with allowed ingredients • Plain artificial sweeteners • Homemade sweets with allowed ingredients	• Flavored syrups • Prepared dessert fillings • Prepared icings/frostings • Spreads with restricted ingredients • Cake decorations • Commercial confectionery • Commercial candies
Beverages	• Plain milk • Pure juices of allowed fruits and vegetables • Plain and carbonated mineral water • Coffee • Herbal teas made from allowed ingredients, without spices (no "zingers" or "zests")	• Flavored milks • Fruit drinks and cocktails with restricted ingredients • Cola-type carbonated drinks • Flavored coffees • Tea, regular or green • All drinks with "flavor" or "spices" • All alcoholic beverages • "De-alcoholized" beers, wines, and other beverages
Other	• Baking powder • Baking soda • Cream of Tartar • Plain gelatin • Homemade relishes with allowed ingredients	• Chocolate and cocoa • Flavored gelatin • Mincemeat • Prepared relishes • Olives • Soy sauce • Miso • Commercial ketchup • Pickles

TYRAMINE SENSITIVITY

A sensitivity to tyramine is most common in individuals who

1. Are taking monoamine oxidase (MAO) inhibiting drugs
2. Suffer from migraine headaches
3. Suffer from chronic urticaria

For persons who are taking monoamine oxidase inhibiting drugs, a tyramine-restricted diet is essential. However, these people will not have a lot of food restrictions if they have no previous history of tyramine sensitivity.

TYRAMINE IS PRESENT IN A NUMBER OF FOODS, PARTICULARLY:

- Aged cheeses
- Raspberries
- Yeast extract
- Bananas
- Chicken liver
- Red plums
- Wines (especially red)
- Avocados
- Beer
- Eggplant
- Other fermented beverages
- Tomatoes
- Vinegar and pickles

Cause of Tyramine Sensitivity

Suppression or relative deficiency of the monoamine oxidase enzyme system that normally breaks down tyramine in the body allows tyramine to rise to a level that results in symptoms. It is excessive undegraded tyramine that causes the symptoms.

A tyramine-restricted diet is especially important for persons taking monoamine oxidase (MAO) inhibitors as therapy. Symptoms indicating excessive tyramine in these people include:

- Hypertension (increased blood pressure)
- Tachycardia (increased heart rate)

◆   Severe headache
◆   Cardiac failure

Medications that are MAOs include:

◆   Hydrazines (used as antidepressants)
    – Isocarboxazid (Marplan)
    – Phenelzine (Nardil)
◆   Nonhydrazines
    – Pargyline (Evtatin, Eutanyl)
    – Tranylcypromine (Parnate)
    – Selegiline (Deprenil, Deprenyl, Eldepryl) (used for treatment of Parkinson's disease)
◆   Antibiotics
    – Isoniazid (anti-tuberculosis drug)

Note: Only Parnate, Nardil, and Marplan are in common use at present. The requirement for a tyramine-restricted diet for persons using other MAO inhibiting drugs will be decided by the physician on an individual basis.

**OTHER SYMPTOMS REPORTED TO BE DUE TO
A SENSITIVITY TO TYRAMINE INCLUDE**

◆ Rapid heartbeat

◆ Clamminess

◆ Itchiness

◆ Migraine headache

◆ Hot feeling

◆ Non-migraine headache

◆ Redness of skin (flushing)

◆ Light-headedness

◆ Sweating

◆ Hives

◆ Chills

THE TYRAMINE-RESTRICTED DIET

For those who are experiencing chronic urticaria or migraine headaches that are considered to be the result of tyramine sensitivity, a reduced tyramine diet is advisable: The response to tyramine is dose-dependent, and the amount of tyramine in foods that causes an adverse reaction will depend on individual tolerance. The number of foods to be restricted initially for these people is usually more extensive than for those who are taking MAO inhibiting drugs, since foods containing lower levels of tyramine are included. Table 19-2 provides details of a tyramine-restricted diet for people who suspect they are intolerant of tyramine.

THE HISTAMINE- AND TYRAMINE-RESTRICTED DIET

Some people find that their migraine headaches diminish significantly in severity and frequency when they avoid **all** food sources of **both** histamine and tyramine. Table 19-3 provides information for such a diet. Four weeks on this diet should be sufficient for a person to determine whether this will provide relief of his or her migraines.

Table 19-2
THE TYRAMINE-RESTRICTED DIET

Type of Food	Foods Allowed	Foods Restricted
Milk and Milk Products	• Plain pasteurized milk • Ricotta cheese • Plain cream cheese	• All other dairy products
Breads and Cereals	• Any pure flour or grain • Limited amounts of yeast-risen breads, including bread, pita, buns, croissants, pizza, English muffins, and crumpets • Baking-powder-leavened products such as biscuits, quick breads, soda bread, scones, and muffins • Cookies, pies, etc., made with allowed ingredients	• Products made with restricted ingredients • Excessive quantities of baked goods with yeast
	• Breakfast cereals with allowed foods, including – Puffed rice and wheat – Corn flakes – Shreddies® – Shredded Wheat® – Plain oats and oatmeal – Plain Cream of Wheat® – All plain grains	• Breakfast cereals, like muesli and granola, with restricted nuts and fruit
	• Plain crackers with allowed ingredients: – Grissol Melba Toast® – RyVita® – Rye Krisp®	• Plain crackers with restricted ingredients
	• Rice and pasta dishes with allowed ingredients	• All packaged rice and pasta meals with "flavor packets"
Vegetables	• All pure fresh and frozen vegetables and juices except those listed at right	• Any over-ripe vegetables • Any pickled vegetables • Avocado • Broad beans • Green peas • Potato • Sauerkraut • Spinach • Sweet potato • Tomato • All prepared vegetables with restricted ingredients • Most commercial salad dressings

Note: This list is not exhaustive. Other foods may contain tyramine and not be listed here. It is up to the reader to read all ingredient labels carefully and to contact the manufacturer if there is any doubt.

Table 19-2 (continued)
THE TYRAMINE-RESTRICTED DIET

Type of Food	Foods Allowed	Foods Restricted
Fruit	• All pure fresh and frozen fruit and juices, except those listed at right • Fruit dishes made with allowed ingredients	• Any over-ripe fruit • Banana • Plums • Prunes • Raisins • Raspberries • Fruit dishes, jams, juices with restricted ingredients
Meat, Poultry, and Fish	• All pure, freshly cooked meat, poultry, and fish except what is listed at right	• Any leftover meat, poultry, or fish and foods containing them • Dry fermented sausages: – Bologna – Pepperoni – Salami • Oysters • Smoked or pickled fish or fish roe (eggs) • Smoked salmon • Pickled herring • Lox • Caviar
Eggs	• All plain eggs	• All prepared with restricted foods
Legumes	• All plain legumes except those listed at right • Pure peanut butter	• Soy beans, tofu • Fermented soy products: – Soy sauce – Fermented bean curd – Soybean paste – Shrimp paste – Chili soybean paste
Nuts and Seeds	• All plain nuts and seeds except those at right	• Walnuts Pecans
Fats and Oils	• Pure butter • Margarine • Pure vegetable oils • Homemade salad dressing with allowed ingredients • Lard and meat drippings • Homemade gravy	• Commercial salad dressings with restricted ingredients • Commercial gravies

Table 19-2 (continued)
THE TYRAMINE-RESTRICTED DIET

Type of Food	Foods Allowed	Foods Restricted
Spices and Herbsd	• All fresh, frozen, or dried herbs and spices	• Seasoning packets • Commercial packaged foods labeled with "spices" or "flavoring"
Sweets and Sweeteners	• Sugar, honey, molasses • Maple syrup, corn syrup • Icing sugar • Pure jams, jellies, marmalades, and conserves made with allowed ingredients • Plain artificial sweeteners • Homemade sweets with allowed ingredients	• Chocolate • Cocoa beans • Cocoa • Spreads with restricted ingredients

Other	• Baking powder
	• Baking soda
	• Cream of Tartar
	• Plain gelatin
	• Homemade relishes with allowed ingredients
	• Small amounts of baker's yeast
	• All vinegars
		• Flavored gelatin
		• Prepared pickles and relishes with vinegar
		• Yeast and meat extracts:
		  – Bovril®
		  – Oxo®
		  – Vegemite®
		  – Brewer's yeast
		  – Nutritional yeast

Beverages	• Plain milk • Pure juices of allowed fruits and vegetables • Plain and carbonated drinks • Tea, herbal tea • Coffee	• Other dairy drinks • Fruit drinks, and cocktails with restricted ingredients • Cola drinks • Cider • Beer, including nonalcoholic beer • Wine (especially red) • Vermouth Note: Some alcoholic drinks tested had no detectable tyramine. These include whiskey, gin, and vodka, but not all brands have been tested. The recommendation is to eliminate *all* alcoholic beverages to see if symptoms will subside with their removal.

Table 19-3
THE HISTAMINE- AND TYRAMINE-RESTRICTED DIET

Type of Food	Foods Allowed	Foods Restricted

Milk and Milk Products	• Plain pasteurized milk from any animal
	• Milk products made without microbial cultures such as
	  – Panir
	  – Mascarpone *
	  – Ricotta*
	  * *Read the labels carefully to ensure no microbial cultures are included.*
	• Ice cream free from any restricted ingredient
	• Cream
		• Fermented milk products from any animal, such as
		  – Cheese of all types
		  – Cottage cheese
		  – Processed cheese
		  – Cream cheese
		  – Sour cream
		  – Buttermilk
		  – Yogurt
		  – Kefir
		• And any other fermented milk products
		• Foods made with milk products other than those allowed

Grains, Cereals, Breads, and Other Baked Products	• Any pure, unbleached flour or grain
	• Baking-powder-leavened products such as
	  – Biscuits
	  – Quick breads
	  – Soda bread
	  – Scones
	  – Muffins
	• Homemade or purchased baked goods made with allowed ingredients
	• Crackers without yeast, such as Triscuits™
	• Breakfast cereals with allowed ingredients including any grain without artificial colors or preservatives
		• Yeast-risen breads and baked products such as:
		  – Bread
		  – Pizza dough
		  – Buns
		  – Pita bread
		  – Croissants
		  – English muffins
		  – Crumpets
		  – Crackers with yeast (read labels) such as Ritz™, Saltines™
		• Products made with restricted ingredients, such as
		  – Anise
		  – Artificial colors
		  – Artificial flavors
		  – Bleached flour
		  – Cheese
		  – Chocolate
		  – Cinnamon
		  – Cloves
		  – Cocoa
		  – Margarine
		  – Preservatives
		  – Restricted fruit including jams and jellies made with these fruits

Note: This list is not exhaustive. Other foods may contain histamine and tyramine and not be listed here. It is up to the reader to read all ingredient labels carefully and to contact the manufacturer if there is any doubt.

Table 19-3 (continued)
THE HISTAMINE- AND TYRAMINE-RESTRICTED DIET

Type of Food	Foods Allowed	Foods Restricted
Grains, Cereals, Breads, and Other Baked Products (continued)		• Baking mixes • Dry dessert mixes • Any food made with or cooked in oils with hydrolyzed lecithin, BHA, BHT • Breakfast cereals containing restricted ingredients
Vegetables	• All pure, fresh, or frozen vegetables and their juices except those in the "restricted" columns	• Potato • Avocado • Broad beans • Green beans • Eggplant (aubergine) • Pumpkin • Sauerkraut • Spinach • Sweet potato • Tomato • Over-ripe vegetables • Pickled vegetables • Packaged salad mixes • Packaged peeled vegetables • Most commercial salad dressings with vinegar, artificial color, flavor, or preservatives

Fruit	• All pure, fresh, or frozen fruit and their juices except those in the "restricted" columns
	• Allowed fruits include
	  – Melons such as cantaloupe (rock melon), honeydew, watermelon
	• Other fruits such as
	  – Apple
	  – Pear
	  – Fig
	  – Kiwi
	  – Mango
	  – Passion fruit
	  – Rhubarb
	  – Starfruit
	  – Longans
	  – Lychees
	• Fruit dishes made with allowed ingredients
		• Lemon
		• Lime
		• The following fresh, frozen, and canned fruits and their juices:
		  – Berries such as blackberrles, blueberries, cranberries, gooseberries, loganberries, raspberrires, strawberries
		  – Stone fruits such as apricots, cherries, nectarines, peaches, plums, prunes
		  – Citrus fruits such as oranges and grapefruits
		  – Other fruits such as bananas, grapes, currants, dates, papayas (pawpaws), pineapples, raisins
		• Fruit dishes, jams, or juices made with restricted ingredients
		• Any over-ripe fruit

Table 19-3 (continued)
THE HISTAMINE- AND TYRAMINE-RESTRICTED DIET

Type of Food	Foods Allowed	Foods Restricted

Meat, Poultry, and Fish	• Pure, freshly cooked meat or poultry *except those* in the "restricted" column
	• Any freshly caught, gutted, and cooked fish
	• If raw meat is not cooked immediately, store it in the freezer
		• All shellfish, roe, and caviar
		• Any fish that has not been gutted and cooked immediately after being caught
		• Commercially canned fish
		• All processed meats such as
		  – Pepperoni
		  – Salami
		  – Bologna
		  – Weiners (hot dog)
		• All pickled meats, eggs, fish

Legumes	• All plain legumes *except those in the "restricted" column,* such as
	  – Lima beans
	  – Green peas
	  – Sugar peas
	• Dried beans and peas, such as
	  – Chickpeas (garbanzo beans)
	  – Pinto beans
	  – White beans
	  – Navy beans
	  – Black-eyed peas
	  – Black beans
	  – Lentils (red, yellow, brown)
	  – Split peas
	  – Peanuts
	  – Pure peanut butter
		• Red beans
		• Soybeans
		• Tofu
		• Fermented soy products such as:
		  – Soy sauce
		  – Fermented bean curd
		  – Soybean paste
		  – Shrimp paste
		  – Chili soybean paste
		  – Miso

Nuts and Seeds	• All plain nuts and seeds and their flours and butters *except those in the "restricted" column*	• Walnuts • Pecans
Fats and Oils	• All cold-pressed oils stored in the refrigerator	• Processed oils containing preservatives such as BHA and BHT
Spices and Herbs	• All fresh, frozen, or dried herbs and spices *except those in the "restricted" column*	• Anise • Cinnamon • Cloves • Curry powder • Hot paprika (cayenne)

Table 19-3 (continued)
THE HISTAMINE- AND TYRAMINE-RESTRICTED DIET

Type of Food	Foods Allowed	Foods Restricted
Spices and Herbs (continued)		• Nutmeg • Seasoning packets with restricted ingredients • Commercial packaged foods labeled with "spices" or "flavoring"
Sweets and Sweeteners	• Pasteurized honey, sugar • Icing sugar • Maple syrup • Corn syrup • Pure jams, jellies, marmalade, and conserves made with allowed ingredients • Plain, artificial sweeteners • Homemade sweets with allowed ingredients	• Unpasteurized honey • Chocolate • Cocoa beans • Cocoa • Flavored syrups • Prepared dessert fillings • Prepared icings/frostings • Spreads with restricted ingredients • Cake decorations • Confectionery • Commercial candies
Beverages	• Plain milk • Pure juices of allowed fruits and vegetables • Plain and carbonated mineral water • Coffee	• Fruit drinks and cocktails with restricted ingredients • Cola-type carbonated drinks • Apple cider • All teas, including green tea • All alcoholic beverages • Nonalcoholic beers and wines • All drinks with "flavor" or "spices" on the label
Other	• Baking powder • Baking soda • Cream of Tartar • Plain gelatin • Homemade relishes with allowed ingredients	• Baker's yeast • All vinegars • Prepared pickles, relishes, ketchup, and mustard containing vinegar • Flavored gelatin • Chocolate and cocoa • Mincemeat • Yeasts of the species *Saccharomyces* • Brewer's yeast • Nutritional yeast • Yeast and meat extracts, e.g., Bovril™, Marmite™, Oxo™, Vegemite™

— CHAPTER 20 —

SALICYLATE INTOLERANCE

The only form of salicylate *proven* to be the cause of symptoms is acetylsalicylic acid (a drug known as "aspirin" in the United States, although this term is a registered trade name in Canada). Sensitivity to acetylsalicylic acid is more common in persons with asthma than in those without it. Furthermore, up to 25% of people who are sensitive to acetylsalicylic acid also react adversely to the azo dye tartrazine (see Chapter 21, page 268 for details), but it is not known whether the two chemicals act in a similar way in the body. Sensitivity to acetylsalicylic acid has also been linked to sensitivities to benzoates and sulfites, but cross-reactivity to these substances has not yet been confirmed by research studies.

Salicylates (but not acetylsalicylic acid) occur naturally in many foods, including fruit, vegetables, herbs, spices, nuts, and seeds. However, research studies have not proven that this source of salicylates causes adverse reactions even in people who are sensitive to acetylsalicylic acid. The *level* of salicylic acid may be the determining factor in salicylate sensitivity. Dietary consumption of salicylate is estimated to be from 10 to 200 mg daily, whereas one dose of regular-strength aspirin provides 300 to 325 mg of acetylsalicylic acid and extra-strength aspirin provides 600 to 650 mg. So, a diet with the highest level of salicylate-rich foods is unlikely to provide as much salicylate as one tablet of regular-strength aspirin.

Sensitivity to acetylsalicylic acid has been implicated in causing urticaria (hives) and angioedema (tissue swelling) and in leading to an asthmatic attack in persons with asthma. However, people with asthma who are sensitive to acetylsalicylic acid can usually ingest the salicylates in foods without difficulty. No controlled research has been undertaken to study the effect of reducing dietary salicylates on the course of asthma.

WHAT CAUSES SALICYLATE SENSITIVITY?

Acetylsalicylic acid inhibits the cyclo-oxygenase pathway of arachidonic acid metabolism, thus reducing the production of certain **prostaglandins** (hormone-like chemicals) that mediate the sensation of pain (for more details of this pathway, refer to Chapter 3, page 43). This reduction accounts for the analgesic (pain-reducing) properties of aspirin. Another result of this inhibition is increased production of **leukotrienes**, hormone-like chemicals that mediate the smooth muscle contraction that causes the bronchospasm of asthma (for more information, refer to Chapter 3, page 43). This effect explains why many persons who are sensitive acetylsalicylic acid suffer from asthma.

Symptoms of Salicylate Sensitivity

Wheezing, urticaria (hives), and angioedema (tissue swelling) are reported symptoms of salicylate sensitivity. Some investigators think that the hyperactivity experienced by some children is due to salicylate sensitivity; however, the role of salicylates in attention-deficit hyperactivity disorder (ADHD) has not been proven by controlled studies. Investigations of the role of food components and additives in this disorder are currently in progress.

Some practitioners in the field of food intolerance believe that, although avoiding foods high in salicylates is unlikely to diminish the symptoms of most persons sensitive to acetylsalicylic acid, a trial on a salicylate-restricted diet may benefit those individuals who have severe symptoms and get no relief from other treatments. For those who wish to investigate the effects of limiting salicylates, the diet in Table 20-2 is suggested. It restricts the foods with the highest levels of salicylates and provides suggestions for low-salicylate substitutes. The diet should not be followed for longer than four weeks initially.

FOOD SOURCES OF SALICYLATES

Salicylates are a natural component of many food plants. Several researchers have developed tables to indicate the level of salicylate in foods.[1] However, none is entirely accurate, because the level of salicylate in a food varies according to plant variety and conditions in the growing environment. It would be extremely

---

[1] J.M.V. Joneja, "Level of Salicylates in Some Common Foods and Beverages," *Dietary Management of Food Allergies and Intolerances: A Comprehensive Guide*, 2nd ed. (Vancouver: J. A. Hall Publications, 1988), pp. 190–199.

difficult, if not impossible, to come up with a nutritionally adequate diet that does not include any foods that contain salicylate. However, some foods have lower levels than others. Table 20-1 lists foods high in salicylates and those with lower, "acceptable" levels of salicylates to give you an idea of how these compare.

THE SALICYLATE RESTRICTED DIET

Table 20-2 provides you with a list of the foods allowed and those restricted on a diet that will limit your intake of salicylate—and still supply you with the nutrients essential for a well-balanced diet. No diet is completely "salicylate-free" unless it is also "food-free," but this comes very close!

Table 20-1
EXAMPLES OF FOODS WITH "HIGH" AND "LOW" LEVELS OF SALICYLATE

Food Category	High Salicylate Content	Low or No Salicylate Content
Herbs	Mint Thyme Tarragon Rosemary Dill Sage Oregano Marjoram Basil Celery seed Sesame seed	Poppy seed Chives (fresh) Parsley
Spices	Aniseed Cayenne Cinnamon Cumin Curry powder Fenugreek Mace Mustard Paprika Turmeric	Saffron (dry powder)

Fruits	Most; especially high levels in
	  Pineapple
	  Apricot
	  Raspberry
	  Loganberry
	  Cherry
	  Dates
	  Dried currants
	  Raisins
		Banana
		Pears (peeled)
		Pomegranate
		Mango
		Papaya
		Golden Delicious apple

Vegetables	Most; especially high levels in
	  Cucumber
	  Gherkin
	  Olives
	  Endive
	  Potato skin
	  Sweet corn
	  Sweet potatoes
		Cabbage (green)
		Cabbage (red)
		Brussels sprouts
		Bean sprouts
		Celery
		Leeks
		Lettuce
		Peas
		Potato (skin has a high level)
		Bamboo shoots (canned)
		Chayote squash
		Shallots

Note: This list is not exhaustive. Other foods may contain salicylate and not be listed here. It is up to the reader to read all ingredient labels carefully and to contact the manufacturer if there is any doubt.

Table 20-1 (continued)
EXAMPLES OF FOODS WITH "HIGH" AND "LOW" LEVELS OF SALICYLATE

Food Category	High Salicylate Content	Low or No Salicylate Content
Nuts	Almonds Brazil nuts Macadamia nuts Peanuts Pine nuts Pistachios Walnuts Water chestnuts Coconut	Cashew
Beverages	Coffee Tea Cola drinks Peppermint tea Fruit juices Most alcoholic drinks	Gin Vodka Whiskey Cocoa (powder) Decaffeinated coffee powder Ovaltine powder Camomile herbal tea (bag)
Confectioneries and Sweeteners	Honey Licorice Peppermints	Granulated sugar Maple syrup
Flavorings, Condiments, and Sauces	Yeast-rich products Marmite Stock cubes Tomato sauce Worcestershire sauce	Soy sauce Malt vinegar
Other	Processed foods Instant (prepared) meals	
Meats and Fish	None	Meat Fish Shellfish Eggs
Milk and Milk Products	None	Milk Cheese
Grains	None	Wheat Rye Oats Barley Rice
Legumes: Dried Peas and Beans	Broad beans (fava beans)	Yellow split peas Brown beans Soy beans Mung beans Lima beans Green split peas Chick peas Brown lentils Red lentils Black-eyed peas

Table 20-2
THE SALICYLATE-RESTRICTED DIET

Type of Food	Foods Allowed	Foods Restricted

Milk and Milk Products	• Plain milk, buttermilk, cream, sour cream, and yogurt
	• All plain uncolored cream cheese, cheddar, mozzarella, cottage cheese, Quark®
	• Parmesan
	• Additive-free ice cream made with allowed ingredients
	• Butter
		• Chocolate-flavored milk
		• Milkshakes
		• Flavored yogurt
		• Prepared
		  – Cheese foods
		  – Cheese slices
		  – Dips
		  – Spreads
		• Other ice cream and frozen treats

Breads and Cereals	• Any pure flour or grain except cornmeal
	• Any prepared, plain bread, buns, biscuits, pizza dough with allowed ingredients
	• Homemade or purchased baked cookies, pies, etc., made with allowed ingredients
	• Prepared breakfast cereals with allowed ingredients
	• Oats and oatmeal
	• Red River Cereal®
	• Plain oat bran
	• All plain grains and their flakes, except cornmeal
	• Plain crackers such as
	  – Grissol Melba Toast®
	  – RyVita®
	  – Rye Krisp®
	  – Wasa® Light or Golden Crackers
	• Homemade crackers
	
	• Plain pasta
	• All homemade crackers, cereals, and pasta dishes with allowed ingredients
	• Plain and wild rice
	• General Foods Minute Rice®
		• Products made with restricted items
		• Cornmeal
		
		• Crackers with color, flavor, or restricted ingredients
		• Read labels on all packaged crackers
		
		• Pasta or rice dinners

Vegetables	• Bamboo shoots, canned* • Beans, fresh, green • Brussels sprouts, fresh • Carrots, fresh	All others

Note: This list is not exhaustive. Other foods may contain salicylate and not be listed here. It is up to the reader to read all ingredient labels carefully and to contact the manufacturer if there is any doubt.

Table 20-2 (continued) THE SALICYLATE-RESTRICTED DIET		
Type of Food	**Foods Allowed**	**Foods Restricted**
Vegetables (continued)	• Cauliflower, fresh • Celery, fresh* • Cabbage, green, fresh* • Cabbage, red, fresh • Corn, niblets, canned • Corn on the cob • Leeks, fresh • Lettuce • Mushrooms, fresh • Onion, fresh • Peas, green, fresh • Potato, white, peeled, fresh • Pumpkin, fresh • Shallots, fresh • Spinach, frozen • Tomato, fresh • Turnip, fresh • Watercress, fresh	
Fruit	• Apple, Golden Delicious • Banana, fresh* • Figs, fresh* • Figs, kadota, canned • Lemon, fresh • Mango, fresh • Papaya (pawpaw) fresh • Passionfruit (granadilla), fresh • Pear, Bartlett, canned* • Pear, Packham, peeled, fresh* • Pineapple juice • Pomegranate, fresh • Rhubarb, fresh	All others
Meat, Poultry, and Fish	• All pure fresh, frozen, or canned meat, poultry, or fish • Processed meat made with allowed ingredients	• Processed with restricted ingredients, such as spices
Eggs	• All	• All prepared with restricted foods
Legumes	• Black-eyed peas* • Brown beans* • Brown lentils*	All others

Table 20-2 (continued)
THE SALICYLATE-RESTRICTED DIET

Type of Food	Foods Allowed	Foods Restricted
Legumes (continued)	• Chickpeas (garbanzos)* • Green split peas* • Lima beans* • Mung beans* • Red lentils* • Soy beans* • Yellow split peas • Pure, natural peanut butter	
Nuts and Seeds	• Brazil nuts, fresh • Cashew nuts, fresh • Coconut, dry, desiccated • Hazelnuts, fresh • Macadamia nuts, fresh • Pecan nuts, fresh • Pine nuts, fresh • Pistachio nuts, fresh • Poppy seed, dry* • Sesame seeds, dry • Sunflower seeds, dry • Walnuts, fresh	• All other nuts and seeds • Any with spices or seasoning
Fats and Oils	• Pure butter, cream, shortening • Pure vegetable oils including canola, olive, sunflower, soy, peanut • Homemade salad dressings with allowed ingredients • Lard and meat drippings • Homemade gravy with allowed ingredients	• Margarine • Prepared salad dressings with restricted foods • Commercial gravies and sauces
Dry Spices and Herbs	• Allspice, dry powder • Basil, dry powder • Bay leaf, dry leaf • Caraway, dry • Cardamom, dry powder • Chili, powder and flakes • Cloves, whole, dry • Fennel, dry powder • Nutmeg, dry powder • Paprika, sweet, dry powder • Pepper, black and white, dry powder • Saffron	• All others • Seasoning salts • Flavoring extracts • Flavoring packets • Any product labeled with "spices"

Table 20-2 (continued) THE SALICYLATE-RESTRICTED DIET		
Type of Food	**Foods Allowed**	**Foods Restricted**
Herbs and Seasonings	• Chili peppers, green, red and yellow, fresh • Chives, fresh • Coriander, fresh leaves • Dill, fresh • Garlic, fresh bulbs • Ginger root, fresh • Horseradish	• All others
Sweets and Sweeteners	• Sugar, molasses • Maple syrup, corn syrup • Icing sugar • Pure jams, jellies, • Marmalades and conserves made with allowed fruit and without added color or flavor • Plain artificial sweeteners • Homemade sweets with allowed ingredients	• Honey • Prepared dessert fillings • Prepared icings and frostings • Spreads with restricted foods • Prepared candies • Cake decorations • Other confectionery • Commercial candies • Fruit Rollups® • Fun Fruits® • Fruit peel • Glacé fruit • Flavored syrups • Licorice • Peppermints
Other	• Baking powder • Baking soda • Cream of Tartar • Distilled white vinegar • Malt vinegar • Baking chocolate • Pure cocoa • Plain gelatin • Pure vanilla extract • Relishes with allowed ingredients • Black and green olives • Pure soy sauce made with allowed ingredients • Vegemite® and Marmite®	• Whipped toppings • Topping mixes • All other vinegars with "flavorings" • Chocolate candy, sprinkles, and syrup • Flavored gelatin • Prepared pickles • Other relishes • Worcestershire sauce • Mustard
Beverages	• Plain and carbonated mineral water • Plain coffee	• All other carbonated drinks and soft drinks • Flavored coffee and coffee mixes

Table 20-2 (continued)
THE SALICYLATE-RESTRICTED DIET

Type of Food	Foods Allowed	Foods Restricted

Beverages	• Ovaltine® powder*
	• Tetley® tea
	• Twinings® teas:
	  – Lemon-scented
	  – Irish Breakfast
	  – English Breakfast
	  – Orange Pekoe
	• Indian/Burmese green tea
	• Jasmine tea
	• Rosehip herbal tea
	• Chamomile herbal tea*
	• Alcohol:
	  – Sherry
	  – Dry vermouth
	  – Hennessey Brandy®
	  – Smirnoff Vodka®
	  – Johnnie Walker Whiskey®
	  – Gilbey's Gin®
		• Other teas
		• Fruit-flavored powders and concentrates
		• All drinks with color, flavor, or spices
		• Diet drinks and diet shakes
		• Meal-replacement drinks
		
		• Liqueurs and coolers
		• Drink mixes and pre-mixed drinks

* These fruits, vegetables, legumes, seeds, and herbs contain no salicylates.

— CHAPTER 21 —

TARTRAZINE INTOLERANCE AND OTHER ARTIFICIAL COLOR INTOLERANCE

Color is one of the most important aspects of food presentation. Unless foods are the right color, they are unacceptable to many people. As a result, manufacturers add colors to foods to enhance their market appeal and consumption. This means that we are eating many different chemicals that would probably never enter our bodies, except as additives to manufactured foods. Most of these chemicals do not result in any harmful effects, but some people do react adversely to them. This chapter provides information for those people who are sensitive to the chemicals used for coloring our foods. It also gives details of a diet that such people can follow to avoid all artificial food coloring agents and still obtain complete balanced nutrition from their food.

In addition to artificial colors, many manufacturers use colors derived from *natural sources*, for example:

◆ Saffron and turmeric as a source of yellow
◆ Beetroot as a red color
◆ Caramel from burned sugar as a brown color
◆ Titanium oxide as a white color
◆ Silver, gold, and aluminum as their natural colors
◆ Chlorophyll from green vegetables as a green color

Colors derived from natural sources are not included in this discussion of causes of food intolerance. Certain sensitive people may experience an allergic reaction to the *source* of the natural color, for example, an allergic reaction to the plant from which the color was derived. This is then treated as an allergy, details of which can be found in Part I of this book.

265

ARTIFICIAL FOOD DYES

In the United States, the Department of Agriculture allows ten artificial colors derived from coal tar under the Food Dye and Coloring Act (FD&C). These are listed in Table 21-1. Many other countries including Canada have similar regulations.

Citrus Red #2 is restricted to coloring orange skins in fruit not used for manufacture of food products (such as orange juice). Orange B is similar in chemical structure to Amaranth, which is not allowed in the United States but is permitted for use in Canada. Orange B is restricted to the casings and surfaces of frankfurters and sausages. However, because of health risks the sole manufacturer in the United States has stopped producing this dye.

In Canada, a number of colors are listed as "permitted" for use in foods. These are listed in Table 21-2.

Artificial Food Dyes in Britain and European Countries

In Britain and Europe, it is somewhat easier for the consumer to identify artificial ingredients on food labels because an efficient system of numbering ("E" numbers) has been developed. Each food additive has a designated number, and a person who knows which food ingredient to avoid simply needs to identify its specific number on the label, which is much easier than looking through a long list of unpronounceable chemical terms. Table 21-3 lists the most common artificial food colors and their E-numbers in the European system.

Table 21-1 ARTIFICIAL FOOD-COLORING AGENTS IN GENERAL USE IN THE UNITED STATES	
FDA Name	**Common Name**
FD&C Yellow #5	Tartrazine
FD&C Yellow #6	Sunset Yellow
FD&C Red #3	Erythrosine
FD&C Red #4	Ponceau
FD&C Red #40	Allura Red
FD&C Citrus Red #2	Citrus Red #2
Orange B	Orange B
FD&C Blue #1	Brilliant Blue
FD&C Blue #2	Indigotine
FD&C Green #3	Fast Green

Table 21-2
ARTIFICIAL FOOD DYES PERMITTED IN CANADA

Alkanet	Fast Green FCF*
Allura Red*	Indigotine*
Aluminum metal	Iron oxide
Amaranth	Orchil
Anthocyanin	Ponceau SX*
Brilliant Blue FCF*	Saunderswood
Canthaxanthine	Sunset Yellow FCF*
Carbon black	Tartrazine*
Citrus Red #2*	
Cochineal	
Erythrosine*	

*Corresponds to FD&C list in Table 21-1.

Table 21-3
ARTIFICIAL FOOD COLORS IN THE EUROPEAN SYSTEM

E Number	Name	E Number	Name
E102	Tartrazine	E129	Allura Red
E104	Quinoline Yellow	E131	Patent Blue V
E107	Yellow 2G	E132	Indigo Carmine
E110	Sunset Yellow	E133	Brilliant Blue FCF
E120	Cochineal	E142	Green S
E122	Carmoisine	E151	Black PN
E123	Amaranth	E153	Carbon Black
E124	Ponceau 4R	E154	Brown FK
E127	Erythrosine BS	E155	Brown HT
E128	Red 2G	E180	Pigment Rubine

Examples of the Use of Artificial Colors in Foods

Table 21-4 is meant only as an example of the use of artificial colors in commercial food products. Not all manufacturers of the foods use the artificial colors indicated. Some countries ban the use of certain colors. The regulations change frequently, so this table may not be entirely accurate at the date it is being read.

TARTRAZINE

Most of the colors listed in Table 21-4 are considered "safe" (Generally Regarded as Safe, or GRAS, designation) by the U. S. Department of Agriculture and have not been cited as a cause of adverse reactions. However, tartrazine and some other azo (nitrogen-containing) dyes have been implicated in adverse reactions. As a result, regulations in the United States require that tartrazine added to foods or medications should be listed separately on the product label. In Canada, at present, this listing is voluntary.

Food manufacturers are *not* required to give the chemical names or common names of the individual artificial colors used in a food product, except for tartrazine in the United States. As a result, colors usually appear on labels as "artificial color" or simply as "color."

Conditions Caused by Tartrazine in Sensitive People

Tartrazine (FD&C #5) can cause symptoms resembling an allergic reaction. Tartrazine-sensitive asthmatics tend to experience triggering or worsening of asthma. Hives, itching, nasal congestion and runny nose, blurred vision, purple patches on the skin, and migraine headaches have all been reported as symptoms of tartrazine sensitivity. However, only a few **double-blind placebo- controlled** trials have indicated that tartrazine is a *direct* cause of these symptoms.

Tartrazine has been demonstrated to cause a rise in plasma histamine levels even in normal healthy adults when they consume more than 50 milligrams of the dye. Histamine-sensitive individuals react at much lower levels of tartrazine. The mechanism for the release of histamine by tartrazine has yet to be discovered. There is no evidence that an immunologically mediated allergic reaction is involved in this process. (Details of histamine intolerance can be found in Chapter 19.)

Some people who are sensitive to acetylsalicylic acid (aspirin) also experience an adverse reaction to tartrazine. It is unclear whether dietary salicylates, which are naturally present in a large number of foods (primarily fruits and vegetables), also are involved in this **cross-reactivity** (Refer to Chapter 20 for more information on salicylates.) Other azo (nitrogen-containing) dyes have also been implicated in adverse reactions.

How Tartrazine Affects the Body

Evidence indicates that tartrazine may initiate the release of histamine from **mast cells** (refer to Chapter 3, page 42, for a discussion of mast cells and their role in allergy). Because tartrazine-induced symptoms are similar to those induced by acetyl-salicylic acid, tartrazine may inhibit the cyclo-oxygenase pathway for converting arachidonic acid to prostanoids (refer to Chapter 20 for details of this process). However, this mechanism of action has not been proven.

Table 21-4
USE OF ARTIFICIAL COLORS IN COMMERCIAL FOOD PRODUCTS

Color Name	Examples of Foods Containing the Color
Tartrazine (Prohibited in Norway and Austria)	Fruit squash and cordials; colored fizzy drinks Instant puddings Packet convenience foods Cake mixes Soups (packets and cans) Bottled sauces Pickles Commercial salad dressings Ice creams and sherbets Candies Chewing gum Jams and jellies Smoked fish Jello Mustard Yogurt
Sunset Yellow (Prohibited in Norway and Finland)	Especially useful for fermented foods that must be heat-treated: Hot chocolate mix Packet soups Candies Yogurts Commercial bread crumbs Cheese sauce mixes Jams and marmalades Canned shrimps and prawns Pickled cucumbers (dill pickles)
Erythrosine (Prohibited in Norway and the USA)	Glacé cherries Canned red cherries, strawberries, and rhubarb Scotch eggs Packet dessert mixes Stuffed olives Chocolates Dressed crab Salmon spread and paté Garlic sausage Luncheon meat Danish salami
Ponceau (Prohibited in Norway and the USA)	Packet soups Seafood dressings Cake mixes

Table 21-4 (continued) USE OF ARTIFICIAL COLORS IN COMMERCIAL FOOD PRODUCTS	
Color Name	**Examples of Foods Containing the Color**
Ponceau (Prohibited in Norway and the USA)	Desert toppings Canned strawberries Canned cherry, raspberry, and red-currant pie fillings Quick-setting jelly mixes ("Jello") Salami
Allura Red (Prohibited in Austria, Norway, Sweden, Japan, Finland)	Allura Red and Amaranth are used in similar products, such as Packet soups Packet cake mixes
Amaranth (Prohibited in Norway and the USA; in France and Italy it can be used only in caviar)	Gravy mixes Canned pie fillings "Jello" style jelly mixes Jams and jellies Canned apple sauce Canned shrimps and prawns Canned pears Liquid vitamin C preparations
Indigotine (Prohibited in Norway)	Cookies Candies Savory convenience food mixes
Brilliant Blue (Prohibited in Austria, Belgium, Denmark, France, Germany, Greece, Italy, Spain, Switzerland, Norway, Sweden)	Canned processed peas

Symptoms of Tartrazine Sensitivity

Symptoms reported to be caused or made worse by tartrazine and other azo dyes are

◆ Asthma
◆ Urticaria (hives)
◆ Nausea
◆ Migraine headaches
◆ Allergic vasculitis (purpura)
◆ Hyperkinesis (hyperactivity disorder)
◆ Contact dermatitis

At present, there are no double-blind placebo-controlled trials proving that any of these conditions are caused by tartrazine.

Tartrazine in Foods

Although tartrazine is yellow, it is also used to produce other colors such as orange, turquoise, green, maroon, and brown, so it is not enough to avoid only yellow-colored foods.

Tartrazine-sensitive persons need to avoid

◆ Any food or medication listing tartrazine as an additive.
◆ Any food described as containing color or artificial color unless it is specifically labeled tartrazine-free. This is particularly important for medications.
◆ A food or medication with "tartrazine-free" on the label is safe for a person who is sensitive to tartrazine, but it is no guarantee that the product does not contain *other* food dyes.

TARTRAZINE IN MEDICATIONS, SUPPLEMENTS, AND OTHER ITEMS

Tartrazine is in some medications (both prescription and nonprescription) and in some vitamin and mineral supplements. Essential medications should be tartrazine-free. Pharmacies keep a list of manufacturers who produce tartrazine-free products. Some toiletries and cosmetics containing colors may cause contact dermatitis.

DIET RESTRICTED IN TARTRAZINE AND OTHER FOOD-COLORING AGENTS

The eating plan in Table 21-5 is designed to eliminate tartrazine and other food dyes from the diet and medications. Labeling tartrazine by name, rather than as merely "color," is mandatory in the United States, but is voluntary in Canada, which means that in Canada, people who are sensitive only to tartrazine must also avoid all commercial foods that have "color" or "artificial color" on the label.

Table 21-5
DIET FREE FROM TARTRAZINE AND OTHER ARTIFICIAL FOOD COLORING AGENTS

Type of Food	Foods Allowed	Foods Restricted
Milk and Milk Products	• Plain milk, buttermilk, cream, sour cream, and yogurt • All plain uncolored cream cheese, cheddar, mozzarella • Parmesan • Quark® • Additive-free ice cream • Butter	• Chocolate-flavored milk • Milkshakes • Flavored yogurt • Commercially prepared — Cheese foods — Cheese slices — Dips — Spreads • Frozen ice cream, sherbet, yogurt, ice milk, dairy treats with color added
Breads and Cereals	• Any pure flour or grain • Any prepared, additive-free, plain bread, buns, biscuits, pizza dough with allowed ingredients • *Bread machines are useful in making additive-free bread products.* • Homemade or purchased baked cookies, pies, etc. made without additives	• Commercial products made with food coloring • Commercial icings and frostings • Most commercial baked goods • Baking mixes
	• Breakfast cereals without color added, such as — Homemade granola — Oats and oatmeal — Plain oat bran — Plain Cream of Wheat® — Puffed wheat — Puffed rice — Red River Cereal® — Shredded Wheat® — Shreddies® — Some corn flakes • All plain grains and their flakes	• Commercial breakfast cereals with added color • Flavored instant oatmeal • Flavored instant Cream of Wheat®
	• Crackers without color added such as — Grissol Melba Toast® — RyVita Rye Krisp® — Wasa®, Light or Golden Crackers — Homemade crackers	• Crackers with color or flavor added

Note: This list is not exhaustive. Other foods may contain food coloring and not be listed here. It is up to the reader to read all ingredient labels carefully and to contact the manufacturer if there is any doubt.

Table 21-5 (continued)
DIET FREE FROM TARTRAZINE AND OTHER ARTIFICIAL FOOD COLORING AGENTS

Type of Food	Foods Allowed	Foods Restricted
Breads and Cereals	• Plain pasta • All homemade crackers, cereals, and pasta dishes without food colors • Plain and wild rice • General Foods Minute Rice®	• *Read all labels carefully on all packaged pasta* • Colored pasta • Macaroni and cheese dinners • Pasta or rice dinners with color or flavor packets
Vegetables	• All pure fresh and frozen vegetables and juices	• Vegetable cocktails such as V8® • Vegetables in sauces and/or seasoning packets • Most pasta sauces unless additive-free • Prepared salads with commercial dressing
Fruits	• All pure fresh, frozen, or canned fruit • Pure frozen and canned juices • Fruit dishes made without added colors	• Fruit cocktail with maraschino cherries • Maraschino cherries • Prepared fruit drinks, other drinks, and cocktails, with any additives • Fruit Rollups • Fruit-flavored gelatin such as Jell-O® • Fruit dishes and preserves with color

Meat, Poultry, and Fish	• All pure fresh, frozen, or canned meat, poultry, or fish
	• Processed meat made without added color
		• Commercially prepared with added color:
		  – Fish pastes, fish roe
		  – Imitation crab
		  – Smoked fish
		• Processed meats with added color
		• Commercial gravies and sauces

Eggs	• All	• All dishes prepared with ingredients with added color
Legumes	• All plain legumes • Pure peanut butter without additives	

Table 21-5 (continued)
DIET FREE FROM TARTRAZINE AND OTHER ARTIFICIAL FOOD COLORING AGENTS

Type of Food	Foods Allowed	Foods Restricted
Nuts and Seeds	• All plain nuts and seeds	• All with added color
Fats and Oils	• Pure butter • Cream • Shortening • Pure vegetable oils • Homemade salad dressings not made with "flavor packages" • Lard and meat drippings • Homemade gravy	• Margarine • Commercially prepared salad dressings with added color • Commercial sauces and gravies
Spices and Herbs	• All pure fresh, frozen, or dried herbs and spices • Seasoning salts including turmeric, paprika, and saffron	• Flavor packets • Flavoring extracts
Sweets and Sweeteners	• Sugar, honey, molasses • Maple syrup, corn syrup • Icing sugar • Pure jams, jellies, marmalades, and conserves without added color • Plain artificial sweeteners • Homemade sweets without artificial color	• Flavored syrups • Prepared dessert fillings • Prepared icings • Spreads with restricted ingredients • Commercial candies • Cake decorations and other confectionery • Fruit Rollups® • Fun Fruits® • Fruit peel, citrus peel • Glacé fruit
Other	• Baking powder • Baking soda • Cream of Tartar • Pure white cider or wine vinegar • Baking chocolate • Pure cocoa • Plain gelatin • Homemade pickles, ketchup, and relishes without added color • Pure soy sauce without added color	• Whipped toppings • Topping mixes • All vinegars with "flavorings" • Chocolate candy • Cake sprinkles • Flavored gelatin • Commercial pickles, relishes, and olives • Some soy sauces • Commercial ketchup • Colored chewing gum • Snacks like Cheese Puffs®

Table 21-5 (continued)
DIET FREE FROM TARTRAZINE AND OTHER ARTIFICIAL FOOD COLORING AGENTS

Type of Food	Foods Allowed	Foods Restricted
Beverages	• Plain milk and buttermilk • Pure juices of fruits and vegetables • Plain and carbonated mineral water • Plain coffee and tea • Beer, wine, plain distilled alcoholic beverages	• Flavored milks • Fruit drinks, other drinks, and cocktails, with any additives • All other carbonated drinks and soft drinks • Liqueurs and coolers • Drink mixes or pre-mixed drinks • Fruit-flavored drink powders and concentrates • All drinks with "flavor," "spices," or "color" • Diet drinks and shakes • Meal-replacement drinks

— CHAPTER 22 —

BENZOATE INTOLERANCE

Benzoic acid, sodium, potassium, and calcium benzoate, and a variety of forms of these chemicals, are used in many different manufactured food products. They have a wide range of uses, such as keeping our food free from contaminating microorganisms, preserving food color, and preventing separation of oils and water (emulsifying). In addition, benzoates occur naturally in some foods, including berries, prunes, tea, and cinnamon. For most people, benzoates pose no threat and cause no adverse symptoms when eaten even in relatively high doses. However, there is a small group of people who do react adversely to benzoates. This chapter is addressed to that small group and provides information on the what, where, and why of benzoate sensitivity, as well as instructions on avoiding all forms of benzoates in the diet, while still obtaining complete balanced nutrition.

BENZOIC ACID AND SODIUM BENZOATE

Both benzoic acid and sodium benzoate are chemicals that manufacturers use to prevent spoilage by microorganisms in a wide variety of processed foods, beverages, and pharmaceuticals, thus extending their shelf life. Benzoic acid is a common ingredient in flavorings (specifically, chocolate, lemon, orange, cherry, fruit, nut, and tobacco) that are used in carbonated and noncarbonated beverages, ice cream, ices, candies, baked goods, pie and pastry fillings, icings, and chewing gum. It may also be used in pickles and margarines. In such processed foods, benzoic acid is used up to a level of 0.1%.

Benzoic acid occurs naturally in foods at varying levels[1] (Table 22-1). *High* levels occur in

◆   Most berries, especially strawberries and raspberries
◆   Prunes
◆   Tea
◆   Spices such as cinnamon, cloves, and anise
◆   Cherry bark and cassia bark

Sodium, potassium, and calcium benzoate are used as preservatives in margarine, codfish, bottled soft drinks, maraschino cherries, mincemeat, fruit juices, pickles, fruit jelly preserves, and jams. In addition, these chemicals may be added to the ice used for cooling fish, and they may be ingredients in eye creams, certain skin creams, and toothpastes.

What Happens to Benzoates in the Body?

Benzoic acid, sodium, potassium, and clacium benzoate are rapidly absorbed into the body from the digestive tract. They are then taken up and circulated in blood. Upon reaching the liver they combine with the amino acid glycine and are excreted from the body through the kidneys in urine. As long as liver function is healthy, and adequate glycine is available, these chemicals are completely eliminated from the body.

BENZOYL PEROXIDE

Benzoyl peroxide is used primarily as a bleaching agent in the manufacture of

◆   White flour
◆   Some cheeses (especially blue cheeses such as Gorgonzola)
◆   Lecithin

Lecithin is an emulsifier, which allows dissimilar food ingredients such as oil and water to stay mixed and not separate on standing. It is used in manufactured foods containing fats and oils. Lecithin's action is improved when benzoyl

---

[1] J. M. V. Joneja, "Level of Benzoates in Common Foods," in *Dietary Management of Food Allergies and Intolerances: A Comprehensive Guide*, 2nd ed. (Vancouver: J. A. Hall Publications, 1998), pp. 208-212.

peroxide, hydrogen peroxide, acetic or lactic acid, or sodium hydroxide is added to produce hydroxylated lecithin, which disperses more readily in water and acts as a better emulsifier than pure lecithin. Certain vitamins can be destroyed by the addition of benzoyl peroxide to food. Where the loss could be significant, such as in the destruction of beta carotene in milk, U.S. government regulations require that the vitamin be replaced, such as in the addition of vitamin A to cheese made from bleached milk.

Most benzoyl peroxide added to food has been converted to benzoic acid by the time the food is eaten. Only a small fraction of the bleach is ingested, most of which is converted in the intestine to benzoic acid or a similar product that is readily excreted in the urine.

ADVERSE REACTIONS TO BENZOATES

The mechanism of adverse reactions to foods containing benzoate is unknown, but evidence suggests that the cyclo-oxygenase pathway of arachidonic acid metabolism may be affected, in a way similar to the activity of salicylates, discussed in Chapter 20. People who are sensitive to acetysalicylic acid (aspirin) are particularly likely to be sensitive to benzoates.

Symptoms of Benzoate Sensitivity

The following symptoms have been reported by people who are sensitive to benzoates:

◆ Asthma
◆ Urticaria (hives)
◆ Angioedema (tissue swelling)
◆ Headaches

Those who have experienced Type I hypersensitivity reactions (atopic allergy), such as respiratory-tract symptoms including asthma or skin reactions (e.g., hives and eczema), may be particularly likely to react to benzoates.

Benzoic acid can act as a mild irritant to the skin, eyes, and mucous membranes. Its adverse effects often increase when the chemical is combined with other additives.

MANAGING BENZOATE SENSITIVITY

People differ in their sensitivity to chemicals like benzoates. Consequently, it is impossible to define a limit of benzoate intake that applies to everyone who is sensitive to benzoate. The general recommendation is to reduce benzoate intake by avoiding foods known to contain added benzoates.

Therefore, benzoate-sensitive persons should avoid

◆ Natural sources of benzoic acid (see Table 22-1).

◆ Any processed foods containing benzoic acid, sodium benzoate, potassium benzoate, or calcium benzoate (*read labels carefully*). In the United States and Canada, these names will appear on food labels; in European countries, benzoic acid will be listed as E210, sodium benzoate as E211, potassium benzoate as E212, and calcium benzoate as E213.

◆ Bleached flour.

◆ Products containing hydrolyzed lecithin, such as margarines, salad and cooking oils, frozen desserts, chocolate, and baked goods.

BENZYL AND BENZOYL COMPOUNDS

A large number of benzyl and benzoyl compounds are allowed in foods. Examples are benzyl acetate, benzyl alcohol, benzyl ether, benzyl butyrate, benzyl cinnamate, benzyl formate, benzyl propionate, and benzyl salicylate. On food labels, this ingredient will include the word "benzyl" or "benzoyl." Most of these compounds are used as synthetic flavorings and perfumes in a wide variety of processed and manufactured foods, beverages, chewing gum, soaps, hair sprays, hair dyes, skin creams, sunscreens, perfumes, and cosmetics.

Some of these compounds are skin irritants and can cause hives and contact dermatitis. Others are digestive-tract irritants and can cause intestinal upset, vomiting, and diarrhea. In very high concentrations, they can have a narcotic effect. A few irritate the eyes and cause respiratory symptoms when inhaled.

PARABENS

Parabens, a class of derivitives of benzoic acid, are sometimes used as preservatives in foods. People who are sensitive to benzoates may also react to parabens because paraben metabolism mimics that of benzoates in the later stages. There are no naturally occurring parabens. On food labels, parabens are indicated by the term "ethyl p-hydroxybenzoate," "methyl p-hydroxybenzoate," or "propyl p-hydroxybenzoate." In European countries, these will appear on labels as E214, E218, and E216, respectively (see Table 22-1).

Parabens are used in processed fruits and vegetables, baked goods, fats, oils, and seasonings. They may be present in cakes, pies, pastries, icings, fillings, fruit products (e.g., fruit sauces, fruit juices, fruit salads, syrups, preserves, jellies), syrups, olives, pickles, beers, ciders, and carbonated beverages.

Table 22-1
BENZOATES: EXAMPLES OF THEIR SOURCES AND USE AS ADDITIVES

Benzoate	E Number	Found in	Added to
Benzoic acid	E210	Edible berries Fruits Vegetables	• Jams • Beer • Dessert sauces • Flavored syrups • Fruit pulp and purée • Fruit juice • Marinated fish (herring and mackerel) • Pickles • Salad dressings • Yogurt • Flavored coffees • Margarine • Table olives • Concentrated juices • Soft drinks
Sodium benzoate	E211	No natural source	• Caviar • Prawns • Candies • Margarine • Fruit pies • Soft drinks • Oyster sauce • Salad dressings • Barbecue sauce • Taco sauce • Cheesecake mix • Soy sauce • Jams and jellies • Dill pickles • Table olives • Concentrated pineapple juice
Potassium benzoate	E212	No natural source	• Margarines • Table olives • Dill pickles • Concentrated pineapple juice
Calcium benzoate	E213	No natural source	• Concentrated pineapple juice
Ethyl-hydroxybenzoate	E214	No natural source	• Beer • Cooked packed beetroot • Coffee and chicory essence

Table 22-1 (continued)
BENZOATES: EXAMPLES OF THEIR SOURCES AND USE AS ADDITIVES

Benzoate	E Number	Found in	Added to
Propyl-hydroxybenzoate	E216	No natural source	• Coloring dyes in solution • Dessert sauces • Flavored syrups
Methyl-hydroxybenzoate	E218	No natural source	• Frozen drink concentrates • Fruit-based pie fillings • Fruit pulp or purée • Glucose • Marinated fish (herring and mackerel) • Pickles • Salad dressings

Table 22-2		
THE BENZOATE-RESTRICTED DIET		
Type of Food	**Foods Allowed**	**Foods Restricted**
Milk and Milk Products	• Plain milk, buttermilk, cream, sour cream, and yogurt • All plain cheese, cottage cheese, ricotta, Quark®, feta • Ice cream made with allowed ingredients	• All prepared milk products made with restricted ingredients • Blue cheese • Gorgonzola cheese
Breads and Cereals	• Any pure *unbleached* flour or grain • Any plain fresh bread, buns, biscuits, pizza dough, with allowed ingredients • Homemade or purchased baked cookies, pies, etc., made with allowed ingredients • Baking chocolate and pure cocoa	• Products made with bleached flour • Restricted fruit • Cinnamon • Cloves • Anise • Artificial flavors • Margarine • Maraschino cherries • Some fruit juices • Some jam and jellies • Some cheeses • Chocolate that is not baking chocolate or pure cocoa • Oils with hydrolyzed lecithin • Some commercial pie and pastry fillings

	• Breakfast cereals with allowed foods, including
	  – All plain grains
	  – Corn flakes
	  – Oats and oatmeal
	  – Plain Cream of Wheat®
	  – Shreddies®
	• Plain crackers without benzoates
		• All others
		
		• *Read all labels carefully*

	• Plain pasta • All homemade crackers, cereals, and pasta dishes with allowed ingredients	• *Read labels carefully* on all packaged pasta meals.
Vegetables	• All pure fresh and frozen vegetables, except those listed at right	Avocado Pumpkin Red beans Soybeans Spinach

Note: This list is not exhaustive. Other foods may contain benzoates and not be listed here. It is up to the reader to read all ingredient labels carefully and to contact the manufacturer if there is any doubt.

Table 22-2 (continued)
THE BENZOATE-RESTRICTED DIET

Type of Food	Foods Allowed	Foods Restricted
Vegetables		• All prepared vegetables with restricted ingredients • Most commercial salad dressings
Fruit	• All pure fresh or frozen fruits except those listed at right • Pure frozen and canned allowed fruit juices • Fruit dishes made with allowed ingredients	• Berries, especially strawberries and raspberries • Prunes • Peaches • Papaya (pawpaw) • Nectarines • Fruit dishes, jams, and juices with benzoates or "flavoring"
Meat, Poultry, and Fish	• All pure fresh, frozen, or canned meat, poultry, or fish • Processed meat made with allowed ingredients	• Meat, poultry, or fish processed with restricted ingredients • Cod • Pickled products
Eggs	• All	• All dishes prepared with restricted foods
Legumes	• All plain legumes except those on restricted list • Pure peanut butter	• Red beans • Soybeans
Nuts and Seeds	• All plain nuts and seeds	• All with restricted ingredients
Fats and Oils	• Pure butter and cream • Shortening • Pure vegetable oils • Homemade salad dressings with allowed ingredients • Lard and meat drippings • Homemade gravy	• All fats and oils with hydrolyzed lecithin • Margarine • Prepared salad dressings with restricted ingredients
Spices and Herbs	• All fresh, frozen or dried herbs and spices except those listed at right	• Anise • Cinnamon • Cloves • Seasoning packets with restricted foods • Foods labeled with "spices"
Sweets and Sweeteners	• Sugar, honey, molasses • Maple syrup, corn syrup • Icing sugar	• Flavored syrups • Prepared dessert fillings • Prepared icings and frostings

Table 22-2 (continued) THE BENZOATE-RESTRICTED DIET		
Type of Food	**Foods Allowed**	**Foods Restricted**
Sweets and Sweeteners (continued)	• Pure jams, jellies, marmalade, and conserves made with allowed ingredients and without added benzoates • Plain artificial sweeteners • Homemade sweets with allowed ingredients	• Spreads with restricted ingredients • Prepared icings and frostings • Prepared candies • Cake decorations and other confectionery • Commercial candies
Other	• Baking powder • Baking soda • Cream of Tartar • Distilled white, cider, or wine vinegars • Baking chocolate • Pure cocoa • Plain gelatin • Homemade pickles and relishes with allowed ingredients • Homemade ketchup with allowed Ingredients	• All other vinegars with flavorings" • Chocolate candy, sprinkles, and syrup • Flavored gelatin • Mincemeat • Prepared pickles, relishes, and olives • Soy sauce • Commercial ketchup • Chewing gum
Beverages	• Plain milk, and buttermilk • Pure juices of allowed fruits and vegetables • Plain and carbonated mineral water • Coffee	• Flavored milks • Fruit drinks and cocktails with restricted ingredients • All other carbonated drinks • Flavored coffee • All tea • All drinks with "flavor" or "spice" • Some ciders and beers

— CHAPTER 23 —

SULFITE ALLERGY AND INTOLERANCE

Sulfite sensitivity affects only a small group of people, but its effects can be devastating. The people most affected are asthmatics, and a significant number of deaths from a sulfite-induced attack have had a direct impact on the use of sulfites in foods and drugs. Consequently, the use of sulfites in foods and drugs has changed considerably over the past ten years. Whereas previously sulfites were used extensively as preservatives, keeping manufactured and natural foods free from disease-causing microorganisms and preventing spoilage, now they have been replaced by other preservatives in many products, and where no effective replacement is available, labeling laws have become stricter. Nevertheless, the sulfite-sensitive person needs to remain vigilant an identifying the foods, beverages, and drugs that may contain sulfites and to carefully avoid them. This chapter will provide you with details of why sulfites cause adverse reactions, where sulfites can be found, and how to avoid all sources of sulfites in your diet, without compromising your nutrition.

Sensitivity to sulfites is most common in people with asthma. Of these people, individuals who are dependent on steroids to control their asthma are considered most at risk for sulfite sensitivity. Although the incidence of adverse reactions to sulfites is estimated to be as high as 1% of the U.S. population, sulfite sensitivity in people *without asthma* is considered rare. Reported symptoms have occurred in most organ systems, including the lungs, gastrointestinal tract, and skin and mucous membranes. Reports of life-threatening anaphylactic reactions in persons with asthma are very rare. *The major risk is a life-threatening asthma attack.*

287

Symptoms reported to be due to sulfite sensitivity include

◆ Asthma in asthmatics
◆ Severe respiratory reactions, including bronchospasm, wheezing, and a feeling of tightness in the chest
◆ Flushing, feeling of temperature change
◆ Onset of hypotension (low blood pressure)
◆ Gastrointestinal symptoms (abdominal pain, diarrhea, nausea, vomiting)
◆ Difficulty in swallowing
◆ Dizziness, loss of consciousness
◆ Urticaria (hives); angioedema (swelling, especially of the mouth and face)
◆ Contact dermatitis
◆ Anaphylaxis (in persons with asthma); anaphylactoid reaction (in persons without asthma)

There is no evidence that avoiding *all* dietary sources of sulfites improves asthma. For people who are not sensitive to sulfites, exposure to sulfites poses very little risk. Toxicity studies in volunteers showed that ingestion of 400 milligrams of sulfites daily for 25 days produced no adverse effects.

People with impaired kidney and liver function should avoid sulfites because the enzymes in the kidney and liver that are required to break down sulfites will be inadequate, resulting in sulfite excess and development of symptoms of sulfite intolerance listed above.

How Sulfites Cause Adverse Reactions

Respiratory symptoms caused by sulfites are thought to be caused by sulfur dioxide, which acts as a direct irritant on hypersensitive airways. Sulfur dioxide is released from sulfurous acid, which forms when sulfites dissolve in water. This effect is enhanced when the sulfite is present in an acidic food. Persons with asthma can have severe bronchospasm after inhaling as little as one part per million of sulfur dioxide. Wheezing, flushing, and other symptoms of asthma have been brought on by the inhalation of the vapors from a bag of dried apricots.

Research suggests an IgE-mediated reaction in which sulfite acts as a **hapten**, combining with protein to form a neoantigen that prompts the immune system to make antigen-specific IgE. However, because the levels of IgE, eosinophils, and histamine are normal in most people who have symptoms of sulfite sensitivity and because sulfite-specific IgE has not been demonstrated in most sensitive people listed, scientists consider that IgE-mediated reactions are very rare, or at least unlikely, as a cause of sulfite sensitivity.

When sulfite enters the body, it is converted quite quickly to sulfate by enzymes. Sulfates are not reactive and thus do not cause any symptoms.

A deficiency in the enzyme sulfite oxidase, which converts sulfite to sulfate, has been suggested as a possible cause of abnormally high levels of sulfites, which may provoke a reaction. However, this hypothesis has not yet been definitively proven to be the main mechanism causing sulfite sensitivity in research studies.

USE OF SULFITES IN FOODS AND MEDICATIONS

Sulfites are used as preservatives in beverages, fruits, vegetables, prepared and pre-sliced foods, and packaged snack foods. The active component is sulfur dioxide, which has been used as a preservative since Roman times, especially for wine. Today it is the most versatile food additive in use.

USES OF SULFUR DIOXIDE (SULFITES) INCLUDE

◆ Prevention of food spoilage by
  – Inhibiting the growth of microorganisms, especially enterobacteria such as *Salmonella*
  – Inhibiting enzymatic and nonenzymatic browning in food plants
  – **Antioxidant** effects (keeping oxygen from changing the food's color or flavor)
  – Preserving the red color of meat by preventing oxidation of myoglobin to metamyoglobin
  – Preventing discoloration of shrimps and lobsters by inhibiting the enzyme tyrosinase
◆ Bleaching of flour, maraschino cherries, citrus peel
◆ Physical modification of dough by modifying the gluten of the flour. This reduces the elasticity of the dough and reduces the time required for mixing and standing of the dough in making batches of baked goods.
◆ Stabilization of vitamin C
◆ Inhibition of nitrosamine formation (e.g., in cooking barley to make malt)

Sulfites are also used as preservatives in some medications, including inhalable and injectable drugs, where they act as antioxidants. Some forms of epinephrine (adrenaline) contain sulfite as a preservative. However, the action of epinephrine appears to overcome any adverse effects of sulfite, and administration of epinephrine in anaphylactic emergencies is the recommended treatment.

Cooking foods does not cause sulfites to lose their effect. In addition, because sulfites bind to several substances in foods, such as protein, starch, and sugars, washing foods, even if a detergent is used, will not remove all traces of sulfites.

Sulfates in foods do not cause the same adverse reactions as sulfites. Persons who are sensitive to sulfites need not avoid sulfates.

Detection of Sulfites in Foods

Chemically treated strips have been developed to test foods for the presence of sulfites. However, because of the high number of false-positive and false-negative results obtained with these test strips, their use is not recommended.

Government Regulations on the Use of Sulfites

"Sulfiting agents or sulfites, traditionally used as food preservatives, are causing concern among consumers. For most Canadians, this use of sulfites is harmless to health. For a few individuals, these substances can cause a severe adverse reaction."[1]

The use of sulfites on *fresh fruit and vegetables*, except sliced potatoes and raw grapes, has been banned in the United States by Food and Drug Administration regulation since 1986 and in Canada since 1987. Canadian regulations state that "no person shall sell any fresh fruit or vegetable that is intended to be consumed raw, except grapes, if sulfurous acid or any salt thereof has been added thereto."

Sulfites **are** *permitted for use in the form of*

Sodium metabisulfite
Potassium metabisulfite
Sodium bisulfite
Potassium bisulfite
Sodium sulfite
Sodium dithionite
Sulfurous acid
Sulfur dioxide

A *specified level* of sulfites (calculated in parts per million) may be added to the following foods and beverages, because no suitable alternatives are currently available:

---

[1] Health and Welfare, Canada,. *Sorting Out Sulfites*, published by authority of the Minister of National Health and Welfare, 1992.

FRUITS AND VEGETABLES
Dried fruits and vegetables
Fruit juices (except frozen concentrated orange juice)
Frozen sliced apples
Frozen sliced mushrooms
Grapes
Sliced potatoes

BEVERAGES
Alcoholic
De-alcoholized wines and beers

SWEETENERS
Glucose solids and syrup
Dextrose (used in making confectionery)
Molasses

FISH
Crustaceans (shellfish)

OTHERS
Jams, jellies, marmalades (sulfite is in the pectin)
Mincemeat
Pickles and relishes
Tomato paste, pulp, ketchup, purée
Gelatin
Pectin
Snack foods
Candies and confectioneries
Frozen pizza dough
Frozen pastry shells

Note that

◆ Not all manufacturers of these products use sulfites.
◆ Canadian government regulations require that if sulfites are used, they must be listed on the label.
◆ U.S. government regulations state that if any food contains *10 parts per million or more*, the sulfite must be identified in the ingredient list on the label.

*Some foods do **not** require labels.* The presence of sulfites in the following *may not* be listed:

◆ Some bulk foods
◆ Individually sold candies
◆ Individually portioned foods such as those sold in vending machines, mobile canteens, and delis
◆ If the sulfite is in a secondary ingredient in a manufactured food. For example, if one of the ingredients in a prepared cake is jam that contains sulfites, the jam must be listed, but not the sulfite contained in it. This is because the final level of sulfite in the finished product is below the amount required by law to be disclosed.

When eating in restaurants, *ask* whether sulfiting agents are present in the foods.

ALCOHOLIC BEVERAGES

In Canada at present, ingredients of alcoholic beverages, including sulfites, *need not* be listed on the label. In the United States, if sulfite levels are 10 parts per million or more in wine, distilled spirits, and malt beverages, sulfites must be listed on the labels.

MEDICATIONS

Sulfites are used in a wide range of medications and pharmaceuticals. The *Compendium of Pharmaceuticals and Specialties* (CPS) provides a list of sulfite-containing products. Consult your pharmacist about the sulfite content of any medications you require.

OTHER SOURCES OF SULFITES

Food processing equipment and food packaging materials (e.g. plastic bags) may be sanitized with sulfites. These sources of sulfites will not be listed on any labels.

Sulfite-sensitive individuals should avoid opening any packages likely to contain sulfites, especially sealed plastic bags containing dried fruits.

Note: Some food manufacturers publish extensive lists of their products in which they specify ingredients to which food-sensitive and food-additive sensitive consumers might react. People with sulfite sensitivity should obtain these publications if they wish to purchase manufactured foods such as cookies, breakfast cereals, boxed entrées, and so on.

SULFITES AND THIAMINE (VITAMIN B1)

When sulfur dioxide dissolves, the resulting disulfide chemical bonds break up certain protein molecules in food. Food spoilage is caused by **enzymes** present in natural foods (e.g., fruits and vegetables) that act on the plant tissue and cause its destruction; we see this as "browning" and eventual rotting of the food. The enzymes responsible for this process, like all enzymes, are **proteins.** Sulfites act on these proteins and destroy them, thus stopping this enzyme destruction of the healthy plant tissue. However, this action of sulfites also destroys some of the nutrient proteins in the plant or animal. One of the most important of these nutrient proteins is thiamine (vitamin B1), which is particularly affected by sulfites. Therefore, government regulations require that sulfites not be used in high-protein foods that are a significant source of thiamine, especially meat of all types, cereals, and milk products.

Table 23-1 provides details of the types of sulfites in common use, the terms under which they may appear on product labels in the United States and Canada, and the E numbers that indicate their presence in foods sold in European countries.

THE SULFITE-RESTRICTED DIET

Table 23-2 gives you details of the foods allowed and restricted when you are following a sulfite-free diet.

Table 23-1
SULFITES: EXAMPLES OF SOURCES AND USES OF AND EUROPEAN E NUMBERS

Additive	E Number	Function	Foods Likely to Contain Sulfite
Sulfur dioxide	E220	• Occurs naturally • May be produced chemically • Prevents browning by destroying plant enzymes	Fruit juices Fruit pulp Fruit syrup Fruit salad Fruit spreads Packet soups Glacé cherries Dried bananas and apricots Jams and jellies Desiccated coconut Beer Wine Cider Cider vinegar Candied peel Canned crabmeat Fruit-based milk and cream desserts Flavorings Fruit fillings Powdered garlic Gelatin Dry ginger root Glucose Soft drinks Frozen mushrooms Dehydrated vegetables and fruits Sausage meat
Sodium sulfite	E221	• Used in food manufacturing to – Sterilize fermentation equipment – Sterilize food containers – Used as a preservative to prevent browning especially of pre-peeled and sliced apples and potatoes – In some countries, used to control microorganisms such as enterobacteria, especially *Salmonella*	Preserved egg yolk Quiick-frozen shrimp, prawns, lobsters Beer Wine Concentrated pineapple juice

Table 23-1 (continued)
SULFITES: EXAMPLES OF SOURCES AND USES OF AND EUROPEAN E NUMBERS

Additive	E Number	Function	Foods Likely to Contain Sulfite
Sodium sulfite (continued)		– Preservation of the red color of meat and shellfish – Manufacture of caramel	
Sodium hydrogen sulfite	E222	• Preservative for alcoholic beverages • Bleaching of cod • Bleaching of sugar	Beer Wine Cider Quick-frozen shrimp, prawns, lobster Quick-frozen french fries Dehydrated instant mashed potatoes Fruit juices Vegetable juices Relishes and some condiments Gelatin-containing puddings
Sodium metabisulfite	E223	• Antimicrobial preservative • Antioxidant • Bleaching agent	Soft drinks Pickled onions Pickled red cabbage Packet mashed potatoes Quick-frozen shrimp, prawns, lobster Quick-frozen french fries Gelatin puddings Alcoholic beverages Dried fruits and nuts
Potassium metabisulfite	E224	• Antimicrobial preservative, especially in fruit and homemade wine • Used to halt fermentation process in commercial breweries • Anti-browning agent	Quck-frozen french fries Quick-frozen shrimp, prawns, lobster Wine Wine-making tablets (Campden tablets)
Calcium sulfite	E226	• Preservative • Firming agent in canned fruits and vegetables • Disinfectant in brewing vats	Cider Fruit juices Canned fruits and vegetables

Table 23-1 (continued)
SULFITES: EXAMPLES OF SOURCES AND USES OF AND EUROPEAN E NUMBERS

Additive	E Number	Function	Foods Likely to Contain Sulfite
Calcium bisulfite	E227	• Preservative • Prevents secondary fermentation in brewing • Used in washing beer casks to prevent the beer from becoming cloudy or sour • Firming agent in canned fruit and vegetables	Beer Jams Jellies Canned fruits and vegetables

Table 23-2
THE SULFITE-RESTRICTED DIET

Type of Food	Foods Allowed	Foods Restricted
Milk and Milk Products	• Plain milk, buttermilk, cream, sour cream, and yogurt • All plain cheese, cottage cheese, ricotta, Quark® • Ice cream made with allowed ingredients • Butter	• All prepared dairy products made with restricted ingredients
Breads and Cereals	• Any pure flour or grain • Any plain fresh bread, buns, biscuits, pizza dough, with allowed ingredients • Homemade or purchased baked cookies, pies, etc., made with allowed ingredients	• Biscuit dough • Frozen pizza dough • Frozen pastry shells • Any baked goods with dried or glacé fruit, molasses, coconut, dehydrated vegetables, commercial frozen apple slices, or confectionery icing

	• Breakfast cereals without dried fruit or coconut, including
	  — Puffed rice and wheat
	  — Shreddies®
	  — Shredded Wheat®
	  — Corn flakes
	  — Oats and oatmeal
	  — Plain Cream of Wheat®
		• All others, including granola and muesli with dried fruit and/or coconut
		
		• Instant oatmeal and Cream of Wheat® with dried fruit.

	• All plain grains • Plain crackers without sulfites • Plain pasta • All homemade crackers, cereals and pasta dishes with allowed ingredients	• Commercial crackers and cereals • All packaged pasta meals • All canned, frozen, and dried commercial pasta dishes
Vegetables	• All pure fresh and frozen vegetables and their juices, except those listed at right	• Dried vegetables • Frozen sliced mushrooms • Processed sliced potatoes • Pickled vegetables • Tomato paste, pulp, purée • All prepared vegetables with restricted ingredients
Fruit	• All pure fresh or frozen fruit except those listed at right • Frozen orange juice	

Note: This list is not exhaustive. Other foods may contain sulfites and not be listed here. It is up to the reader to read all ingredient labels carefully and to contact the manufacturer if there is any doubt.

Table 23-2 (continued)
THE SULFITE-RESTRICTED DIET

Type of Food	Foods Allowed	Foods Restricted
Fruit (continued)	• All canned and bottled juices, except those listed at right • *Check labels.*	• Grapes • Commercial frozen apple slices • Dried and glacé fruit • Maraschino cherries • All other frozen juices • Grape juice • Cider • Most bottled lime and lemon juice
Meat, Poultry, and Fish	• All unprocessed pure, fresh, or frozen meat, poultry, or fish. • Fish canned with water, or with water and only salt • Freshly caught crab, crayfish, lobster, prawns, shrimp, and squid that has not had a sulfite wash • Processed meat made with allowed ingredients.	• Processed with restricted ingredients • Canned tuna with sulfites • All processed crustaceans • Processed meats with restricted ingredients • Gelatin
Eggs	• All	• Any prepared with restricted ingredients
Legumes	• All plain legumes • Pure peanut butter	• All others
Nuts and Seeds	• All plain nuts and seeds	• Any with restricted ingredients
Fats and Oils	• Pure butter and cream • Shortening, margarine • Pure vegetable oils • Homemade salad dressings with allowed ingredients • Lard and meat drippings • Homemade gravy	• All others
Spices and Herbs	• All fresh, frozen, or dried herbs and spices.	• All herb or spice mixes and seasoning packets with restricted ingredients, such as dehydrated vegetables
Sweets and Sweeteners	• White sugar, honey • Maple syrup, corn syrup • Icing sugar	• Brown sugar, molasses • Glucose solids and syrup • Dextrose (used in sweets)

	Table 23-2 (continued) THE SULFITE-RESTRICTED DIET	
Type of Food	**Foods Allowed**	**Foods Restricted**
Sweets and Sweeteners (continued)	• Pure jams, jellies, marmalade, and conserves made without added pectin or gelatin and with allowed ingredients • Plain artificial sweeteners • Homemade sweets with allowed ingredients	• Spreads with restricted ingredients • Commercial icing and frosting • Cake decorations and other confectionery • Commercial candies
Other	• Baking powder, baking soda, • Cream of Tartar • Distilled white vinegar • Baking chocolate • Pure cocoa • Homemade pickles and relishes • Homemade ketchup with allowed ingredients	• All other vinegars • Chocolate candy, sprinkles, and syrup • Mincemeat • Prepared pickles and relishes • Commercial ketchup • Gelatin and pectin
Alcohol	• None	• All
Medications	• All without sulfites and dextrose • *Check with pharmacist.*	• All others

— CHAPTER 24 —

BHA AND BHT INTOLERANCE

The average North American diet relies heavily on convenience foods in the form of processed and packaged meals, usually rich in fats and oils. In order to keep these foods safe for the consumer, **antioxidants** are used extensively to prevent fats and oils from becoming rancid and giving foods an objectionable taste and odor. BHA (butylated hydroxyanisole) and BHT (butylated hydroxy-toluene) are two of the most powerful antioxidants available for this purpose. Although most people have no trouble in consuming these chemicals, a few people develop symptoms when they eat them. This chapter will provide these sensitive people with the information they require to understand how their body reacts to these chemicals, where they are to be found, and how to safely avoid them in their daily diet, without any risk of nutritional deficiency.

BHA and BHT do not occur in nature. For the information of readers who like to know exactly what the chemicals they are consuming are made from, BHA is a mixture of 2- and 3-tert-butyl-4-methoxy-phenol, made from p-methoxyphenol and isobutene. BHT is made from p-cresol and isobutylene. It was originally developed as an antioxidant for use with petroleum and rubber products. Both products are very effective antioxidants, and for most people they have proven to be safe as food additives.

BHA and BHT are often used in combination with other antioxidants such as propyl gallate (where this is allowed), citric acid, or phosphoric acid. The fact that a large percentage of the antioxidant is lost during the processing of food (potato chips and similar snack foods lose 90% of the antioxidant; cookies lose about 35%) means that the quantity consumed is actually much less than what was added to the product during its manufacture. However, when BHA and BHT are used in the same product, 20 times the usual amount of BHA is stored in the body's fat.

SENSITIVITY TO BHA AND BHT

Extremely high doses of BHA and BHT in experimental animals have consistently resulted in enlargement of the liver. Both kidney and liver functions have been affected. In addition, adverse effects on the brain have resulted in abnormal behavior patterns in experimental animals.

In humans, BHA and BHT have been reported to cause rashes and hives in sensitive individuals. Those most frequently affected are aspirin-sensitive, so it is thought that the intolerance to BHA and BHT may be due to inhibition of the cyclo-oxygenase pathway of arachidonic acid metabolism, similar to that suspected for salicylate sensitivity (see Chapter 20). Some reports have implicated BHA and BHT in childhood hyperactivity disorders.

In 1978 the United Nations Joint FAO/WHO Expert Committee on Food Additives suggested that daily ingestion of these chemicals should not exceed 0.5 milligrams per kilogram of body weight (e.g., 34 mg for a 68 kg adult). However, intake should be much lower for individuals who are sensitive to these chemicals. Their goal should be to eliminate BHA and BHT by reading food labels carefully and avoiding all possible sources of these preservatives. In many countries, BHT is not permitted in foods intended specifically for babies and young children. BHA is not permitted for food use in Japan.

FOOD PRODUCTS CONTAINING BHA AND BHT

Foods likely to contain BHA and BHT are

- Vegetable oils
- Margarines
- Foods cooked in or containing vegetable oils, such as
  - Potato chips
  - Nut meats
  - Doughnuts
  - Pastries and pie crusts
  - Breakfast cereals
  - Baked goods
  - Salted roasted peanuts
- Dehydrated potatoes
- Dry breakfast cereals
- Dried fruits
- Dry yeast
- Packaged convenience foods

Additional foods that may contain BHA and BHT are

- Beverages
- Ice cream
- Candies
- Chewing gum
- Gelatin deserts
- Soup bases
- Potato and sweet potato flakes

- Lard and shortening
- Animal fats
- Unsmoked dry sausage
- Enriched rice
- Cake mixes
- Glacé fruits
- Dry dessert mixes

BHA and/or BHT may be added to the packaging of cereals, crackers, and other convenience foods to help maintain freshness of the food. BHA and BHT will appear on the label if the food contains the preservatives or if they are present in the packaging materials.

THE BHA- AND BHT-RESTRICTED DIET

People who have, or suspect they have, a sensitivity to BHA or BHT should follow the guidelines for restricting their intake of these chemicals that are provided in Table 24-1.

Table 24-1 THE BHA- AND BHT-RESTRICTED DIET		
Type of Food	Foods Allowed	Foods Restricted
Milk and Milk Products	• Plain milk, buttermilk, cream, sour cream, and yogurt • All plain cheese, cottage cheese, ricotta, Quark® • Ice cream made with allowed ingredients • Butter	• All prepared dairy products made with unknown fats or oils, such as – Cheese foods – Cheese spreads – Cream sauces • Drink mixes • Dry dessert mixes • Ice cream
Breads and Cereals	• Any pure flour or grain • Any plain fresh bread, buns, biscuits, pizza labeled "preservative-free" • Check with baker or manufacturer whether oil or packaging contains BHA and/or BHT • Most fat-free baked goods should be safe, but check. • Homemade breads, buns, baked cookies, pies, etc., made with allowed ingredients	• All other grains and baked goods, including those fried in fat, such as doughnuts • Pie crusts • Pastries • Cake and other baking mixes • Dry dessert mixes
	• Breakfast cereals with allowed ingredients and packaging, including – Puffed rice and wheat – Post Bran Flakes® – All plain grains and their flakes – Original Cream of Wheat® – Red River Cereal® – Pure oat bran • *Read all cereal labels.*	• All others
	• Crackers: – Homemade Melba toast – Grissol Melba Toast – RyVita Snackbread – Wasa Light or Golden Crackers® – Almost all rice cakes • *Read cracker labels.*	• All others

Note: This list is not exhaustive. Other foods may contain BHA or BHT and not be listed here. It is up to the reader to read all ingredient labels carefully and to contact the manufacturer if there is any doubt.

Table 24-1 (continued)
THE BHA- AND BHT-RESTRICTED DIET

Type of Food	Foods Allowed	Foods Restricted
Breads and Cereals (continued)	• Plain pasta • Plain and wild rice • General Foods Minute Rice® • All homemade cereals, crackers, and pasta dishes with allowed ingredients	• Enriched rice • *Read labels on all packaged pasta meals and rice meals.*
Vegetables	• All pure fresh, frozen, and canned vegetables and their juices • V-8 Vegetable Cocktail® • Homemade french fries	• Prepared vegetable dishes with unknown fats or oils • Salads with commercial salad dressings • Some commercial french fries • Potato and sweet potato flakes • Dehydrated potatoes
Fruit	• All pure fresh, frozen, or canned fruit and juices • Pure fruit ices, sorbets, and ice pops	• Prepared fruit dishes with unknown fats or oils • Glacé fruits • Dried fruits
Meat, Poultry and Fish	• All pure fresh or frozen meat, poultry, or fish. • Fish canned in broth or water, not in oil. • Processed meat made with allowed ingredients • *Read all meat labels.*	• Processed with unknown oils or fats • Unsmoked dry sausage • Processed meats with restricted ingredients
Eggs	• All	• All prepared dishes with restricted foods.
Legumes	• All plain legumes except those listed at right • Pure, natural peanut butter	• Prepared legume dishes with unknown fats or oils. • Some regular peanut butter.
Nuts and Seeds	• All plain nuts and seeds • Pure almond butter and sesame seed butter (tahini)	• All with restricted ingredients, especially snack nuts and seeds
Fats and Oils	• Pure butter and cream • Vegetable oils • Homemade salad dressings with allowed ingredients • Lard and meat drippings • Homemade gravy	• All fats with BHA and/or BHT • Margarine • Shortening • Lard • Most commercial salad dressings • Prepared gravy

Table 24-1 (continued)
THE BHA- AND BHT-RESTRICTED DIET

Type of Food	Foods Allowed	Foods Restricted
Spices and Herbs	• All fresh, frozen, or dried herbs and spices	• Seasoning packets with BHA and/or BHT
Sweets and Sweeteners	• Sugar, honey, maple syrup • Maple syrup, corn syrup • Icing sugar • Pure jams, jellies, marmalades, and conserves made with allowed ingredients • Plain artificial sweeteners • Homemade sweets with allowed ingredients • Pure baking chocolate and cocoa	• Syrups and sauces with restricted ingredients • Commercial candies • Commercial icings and frostings • Commercial chocolates
Other	• Baking powder • Baking soda • Cream of Tartar • Fleishmann's Quick-Rise Yeast® • Distilled vinegar • Baking chocolate • Pure cocoa • Plain gelatin	• Dry dessert mixes • Cake and baking mixes • Most dry yeast • Glacé and dried fruit • Chocolate candy, sprinkles, and syrup • Flavored gelatin • Soup bases • Chewing gum

— CHAPTER 25 —

NITRATE AND NITRITE SENSITIVITY

Nitrates and nitrites are used in foods as preservatives, particularly as protection against the deadly bacterium *Clostridium botulinum*, the cause of botulism, a frequently fatal neuromuscular disease with paralysis caused by the toxin produced by the bacterium, which multiplies within the food. They are also used to give flavor and color to manufactured foods, especially processed meats.

Nitrites and nitrates represent one of the oldest and most effective ways of preserving meats. Without nitrites and nitrates there would be many deaths from the growth of toxic microorganisms. However, the mechanisms that allow these chemicals to kill bacteria may also cause adverse effects in the human body when the food containing the nitrate or nitrite is consumed in excessive quantities. People who are sensitive to the chemicals react at a lower dosage (level) than others, but anyone can develop symptoms if they consume very high doses.

This chapter will provide you with information on when and how nitrates and nitrites enter our foods and how to avoid excessive intake of both chemicals.

SYMPTOMS OF SENSITIVITY

Nitrites preserve the red color of meat by changing the nature of the hemoglobin of the red blood cells. The function of hemoglobin is to carry oxygen throughout the body. When nitrites enter the bloodstream of persons who have eaten the nitrite-treated meat, their hemoglobin is likewise changed if the nitrite level is excessive. This may lead to a condition known as methemoglobinemia with symptoms such as anemia, breathing difficulty, palor, dizziness, and headaches. Because of their small size, infants and young children are more susceptible to nitrite poisoning than adults, and nitrites are not permitted in foods intended for babies under the age of six months.

Nitrites can react with substances called amines in the digestive tract to form nitrosamines, which may be carcinogenic when exposure to the chemicals is excessive and prolonged. There is evidence that consumption of vitamins A, C, and E (antioxidants) in the form of fresh yellow and green vegetables, fish, and plant oils, protects against stomach and intestinal cancer in this situation. Potassium nitrite has been linked to atrophy of the site in the adrenal gland that is responsible for secreting aldosterone, the hormone that maintains the balance of sodium, potassium, and chloride in the blood.

Prolonged exposure to nitrates may cause anemia and inflammation of the kidneys, and ingestion of a large quantity may result in gastrointestinal inflammation with severe abdominal pain, vomiting, vertigo (a sensation as if the world is revolving around the person, similar, but different from, dizziness), muscular weakness, and irregular pulse (nitrate toxicity). A high intake of sodium nitrate has been associated with inhibition of the functioning of the thyroid gland. Nitrates may be converted to nitrites during food spoilage or by intestinal bacteria after consumption. They then have the same effect as nitrites discussed above.

Other reported symptoms include recurrent hives and migraine and nonmigraine headaches.

NITRATES AND NITRITES IN FOODS

The presence of nitrates or nitrites in manufactured foods will be indicated on the label as sodium nitrate, potassium nitrate, sodium nitrite, or potassium nitrite. High levels are found in processed meats such as pepperoni, frankfurters, weiners, sausages, salami, bologna, other luncheon meats, bacon, and ham, as well as in smoked fish and some imported cheeses.

Plants can contain naturally occurring nitrates derived mainly from nitrate-containing fertilizers.

The following plant species tend to have higher levels of nitrates than others do:[1]

- Beetroot and beet greens
- Cabbage
- Lettuce
- Parsley

---

[1] Allergy Advisor; Zing Solutions (http://AllergyAdvisor.com/)

- Carrot
- Celery
- Collards
- Eggplant
- Fennel
- Leeks

- Potato
- Radishes
- Spinach
- Strawberry
- String beans (green beans; french beans)
- Turnip greens

Table 25-1 provides information about the use of nitrates and nitrites in foods and where you are likely to encounter nitrates and nitrites in your diet. In the United States and Canada, the terms "nitrate" and "nitrite" will appear on product labels; in European countries, the E-numbers will indicate which chemical is present in the food.

People vary in their tolerance of nitrates and nitrites. It is therefore very difficult to give guidelines on how much of a food a sensitive person can eat without having symptoms. The best advice is this: A person who is intolerant to nitrites and nitrates should avoid those foods that have been shown to have the *highest levels of the chemicals*, as indicated in Table 25-2.

Table 25-2 gives you some idea of the actual levels of nitrates and nitrites in certain foods, demonstrating how these vary among different food types and products. Because the levels of nitrates and nitrites vary according to how much is added to a processed meat, or how much is in the soil in which a plant is grown, it is not possible to provide an accurate measure in each food.

Table 25-1
SUMMARY OF THE USE AND EFFECTS OF NITRATES AND NITRITES IN FOODS

Compound	E Number	Effect and Function	Used in
Potassium nitrite • Potassium salt of nitrous acid • Occurs naturally • May be manufactured by reacting nitrous oxide and nitric oxide with potassium hydroxide	E249	• Converts the iron-containing pigments in the flesh to stable bright pink compounds • Preservative in meat, particularly in preventing the development of spores of *Clostridium botulinum*, the bacterium that causes botulism	• Cooked meats • Canned meats • Corned meat • Liver sausage • Meat paté • Pickled meats • Sausages • Smoked fish
Sodium nitrite • Does not occur naturally • Derived from sodium nitrate by bacterial or chemical action	E250	• Preservative, especially by inhibition of *Clostridium botulinum* • Used in meat curing to give a red color to the meat	• Cured meat • Cured meat products • Salted meat • Pork sausage • Bacon • Turkey and ham loaf • Smoked frankfurters • Weiners • Tongue • Pressed meats • Canned meats • Frozen pizza • Smoked fish

Sodium nitrate (Chile saltpeter)
 	
• Naturally occurring mineral, especially in the Chilean desert
• Formed by reaction between nitric acid and sodium carbonate
	E251	• Preservative
		• Added to salt in curing meats
		• Prevents loss of color in meats
			• Bacon
			• Pressed meats
			• Ham
			• Tongue
			• Beef
			• Canned meats
			• Cheese, other than
			  – Cheddar
			  – Cheshire
			  – granapadano
			  – provolone
			• Frozen pizza

Potassium nitrate (Saltpeter) • Naturally occurring mineral	E252	• Inhibition of *Clostridium botulinum* • Added to salt in curing of meat products • Prevents loss of color	• Cured meats • Sausages • Smoked frankfurters • Weiners

Table 25-1 (continued)
SUMMARY OF THE USE AND EFFECTS OF NITRATES AND NITRITES IN FOODS

Compound	E Number	Effect and Function	Used in
Potassium nitrate (Saltpeter), (continued) • Formed by reaction of potassium chloride and concentrated nitric acid • May be manufactured artificially from waste animal and vegetable material			• Bacon • Ham • Tongue • Pressed meats • Canned meats • Dutch cheeses • Fish products • Spirits

Table 25-2
LEVEL OF NITRATES AND NITRITES IN SOME MEATS AND VEGETABLES

FOOD	Mean Level (mg/100 g)
NITRITES	
Meats	
Bacon	1.3
Bacon, smoked	3.1
Luncheon meat	0.3
Ham, smoked	3.0
Salami	0.3
Salami, kosher	38.0
Vegetables	
Cucumber, raw	2.4
Green beans, raw	25.3
Eggplant, raw	30.2
Lettuce, raw	85.0
Lima beans, raw	5.4
Melon, raw	43.3
Onion, raw	13.4
Peas, raw	2.8
Pepper, sweet, raw	12.5
Pickles	5.9
Potato, raw	11.9
Pumpkin, raw	41.3
Sauerkraut	19.1
Spinach, raw	186.0
Sweet potato, raw	5.3
Tomato, raw	6.2
NITRATES	
Vegetables	
Asparagus, raw	2.1
Beet, raw	276.0
Beans, dry	1.3
Broccoli, raw	78.3
Cabbage, raw	63.5
Carrot, raw	11.9
Cauliflower, raw	84.7
Corn, raw	4.5

Note: Nitrates may be converted to nitrites in the mouth and intestine. Thus, the level of the chemical in food does not always reflect the level in the body after digestion.

Source: J. M. V. Joneja, "Level of Nitrates and Nitrites in Some Meats and Vegetables," in *Dietary Management of Food Allergies and Intolerances: A Comprehensive Guide*, 2nd ed. (Vancouver: J. A. Hall Publications, 1998), pp. 243-244.

— CHAPTER 26 —

MONOSODIUM GLUTAMATE (MSG) INTOLERANCE

Monosodium glutamate (MSG), a flavor enhancer common in Chinese cooking, is used increasingly to flavor Western foods. In addition, some foods, such as tomato, mushrooms, and cheese, contain *natural* glutamates that resemble MSG. A **glutamate** is a derivative of the amino acid called glutamic acid that is an essential part of proteins.

Persons sensitive to MSG report a variety of symptoms known as the "Chinese Restaurant Syndrome" or "Kwok's Syndrome." Symptoms may include facial flushing, pain in the face and the back of the neck, headache, tingling and burning sensations, blurred vision, nausea and vomiting, increased heartbeat, chills, and shaking. Several incidents of severe asthma have been attributed to the ingestion of MSG; depression, irritability, and other mood changes have also been reported.

Experts are widely divided on the subject of MSG sensitivity. A recent review stated that results of a number of research studies "led to the conclusion that 'Chinese Restaurant Syndrome' is an anecdote applied to a variety of postprandial [occurring after a meal] illnesses: rigorous and realistic scientific evidence linking the syndrome to MSG could not be found."[1] On the other hand, some clinicians have estimated that the prevalence of Chinese Restaurant Syndrome may be as high as 1.8% of the adult population.[2]

This chapter will provide you with information on what you may experience if you are sensitive to glutamates. It discusses how glutamates may cause your symptoms, and how to reduce your intake of glutamates without causing any nutritional deficiencies in your diet.

---

[1] Tarasoff and M. F. Kelly, "Monosodium L-Glutamate: A Double-Blind Study and Review." *Food Chemistry and Toxicology* 31, no. 12 (1993): 1019-1035.

[2] G. Kerr, M. Wu-Lee, and M. El-Lozy, "Prevalence of the 'Chinese Restaurant Syndrome.'" *Journal of the American Dietetic Association* 75 (1979): 29-33.

How MSG Causes Symptoms

MSG is the sodium salt of glutamic acid, an amino acid. Glutamate is the active ingredient in the compound.

One theory to explain sensitivity to MSG links its action to abnormally high levels of **acetylcholine,** a neurotransmitter that acts on the brain and central nervous system. Because glutamate acts as a building block in the synthesis of acetylcholine, as well as other physiological chemicals, the symptoms of MSG sensitivity may be caused by excessive levels of neurotransmitters that develop in a short period of time. Toxic levels of acetylcholine may explain the symptoms of the Chinese Restaurant Syndrome.

The usual source of glutamate is food proteins, where it is combined with other amino acids. Before glutamate is free to be absorbed by the body, the **peptide** bonds in these proteins must be broken by **enzymes** in the process of digestion. Because this process is gradual, it controls the level of free glutamate in the body. According to the theory of "neurotransmitter toxicity," when MSG is eaten, glutamate enters the bloodstream rapidly because no peptide linkages need to be broken. Clinical studies have shown that an MSG dose of 0.1 gram per kilogram of body weight can induce plasma glutamate levels to rise to 15 times the normal concentration in about one hour. However, a relationship between plasma glutamate levels and symptoms has not been demonstrated in well-conducted research trials.

Some practitioners have noticed a deficiency of vitamin B6 (pyridoxine) in a number of MSG-sensitive persons. This deficiency could reduce the breakdown of glutamate in the liver, thus prolonging high plasma glutamate levels and causing symptoms to worsen.

Symptoms Possibly Caused by MSG

The following symptoms are reported to be caused by MSG:

Flushing
Tightness around face, jaw, and chest; numbness of face
Tingling, burning of face and chest
Rapid heartbeat
Nausea, diarrhea, stomach cramps
Headache, especially at back of head and neck
Weakness, dizziness, balance problems, staggering
Confusion, slurred speech

Blurring of vision, difficulty focusing, seeing shining lights
Chills and shaking, excessive perspiration
Difficulty in breathing
Symptoms of asthma (in persons with asthma)
Water retention, thirst
Insomnia, sleepiness
Stiffness, heaviness of arms and legs
Mood changes, such as irritability
Depression, paranoia

Symptoms of Chinese Restaurant Syndrome are reported to usually occur within 30 minutes of eating a meal high in MSG. Symptoms of *asthma*, however, have been reported to occur 1 to 2 hours after MSG ingestion and even as long as 12 hours later.

MANAGEMENT OF MSG SENSITIVITY

A "safe level" of MSG in foods cannot be set because a number of different factors contribute to plasma levels of glutamate, only one of which is the MSG added to food. Glutamate is a natural component of the body, where it plays an essential role in metabolism. Enzymes called transaminases in the liver allow glutamate to interact in a variety of reactions, and free glutamate is also found in muscle, brain, kidneys, and other organs. A person who weighs 70 kilograms has the equivalent of about 12 grams of MSG in his or her body. Whether or not any particular plasma level can be considered "safe" is not known.

Milk contains natural free glutamate. The daily intake of a 3 kilogram infant obtained from 480 grams of mother's milk is 3.75 grams (1.25 g/kg body weight).

The Joint FAO/WHO Expert Committee on Food Additives has evaluated MSG and has judged that no restriction is necessary for the use of MSG in food. This means that MSG can be added to any prepared food to the level that the manufacturer considers optimum for enhancing the flavor of its product.

Because MSG is a food additive that appears on the Generally Recognized as Safe (GRAS) list, a food manufacturer is not required by law to include MSG in a list of ingredients on product labels. Listing MSG as an ingredient is voluntary on the part of the manufacturer.

MSG-sensitive persons should restrict their intake of MSG as much as possible. Because alcohol seems to increase the rate of absorption of many foods as well as MSG, drinking alcoholic beverages while eating MSG-containing foods probably increases both the severity and rate of onset of symptoms. In addition, eating foods containing MSG on an empty stomach seems to increase the adverse effects of MSG.

SOURCES OF MSG

The following flavorings contain MSG and may appear on food labels:

- Accent
- Ajinomoto
- Zest
- Vetsin
- Gourmet powder
- Subu
- Chinese seasoning
- Glutavene
- Glutacyl
- Hydrolyzed vegetable protein (HVP)
- Hydrolyzed plant protein (HPP)
- Natural flavoring (may be HVP)
- Flavoring
- Kombu extract
- Mei-jing
- Wei-jing
- RL-50

Many prepared foods contain MSG or one of the above flavorings. Foods containing these additives include

Canned meats
Prepared dinners and side dishes
Canned soups
Dry soup mixes
Gravy and seasoning mixes
Cookies and crackers
Cured meats
Smoked meats and sausages
Diet foods
Freeze-dried foods
Frozen foods
Potato chips
Prepared snacks
Prepared salads, salad dressings, and mayonnaise
Croutons
Bottled and canned sauces
Spices and seasonings

Glutamate is also present in monopotassium glutamate, monoammonium glutamate, calcium glutamate, and other salts of glutamic acid. Some MSG-sensitive persons may react to these salts also. Look for these terms on food labels.

Restaurants, Cafeterias, and Fast-Food Restaurants

The majority of eating places in North America include MSG in some form in most of their dishes, unless they specifically state otherwise. However, most reputable establishments can supply a list of the ingredients in their menu items.

Avoiding MSG

Table 26-1 provides you with guidelines to avoid added MSG in your food and to reduce your intake of natural forms of glutamate.

	Table 26-1 THE MSG-RESTRICTED DIET	
Type of Food	**Foods Allowed**	**Foods Restricted**
Milk and Milk Products	• Plain milk, buttermilk, cream, sour cream, and yogurt • All plain cheese, cottage cheese, ricotta, Quark® • Pure vanilla ice cream • Plain salted or unsalted butter	• Flavored milk • Commercial dips • Flavored yogurts • All flavored and smoked cheese, cheese slices, and cheese foods • All other ice cream • All seasoned butter
Breads and Cereals	• Any pure flour or grain • Any bread, bun, pita or pizza dough without flavoring, except plain sourdough	• Bread, baking mixes, or grain mixes with flavoring or seasoning packets • Sourdough bread and buns • All others, such as croutons, stuffing, meat coating mixes

	• Breakfast cereals without flavorings, including
	  – Puffed rice and wheat
	  – Shreddies®
	  – Shredded Wheat®
	  – Corn flakes
	  – Cereals with malt or malt syrup
	  – Pats and oatmeal
	  – Plain Cream of Wheat®
	  – All plain grains
		• All others, especially the colored and flavored cereals made to appeal to children
		• Flavored oatmeal and Cream of Wheat®

	• Plain crackers without flavoring (*read labels*) • Plain pasta • All homemade baked goods, cereals, and pasta dishes with allowed ingredients	• All flavored crackers • All flavored pasta • All canned, frozen, and dried commercial pasta dishes
Vegetables	• All pure fresh and frozen vegetables and their juices	• Canned vegetables and juices • *Read labels on plain frozen vegetables.* • Commercially prepared vegetables with sauces and flavorings
Fruit	• All pure fresh and frozen fruits and their juices • Homemade fruit dishes and drinks with allowed ingredients	• Fruit dishes with flavoring • Fruit drinks and cocktails

Note: This list is not exhaustive. Other foods may contain MSG and not be listed here. It is up to the reader to read all ingredient labels carefully and to contact the manufacturer if there is any doubt.

Table 26-1 (continued)
THE MSG-RESTRICTED DIET

Type of Food	Foods Allowed	Foods Restricted

Meat, Poultry, and Fish	• All unprocessed pure, fresh, or frozen meat, poultry, or fish
	• Fish canned with water or with water and only salt
	• Processed meat such as ham, with "MSG-free" on the label
	• Homemade sausages, etc.
		• Processed or with restricted ingredients, e.g.:
		  – Stuffing
		  – Butter-basted in broth with spices or seasoning
		• Cured or smoked sausages, patties, etc.
		• Canned, except as listed at left

Eggs	• All	• All prepared with restricted foods
Legumes	• All plain legumes • Pure peanut butter	• All others
Nuts and Seeds	• All plain nuts and seeds	• All others
Fats and Oils	• Pure butter and cream • Shortening • Pure vegetable oils • Homemade salad dressing • Lard and meat drippings • Gravy	• All others
Spices and Herbs	• All fresh, frozen, or dried herbs and single spices	• All herb or spice mixes and seasoning packets • *See listing of flavorings containing MSG on page 316.*
Sweets and Sweeteners	• Sugar, honey, molasses • Pure jams and jellies • Pure corn and maple syrup • Plain artificial sweeteners • Homemade sweets and fruit drinks with allowed ingredients	• Artificially flavored and colored sweeteners, jams, jellies, icings, cake decorations, candies, and drink mixes

—PART III—

DETERMINING THE CULPRIT FOODS AND FOOD COMPONENTS: ELIMINATION AND CHALLENGE PROCEDURES

This section provides you with all the information you will need to determine exactly which foods, naturally occurring chemicals in foods, and food additives are making you sick. Determination of the foods responsible for clinical symptoms requires *elimination* of the culprit foods for a trial period in which the symptoms of concern should disappear. This is followed by careful *challenge*, or reintroduction, of each individual food component in a precisely selected and controlled fashion so that its effects on the body can be monitored. This is the only way to accurately determine the role of foods in the disease process.

The elimination and challenge process may be used to confirm or refute any "allergy tests" or to establish the most appropriate therapeutic diet in the management of specific food-related conditions. The process may appear time-consuming and tedious, but the exercise is definitely worthwhile because it will provide you with invaluable information about precisely how your body responds to foods. Every person is unique, and the diet that works for one will not be appropriate for another. This section allows you to explore your own way of processing food, which will serve you well for the rest of your life. Because this process does involve extreme dietary manipulation for a short period of time, it is best carried out with the help of a professional trained in the field. Ideally, you would work with your physician and a registered dietician so that any risk of severe reactions and unsafe diets can be quickly dealt with. For mild, chronic types of symptoms you may be able to carry out the process yourself, but involving a health care professional is always the best and safest route to follow.

Elimination diets remove all of the food components that your food and symptom record suggests could be responsible for your symptoms. Then follows the challenge phase, in which each individual food component is reintroduced in such a way that you can monitor your response not only to the component itself but also to the specific dose of the component that triggers your symptoms. Because most food *intolerances* are dose related—that is, it requires a certain amount of the food to elicit a response in your body—determining your *tolerance* will allow you to eat a small quantity of the food without distress, when a larger quantity could cause a reaction. This is valuable information that allows you to "cheat" a little without undue concern when faced with food so tempting that you cannot resist. This does not apply to food *allergy* when exposure to the tiniest amount of food can elicit an allergic response, especially in a person prone to an anaphylactic reaction (see page 325). In cases of skin-test positive, blood-test positive, and challenge positive allergic reactions, strict avoidance of all forms of the allergen is essential. This difference between food allergy and food intolerance should be very clearly understood. You should return to Part I if this distinction is unclear.

It cannot be stressed strongly enough that if you have any cause to suspect a severe or anaphylactic reaction to a food, any challenge tests should be undertaken only under strict medical supervision in a facility equipped for resuscitation.

Never challenge on your own a food that has caused a severe reaction in the past or has elicited a strong reaction on a skin test, or if you have a high level of IgE to the food on a blood test.

— CHAPTER 27 —

ELIMINATION DIETS: ELIMINATION PHASE

The aim of any elimination diet is to remove the food components that are causing adverse symptoms or making them grow worse. Elimination diets set the stage for subsequent determination of the culprit food components by allowing the allergic person to become symptom-free in order that when the specific reaction triggers are reintroduced, they cause noticeable, and sometimes measurable, symptoms. There are three types of diets in the elimination phase of the management program:

1. Selective elimination diets
2. Few-foods elimination diets
3. Elemental diets

Each diet has a specific function in the management of food sensitivity (Figure 27-1).

CHOOSING THE MOST APPROPRIATE ELIMINATION DIET

In order to determine which elimination diet is the most appropriate for you, the following information is required:

◆ A careful *medical history*. It is especially important to record any *anaphylactic reactions* suspected to be due to food.
◆ Exclusion of *any other cause* for the symptoms, determined by diagnostic tests and procedures, carried out by your medical advisors.

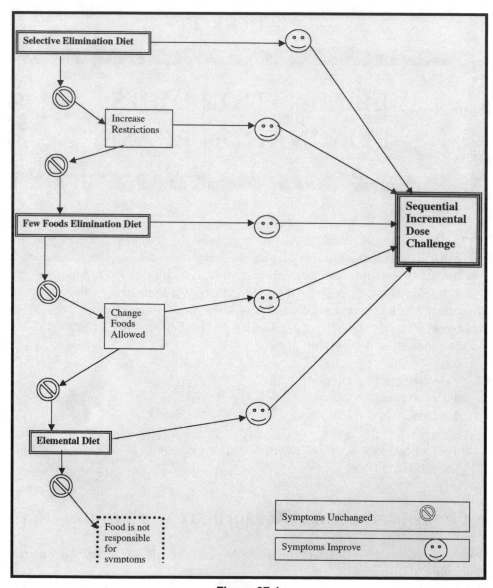

Figure 27-1
Procedure for Elimination and Challenge: Flow Chart for Selection of Appropriate
Elimination Diet

◆ Results of any *allergy tests* previously carried out by qualified practitioners.
◆ A careful record of all foods, beverages, supplements, and medications ingested during a 7-day period, with details of symptoms experienced during this time. This record is called an "exposure diary."

Exposure Diary

Record each day, for a minimum of 7 days:

◆ All foods, beverages, medications, and supplements ingested
◆ Approximate quantities of each (teaspoons, tablespoons, cups, grams, ounces)
◆ Composition of compound dishes and drinks (ingredient list)
◆ The time at which each was taken
◆ All symptoms experienced, graded on severity:
   Scale: 1 (mild); 2 (mild-moderate); 3 (moderate); 4 (severe)
◆ Time of onset of the symptoms
◆ How long the symptoms lasted and whether medications were taken to control the symptoms
◆ Status on waking in the morning (symptom-free? type and severity of symptoms?)
◆ If sleep was disturbed during the night, whether this was due to specific symptoms

THE ELIMINATION DIET

The appropriate elimination diet excludes all suspect allergens and intolerance triggers based on the above information, specifically:

◆ The detailed medical history
◆ Analysis of the exposure diary
◆ Results of any previous allergy tests
◆ Foods that you suspect may be a cause of your symptoms

Each type of elimination diet has a place in determining the culprit foods:

◆ Selective elimination diets: one or a small number of specific foods are eliminated for a specified period of time. For example, milk-free diet, egg-free diet, wheat-free diet, or a combination of these (please refer to Chapters 8 to 15).

◆ Few-foods elimination diets (sometimes referred to as oligo-antigenic diets): only a few (usually fewer than ten) foods are allowed for a specified period of time.

◆ Elemental diets: only an amino-acid-based formula is allowed for the duration of the elimination phase. No solid food is consumed. Sometimes an extensively hydrolyzed formula may be used, especially for babies.

Selective Elimination Diets

Selective elimination diets are usually used when ingestion of a specific food causes a sudden acute reaction and when there is indication of an IgE-mediated hypersensitivity reaction based on skin tests or tests for food-specific antibody. In the case of anaphylaxis, or acute reactions, such diets can be considered therapeutic.

You may also use selective elimination diets to identify specific food triggers in chronic allergic disease, for example, migraine headaches, atopic dermatitis (eczema), urticaria (hives), and angioedema (swelling). In these cases, if the symptoms persist after you eliminate specific foods, the assumption is that the foods avoided are not the cause of the reaction.

Selective and therapeutic diets are normally followed for a period of four weeks. This allows sufficient time for recovery from the initial "withdrawal symptoms" and, in most cases, relief of all symptoms that are due to food components. It also allows sufficient time for a person to adapt to the diet, both physiologically and psychologically, and to make the necessary lifestyle adjustments to accommodate the dietary restrictions. Because selective elimination diets are nutritionally adequate, no risk is associated with prolonged adherence to the diet. Taking into consideration the immunological response, four weeks' freedom from exposure to an allergen is also a suitable time for challenge with the offending allergen. This interval of freedom allows the person to be symptom-free, but the level of antigen-specific IgE will *not* be reduced so that in a Type I hypersensitivity reaction, challenge will elicit a clear, and sometimes enhanced, response.

SELECTIVE ELIMINATION DIETS ARE PARTICULARLY USEFUL IN TWO TYPES OF SITUATIONS:

◆ When specific foods need to be eliminated, usually to confirm the accuracy of allergy tests such as scratch, prick or intradermal skin tests, food-specific antibody tests such as RAST or ELISA, and others (see Chapter 5)

◆ When food components are known or suspected to be the major cause of a certain condition, but allergy to a specific food is not the cause (i.e., specific food intolerance, such as lactose intolerance or intolerance of a known food addtitive)

Specific Food Restrictions

The elimination of specific foods in preparation for challenge, or in situations where the culprit food component has been definitively identified, is a relatively straightforward process. The food-sensitive individual should prepare three important lists:

1. The foods which must be avoided and manufactured foods that commonly contain the subject food
2. A comprehensive list of the terms that identify the food in an ingredient list or on a food label
3. Alternative food sources of *all* the nutrients that may be deficient when the subject food is eliminated, in order to reduce the risk of nutrient deficiency. If alternative food sources are limited, the person will need to take appropriate supplements.

Specific examples of selective elimination diets include diets free from

- Milk
- Egg
- Wheat
- Peanut
- Soy
- Tree nuts
- Fish
- Shellfish
- Lactose
- Sulfites
- Benzoates
- Artificial food colors
- Nickel
- Monosodium glutamate (MSG)

Selective elimination diets are designed to remove all suspect allergens and intolerance triggers, but to include all foods that are not involved in the clinical condition or which have tested negative on earlier diagnostic tests. Instructions for management of selective elimination diets for specific foods and details and discussion of therapeutic diets can be found in Joneja's *Dietary Management of Food Allergies and Intolerances: A Comprehensive Guide* (2nd ed,; Vancouver: J. A. Hall Publications, 1998).

Nutritional Adequacy of Selective Elimination Diets

A person's nutrient needs can be adequately supplied by a selective elimination diet that includes alternative foods which are nutritionally equivalent to those removed. *There is no reason anyone should lose weight or not obtain all of his or her essential nutritional requirements on a selective elimination diet*. If the allowed foods do not provide all the nutrients required, appropriate dietary supplements will supply the deficit. The need for nutrient supplements is determined by the foods being eliminated from the diet. Check with your health care provider, ideally a physician and/or registered dietician, to ensure that all of your nutritional needs are being met during this stage of your management.

Duration of the Selective Elimination Diet

The selective elimination diet is usually followed for four weeks. In cases where the symptoms occur only intermittently (for example, migraine headaches), the diet should be followed until at least three or four episodes would usually have occurred.

If the symptoms have not disappeared or greatly decreased after four weeks, either allergens or intolerance factors remain in your diet, or the symptoms are unrelated to foods. To determine whether foods in the elimination diet are responsible for the remaining symptoms, you should keep another exposure diary for five to seven days while continuing with the elimination diet. Analysis of this second exposure diary should indicate if other foods or chemicals could be causing the remaining symptoms. A further elimination of foods can be carried out for two more weeks if indicated by the second food exposure diary. You should follow the new diet for no longer than two weeks and keep an exposure diary for the second week of the diet.

Elimination Diets and Children

Young children are especially vulnerable to nutritional deficiency because *all* nutrients are needed in the years of maximum growth. It is particularly important that there be careful and frequent evaluation of the elimination diet to ensure that the child's nutritional needs are being met at each stage of the process of determining his or her allergenic foods. For this reason, a few-foods elimination diet is rarely recommended before puberty. If it is really necessary for purposes of identifying extremely extensive food allergy, someone under the age of 13 years can follow the few-foods elimination diet, but *only* under the supervision of a qualified health care practitioner.

When young children are on an elimination diet, it is wise to put forbidden foods in places that are not easily reached. Parents of defiant youngsters have been known to install locks on cupboards and luggage straps on refrigerators and freezers–and even to dress the child in a T-shirt printed with the message "Don't feed me, I'm allergic!"

Follow-Up to the Selective Elimination Diet

Following the four or six weeks on the selective elimination diet, the challenge phase begins. Even if the symptoms have improved only a little, a specific challenge of food components may reveal reactions that are not noticeable when the food is eaten frequently. Some practitioners refer to this as "unmasking a hidden food allergy."

FEW-FOODS ELIMINATION DIET

Sometimes, it is very difficult to determine the foods that should be excluded on a selective elimination diet. When there are multiple symptoms that do not fit into any pattern of reactivity that would suggest a reaction to food allergens, and there are no indicators of intolerance to food additives or sensitivity to natural components of foods, a few-foods elimination diet is useful. Such diets are particularly valuable in the management of chronic allergic conditions.

A few-foods elimination diet differs from a selective elimination diet in that only a small number of foods are allowed. These are the foods that are considered to be the *least likely* to trigger an allergic reaction. Such diets are indicated when there are many symptoms with no clear relationship to specific foods.

Because a few-foods elimination diet is not nutritionally complete, it should never be followed for more than 14 days. Usually, 7 to 10 days is sufficient to show results, and this period **should not** be exceeded for children under 7 years of age. A role for foods in causing the symptoms should become apparent if symptoms disappear or improve significantly within this time period. Extending the few-foods elimination diet beyond 14 days *if the symptoms remain unchanged* is a fruitless exercise and can be detrimental to the health, because the immune system may become depressed on this "semi-starvation" regimen. If symptoms do not clear within 14 days, it is because

1. One or more of the foods included in the diet are allergenic for the person *or*
2. Foods are not contributing to the symptoms

To confirm assumption 1: Replace each food with one from the same food group and continue the elimination for another 7 days.

To confirm assumption 2: initiate sequential incremental dose challenge of each restricted food (see Chapter 28).

Foods Allowed

There are many few-foods elimination diets in use, and each practitioner tends to favor a particular diet. The diet provided here (Table 27-1) includes foods that consistently prove low in allergenicity for the majority of the population, and it is the one most often followed. Adjustments must be made for individuals with unusual reactions who might respond adversely to one or more of the foods included. The most effective of these diets are individualized for each patient because the persistence of symptoms could be due to one or more foods left in the diet. It is important that the foods selected are ones to which the person following the diet has shown no evidence of reactivity in the past. The diet contains no food additives, flavor enhancers, or modifiers, so both allergens and chemical food additives are minimized or eliminated.

General Instructions for the Few-Foods Elimination Diet

1. It is wise to begin the diet trial during a quiet social season, not at Christmas, Hanukkah, or other religious holidays, or around birthday parties, weddings, or other important celebrations. If there is a social event during this diet, take your own food or hold the party in your home so that appropriate foods are available at all times.
2. You will need to shop ahead, having plenty of appropriate foods on hand. The diet may be somewhat boring, but there is no need to go hungry. There is no restriction on calorie intake unless you actually want to lose weight. *Weight loss should not be a primary goal during this test period.* It is important that you remain healthy and as well-nourished as possible while investigating specific responses to foods. The issue of weight loss can be addressed later if necessary.
3. The meals are quite simple, without spices, butter, or condiments.
4. Favor fresh food sources over other sources. Frozen is the next best alternative.
5. Stay on the diet for 10 to 14 days.
6. Keep a diary of the entire experience that includes a record of the food eaten, the date and time of eating, and any reactions that you experience.

7. Wash and cook foods with only *distilled* water. Tap water may contain contaminants that could cause reactions.

8. Use pots, pans, and containers made from iron, aluminum, or glass (such as Pyrex) in food preparation and cooking. Utensils made from stainless steel, or with Teflon or Silverstone coatings, may add reactive chemicals to the foods being cooked in them.

9. Avoid
   ◆ Chewing gum
   ◆ Over-the-counter medications (unless they are essential)
   ◆ Breath mints
   ◆ Coffee
   ◆ Tea (including herbal tea)
   ◆ Diet drinks
   ◆ Mouthwash
   ◆ Cigarettes and other tobacco products

10. Continue taking necessary prescription medications. Consult your doctor about the advisability of discontinuing any prescribed medication.

11. During the first five days on the diet, your symptoms may seem to get worse or you may feel "unwell," with symptoms similar to those of "flu." Lots of rest, alkali salts (see the box), and distilled water will help to minimize these symptoms. By the end of four days, some symptoms should start to clear, and most food reactions should have greatly decreased or disappeared by the fifth or sixth day

12. Because the diet is nutritionally inadequate, it **must not** be continued for more than 14 days.

Recipes and meal planning for a sample few-foods elimination diet are provided in Appendix I.

ELEMENTAL DIETS

When allergy to multiple foods is suspected, and when either selective or few-foods elimination diets have failed to resolve a patient's symptoms, an elemental formula alone for a short period of time (one to four weeks) should determine whether the illness is food related. Elemental formulas are used only in rare cases where all other elimination diets have failed to resolve symptoms, but the suspicion of an allergic etiology for the patient's illness remains high. An elemental diet supplies calories and all essential macro- and micronutrients in the form of an amino-acid-based formula. Such diets are easy to maintain in infancy, but more difficult in adulthood. Most elemental formulas are unpalatable and may be better tolerated by naso-gastric feeding, which is sometimes considered in extreme

---

ALKALI SALTS

Alkali salts often help reduce physical symptoms during the first several days of the diet. Mix together in a glass container:

- 2 tablespoons (25 mL) of sodium bicarbonate
- 1 tablespoon (15 mL) of potassium bicarbonate

Store the mixture in a screw-capped jar.

Sodium bicarbonate is baking soda. Potassium bicarbonate is available in larger drug stores. If the pharmacy does not carry it, potassium bicarbonate can usually be obtained by special order.

Dosage:

- ½ teaspoon (2 mL) of the mixture in ½ cup (125 mL) of warm water

Take one dose as needed when you feel unwell or experience flu-like symptoms while on the diet.

Some specialized pharmacies carry pre-mixed "alkali salts" containing sodium and potassium bicarbonate with or without vitamin C.

---

cases of food allergy. Elemental formulas can be made more palatable by flavoring added by the manufacturer, but this adds the risk for adverse reactions to the chemicals in the flavoring compounds.

There are a number of elemental formulas available. None should be used without the knowledge and approval of your physician, and none continued for any prolonged period of time. EleCare, Vivonex, Tolerex, and Elemental O28-Extra are examples of formulas suitable for adults. Neocate and hydrolyzed casein formulas such as Nutramigen, Alimentum, and Pregestimil are available for infants. Before choosing a specific formula, check with your physician to make sure it will suit your needs. The number of daily calories supplied by the formula must be calculated for each individual so that the required quantity of formula is consumed. In addition, you should confirm the precise composition of the formula with the manufacturer, since sometimes the ingredients are changed without notice.

Table 27-1
FOODS ALLOWED ON THE FEW-FOODS ELIMINATION DIET

Food Category	Food	Specific Food Items
Meat and Alternates	• Lamb • Turkey If lamb and turkey are not tolerated: • Fish	 – Perch – Red snapper – Sea bass
Grains	• Rice • Tapioca • Millet	• Whole grains, flours, and pure cereals made from these grains
Vegetables	• Squash	• All kinds including: – Acorn – Butternut – Chayote – Hubbard – Winter squash – Pattypan – Spaghetti squash – Yellow squash – Summer squash – Crookneck – Zucchini – Pure infant squash in jars
	• Parsnips • Sweet potatoes • Yams • Lettuce	 • Pure infant sweet potatoes in jars • Iceberg (head lettuce) is the least tolerated of the lettuces. If it is not tolerated, other varieties may be acceptable.
Fruits	• Pears • Cranberries	• Pure bottled pear juice • Pure infant pears in jars • Homemade cranberry juice
Oils	• Canola oil • Safflower oil	

Table 27-1 (continued) FOODS ALLOWED ON THE FEW-FOODS ELIMINATION DIET		
Food Category	**Food**	**Specific Food Items**
Condiments	• Sea salt	
Desserts	• Pudding made from tapioca beads or rice, fruit, and fruit juice of allowed fruits • Agar-agar (seaweed) may be used as a thickener	
Beverages	• Distilled water • Juice from the allowed fruits and vegetables	• In glass bottles (available from drug stores), (It is less expensive to use your own containers)

EXPECTED RESULTS OF ALL ELIMINATION DIETS

If food components are indeed responsible for your symptoms, there are a number of things you might experience after the elimination phase:

◆ If all or most of your major reaction triggers have been excluded, you may actually feel *worse* on days 2–4 of the elimination diet. Theoretically, this may be due to a condition of antibody excess, causing a condition known as serum sickness.

◆ By days 5–7 of exclusion, you will begin to feel noticeably better if the allergens and intolerance triggers responsible for your symptoms have actually been eliminated.

◆ Your symptoms should have improved significantly after 10–4 days of exclusion. If all allergens and antagonistic foods have been eliminated, all symptoms should have disappeared after about three weeks.

◆ If substitution of alternative foods for excluded nutrients is adequate, you should not lose any weight in the two or four weeks of the elimination diet.

◆ If your symptoms have not improved significantly, it is likely that you are consuming unidentified allergens or intolerance factors or that foods are not the cause of your symptoms.

◆ The duration of the initial elimination phase will depend on the type of symptoms being managed: For example, reactions that appear only intermittently at widely spaced intervals (such as migraine headaches), or those that may be due to delayed reactions to foods and additives, might require a longer elimination phase. Gastrointestinal symptoms, on the other hand, will usually respond promptly to appropriate dietary measures, and the patient will feel better within seven to ten days.

◆ Most selective elimination diets are followed for four weeks; few-foods elimination diets are usually followed for 10 to 14 days.

◆ An elimination diet should *never* be followed for longer than 10 to 14 days if there is any danger of nutritional deficiency such as may occur on the few-foods elimination diet.

◆ Keep another food and symptoms record for the last week of your elimination diet phase. This will show whether your symptoms have improved. If symptoms still persist, a clear pattern of occurrence might be obvious that could point to a specific food trigger, which you can avoid for a further trial period.

◆ Further elimination of foods can be carried out, in addition to the original list, for another two weeks, based on analysis of the second exposure diary.

◆ Following 14 days on the few-foods elimination diet, or four weeks on a selective elimination diet (or six weeks if more foods have been eliminated for two weeks after the original four), a sequential incremental dose challenge should be started (see Chapter 28).

◆ Even if your symptoms do not seem to have improved a great deal, specific challenge of food components sometimes reveals adverse reactions that are not noticeable when the food is eaten continuously.

REASONS FOR FAILURE IN FOLLOWING AN ELIMINATION DIET (WHY YOU MIGHT GIVE UP!)

There are several key reasons why a person may not adhere to dietary restrictions. These include:

◆ Insufficient knowledge or understanding about the restrictions and why they are necessary. Do read Chapters 1 to 6 again to refresh your memory and reinforce your resolve.

◆ The diet is too intrusive to be acceptable (too many restrictions, or the prescribed diet plan does not take into account your lifestyle and tastes). Try to adjust your lifestyle, or reorganize your diet to fit your lifestyle. You will be unlikely to follow a diet that is drastically different from your normal way of eating, so go over your original exposure diary again, and insert substitute foods rather than trying to develop a totally new diet "from scratch."

◆ The diet fails to reduce or abolish symptoms. This can be due to a number of factors:
  – The diet is frequently abandoned during the first 2 to 4 days because the symptoms have intensified during this period.
  – The diet may have improved the symptoms for which food components are responsible, but the remaining symptoms are caused by factors other than foods, which will not improve by dietary manipulation.
  – Sources of the allergenic foods remain in the diet. Do make sure that you are well-informed about "hidden sources" of the food and that you are familiar with *all* the terms that can indicate the presence of the food on ingredient labels. Reread the chapters on specific food restrictions, Chapters 8 to 26. Lists of terms are provided under each food category
  – Some of the restricted ingredients might have been introduced during manufacture or serving of the allowed foods. For example, there can be contamination of utensils and equipment when several different foods are processed without adequate cleaning in between batches–this is a particular problem with ice cream and bakery products such as cookies.

◆ Excessive expectations of the diet have not been met (a cure rather than mere improvement was expected).

◆ The diet is no longer needed because the symptoms disappeared spontaneously, or, in children, the child "grew out of" the symptoms.

◆ Cost should *not* be an important element in not adhering to a diet, because most of the initial elimination diets are followed only for a short period of time and the savings from the foods eliminated usually offset the cost of the substitute foods. A few comparison studies show that there is not a significant difference in cost between the regular diet and the elimination diet except in the cases where expensive elemental food replacements and supplements have been prescribed.

FOLLOW-UP TO THE ELIMINATION DIET

Following the elimination diet, sequential incremental dose challenge should be initiated in order to identify the specific food(s) responsible for the patient's symptoms (Chapter 28) When the culprit food components have been identified, a selective elimination diet, now referred to as a maintenance diet (Chapter 29) can be continued as long as necessary, without any nutritional risk.

THERAPEUTIC DIETS

The information provided above is designed for the management of the diet when food allergy and intolerance is the suggested cause of a person's symptoms. However, there is another type of selective elimination diet that is used in situations where a diagnosis has been made and the cause of the condition has been identified as a food component. Treatment for these conditions is strict avoidance of the causative food component, and carefully designed "therapeutic diets" are essential in the management of the patient's condition.

Therapeutic diets are usually classified depending on the situation in which they are used:

◆ Inborn errors of metabolism of various types, for example:
 – Errors in carbohydrate metabolism, such as galactosemia, hereditary fructose intolerance, and glycogen storage diseases
 – Errors in amino acid metabolism of which the most well-known is phenylketonuria, in which dietary phenylalanine must be restricted
 – Anomalies in lipid metabolism, of which hyperlipoproteinemia is probably the most frequently encountered example
◆ Metabolic anomalies that are more commonly referred to as food intolerances. Examples include disaccharide deficiency of several types, such as:
 – Lactose intolerance, caused by a deficiency in the enzyme lactase
 – Sucrose intolerance, usually a congenital condition caused by a deficiency in the production of sucrase
 – Glucose-galactose intolerance
◆ Conditions in which food components need to be restricted, although their role in the cause of the disease is as yet unknown. Examples include:
 – Gluten-sensitive enteropathy (celiac disease), in which all gluten-containing foods need to be avoided
 – Cow's milk protein enteropathy, most frequently seen in young infants, in which all cow's milk proteins need to be excluded

A second group of therapeutic diets are used when specific food components are suspected to be a cause, or an exacerbating factor, in a clinical condition in which all other causes have been ruled out. Most of the diets in this category should be considered experimental until further research can confirm their usefulness and possibly determine *how* the suspect food component is causing adverse reactions. Therapeutic elimination diets have been used successfully in the management of conditions such as:

◆ *Idiopathic urticaria and angioedema*, in which dietary sources of histamine are restricted

◆ *Irritable bowel syndrome*, in which foods are modified to promote digestion and absorption in the small intestine, and to reduce the build-up of undigested food in the colon where it promotes microbial fermentation

◆ *Migraine headache*, in which biogenic amines such as histamine, tyramine, phenylethylamine, and octopamine are restricted

◆ *Infant eczema*, in which the major food allergens and all artificial food additives are restricted

Therapeutic diets are designed to *remove* all suspect allergens and intolerance triggers, but to *include* all foods that are not involved in the clinical condition or have tested negative on the diagnostic tests employed. Instructions for management of selective elimination diets for specific foods, and details and discussion of therapeutic diets, can be found in Joneja's *Dietary Management of Food Allergies and Intolerances: A Comprehensive Guide.*

— CHAPTER 28 —

REINTRODUCTION OF FOODS: CHALLENGE PHASE

When the Elimination Test Diet has been completed, the next step in identifying the foods and food additives associated with adverse reactions is to reintroduce each component individually so that those responsible for symptoms can be clearly identified. This is achieved by careful challenge with precise quantities of each food component and careful monitoring of symptom development, looking for immediate reactions (within a four-hour period) or delayed reactions (from one to four days) following ingestion.

Food allergy practitioners use three different types of food challenges:

1. **Double-blind placebo-controlled food challenge** (DBPCFC) is usually used in research studies or specialized clinics. The patient is given a capsule containing the test food or a placebo (usually glucose powder). Neither the supervisor nor the patient knows which is being eaten. The patient's response to each capsule in turn is recorded. After the test, the identity of the material in the capsules is revealed. The placebo should produce no symptoms; the patient's allergenic foods will cause symptoms.

2. **Single-blind food challenge** is usually supervised by a physician or, more commonly, a dietitian or nurse in an office setting. The patient is unaware of the identity of the food. The supervisor does know which food is being challenged. The food is disguised in another, stronger-tasting, food.

3. **Open food challenge** is most frequently carried out by the allergic person at home. The person is aware of the identity of the food and the quantity being consumed in each test.

DOUBLE-BLIND PLACEBO-CONTROLLED FOOD CHALLENGE

The **double-blind placebo-controlled food challenge** (DBPCFC) is regarded as the "gold standard" by most traditional allergists. It is always conducted by a clinician. In this procedure, neither the patient nor the supervisor of the challenge knows the identity of the food.

◆ The food is lyophilized (freeze-dried) and, in powder form, is enclosed in a gelatin capsule.

◆ A placebo, usually glucose powder, is enclosed within a similar capsule and is used as a negative control.

For IgE-mediated reactions, the way the food challenge is carried out tends to vary from clinic to clinic. Two examples reported in the literature are given below; others may be obtained from published data.[1,2]

Method 1

IgE-Mediated Reactions

The challenge is done when the patient is fasting. The first dose is unlikely to cause symptoms (25 to 500 milligrams of lyophilized food).

◆ The dose is usually doubled every 15 to 60 minutes; the interval between doses is dictated by the reported course of the patient's symptoms.

◆ The patient is usually observed for two hours after each dose for the development of symptoms.

◆ If the patient shows no symptoms after consuming 10 grams of lyophilized food (equivalent to about one egg white, or one 4-ounce glass of milk), it is unlikely that he or she is actually allergic to that food.

◆ In most IgE-mediated disorders, challenges to new foods may be conducted every 1 to 2 days.

Non–IgE-Mediated Reactions

◆ In dietary protein-induced enterocolitis, allergen challenges require up to 0.3 to 0.6 grams of food per kilogram of body weight given in one or two doses. The patient is usually observed for 24 to 48 hours for the development of symptoms.

---

[1] H. A. Sampson, "Food Allergy Part 2. Diagnosis and Management." *Journal of Allergy and Clinical Immunology* 103, no. 6 (1999); 981–989.

[2] S. H. Sicherer, "Food Allergy: When and How to Perform Oral Food Challenges." *Pediatric Allergy and Immunology* 10 (1999): 226–234.

♦ In eosinophilic gastroenteritis, several feedings over 1 to 3 days may be required to elicit symptoms; the patient is observed for up to 4 days for the development of symptoms.

♦ With most non–IgE-mediated reactions, challenges need to be at least 3 to 5 days apart.

Method 2

♦ The test dose is 8 to 10 grams of the dry (lyophilized) food, 100 milliliters of wet food, or double these quantities for meat or fish.

♦ The patient consumes the dose at 10- to 15-minute intervals over a total of 90 minutes.

♦ A meal-sized portion of the food is consumed a few hours later.

♦ The clinician records symptoms and makes assessments for reactions in the skin, gastrointestinal tract, and respiratory tract.

♦ Challenges are ended when the patient shows a reaction.

All negative challenges (i.e., the patient shows no reaction) need to be confirmed by eating the food while being observed by the doctor or test supervisor to rule out false-negative responses.

The DBPCFC is expensive and labor-intensive, so most are conducted either in a research setting or in specialized facilities such as allergy clinics or hospitals when knowing the identity of the culprit food is extremely important for the health of the patient.

SINGLE-BLIND FOOD CHALLENGE

In this method of challenge, the suspect allergen is known to the supervisor, but unknown to the patient. The food is disguised in a strongly flavored food such as

♦ Fruit juice (cranberry, apple, or grape)
♦ Infant formulas for babies and children
♦ Elemental formulas, appropriate for children or adults
♦ Meat patties
♦ Cereals
♦ Added ingredients with strong flavors such as mint, fish, or garlic
♦ Lentil soup

Most IgE-mediated reactions, and those resulting in severe allergic symptoms, are conducted under medical supervision, in appropriately equipped facilities. The majority of anaphylactic reactions to foods are not challenged because it is frequently possible to identify the food responsible based on the patient's history. If such challenges are necessary, they should be conducted only under the strictest medical supervision with appropriately qualified and equipped personnel in attendance.

SEQUENTIAL INCREMENTAL DOSE (OPEN) FOOD CHALLENGE (SIDC)

Many adverse reactions to foods do not result in severe reactions and can be safely carried out by a person at home. The methods described here for identifying foods that trigger adverse reactions would be more appropriately considered "reintroduction" rather than challenge and would be carried out on foods not deemed likely to cause a severe reaction. Because unnecessary restriction of foods can be extremely detrimental to nutritional health and emotional and social well-being, it is very important that the foods responsible for adverse reactions be correctly identified, even though they are not life-threatening.

In many types of foods, there are several different components that can be challenged individually. By separating those that can be tolerated from those that need to be avoided, a person's diet can be liberalized to include those that are safe, thereby providing a wider range of food choices as well as ensuring a more complete nutritional intake. Reactivity to a component of a food, but not the whole food, is well-known in the case of lactose intolerance: Only the milk sugar (lactose) needs to be avoided; the milk proteins are tolerated, so lactose-free milk and its products can be included in the diet to supply many essential nutrients. A similar liberalization of dietary restrictions can be achieved when individual food components are reintroduced separately. For example, in milk allergy/intolerance, challenge with casein, whey, and lactose individually will determine a person's reactivity to each; those that cause a reaction will be avoided; those that are tolerated can be included in the regular diet.

Instructions for carrying out the sequential incremental dose challenge (SIDC) are provided below. The initial selective elimination diet, few-foods elimination diet, or elemental formula is continued for the duration of the challenge phase of the program. Foods are not added back into the diet until *all* of the foods within a category have been tested separately, even if they produce no reaction during the challenge. This is to ensure that the quantity of each food component is consistent with the test directives. If foods are added back as they are tolerated, the quantity of a single component will be increased by including previously tested and tolerated foods containing that component. For example, while testing milk components, if the patient tolerates Test 1 for casein proteins, then including cheese in the diet while the subsequent challenges are carried out will increase the quantity of casein in each test.

The instructions provided are designed to allow reintroduction of increasing doses of the test foods so that the clinician can determine the patient's limit of tolerance (quantity allowed) as well as the individual food components that are safe. A chart is provided in Appendix II for recording the outcome of each challenge test.

Any foods that have caused an anaphylactic reaction, have been suspected to be the trigger for an anaphylactic reaction, or have been, or are suspected to be, the cause of a severe allergic reaction (especially in an asthmatic) should be challenged only under medical supervision in a facility equipped for resuscitation.

General Instructions for Conducting the SIDC

◆ The selective or few-foods elimination diet continues for all meals throughout the testing period.
◆ An initial screening challenge provides a measure of safety (labial food challenge):
— The food is placed on the outer border of the lower lip for 2 minutes.
— The site is observed for the development of a local reaction for 30 minutes.
— Signs of a positive reaction are
• Swelling, reddening, or irritation where the food was placed
• Development of a rash on the cheek and/or chin
• Rhinitis (nasal inflammation) or conjunctivitis (eye inflammation)
• A systemic reaction involving several different sites in the body distinct from where the food was placed
◆ If the labial food challenge is negative, the patient will consume each food component three times on the test day at four-hourly intervals and watch for the development of symptoms.
◆ The symptoms that develop will be the same as those that the patient has experienced in the past, but the intensity or severity may be significantly increased. Any new symptoms not previously experienced are unlikely to be due to the food; an unrelated cause should be investigated, and the food challenge repeated in not less than two weeks.

- If symptoms develop at any time, consumption of the test food component stops immediately. The patient continues the basic elimination diet until the symptoms subside completely. Testing of the next food in the sequence can begin 48 hours after the symptoms have disappeared. This interval allows enough time for all of the reactive food to be eliminated from the body before another one is introduced.

- If the test food does not cause an immediate reaction on Day 1 of its introduction, the next day (Day 2) is a monitoring day for delayed reactions. The patient eats the basic elimination diet at each meal, but does not eat any of the test food during Day 2. Symptoms that appear on Day 2 are usually due to a Type III hypersensitivity reaction to an antigen or to a non–immune-mediated reaction to a food additive.

- If no symptoms develop on Day 1 or 2 of the test, the food can be considered safe. Then the next food component in the sequence can be tested.

- Under most circumstances, two days is adequate for reactions to the test food to appear. However, occasionally it is unclear whether the symptoms were due to the food or to some unrelated event, or the reaction may be extremely mild. In such cases, the same food is eaten on Day 3 but in larger quantities than on Day 1, again in three increasing doses. Day 4 would then become a second monitoring day for delayed reactions. If the test food is responsible for a reaction, the symptoms will increase in severity on both Day 3 and Day 4. If the food is not responsible, the symptoms will diminish, or remain unchanged, over Days 3 and 4.

- The food category selected for each test is up to the patient, or sometimes the clinician will decide on a specific sequence of introduction. However, when one category of food is selected, each test in the category, in the prescribed sequence, should be followed in order that the maximum amount of information about the patient's pattern of reactivity can be obtained from the results.

Challenge Tests for Food Additives

The challenge test is designed to determine adverse reactions to foods. Testing for food additives is more difficult, because in most cases it is not easy to obtain the additive in its pure form, or even to find it as a single additive in a manufactured food. Usually several different chemicals, such as flavor and texture modifiers, color, and preservatives, are added simultaneously.

Some research studies have attempted to test food additives. The chemicals were added in their pure form to an orange drink containing no additives, in the following amounts:

Tartrazine	8.5 mg in 250 mL
Sunset yellow	8.5 mg in 250 mL
Sodium metabisulfite	12.5 mg in 250 mL
Sodium benzoate	55.0 mg in 250 mL

However, for challenge tests that the patient does at home, it is probably sufficient to test the foods containing additives in the context within which they would normally be eaten. The patient consumes the food with a high level of the suspect additive, and the reaction is compared with that experienced after eating the same food without the additive. For example:

◆ Many manufactured macaroni-and-cheese dinners (for example, Kraft Macaroni and Cheese) contain tartrazine. The manufactured product should be tested and compared to a similar homemade meal, using cheddar cheese, which has a similar color but contains the natural yellow color annatto and not tartrazine.

◆ Cinnamon contains a high level of naturally occurring benzoates. Eating applesauce with cinnamon, and applesauce without the spice, will indicate whether cinnamon, and therefore benzoate, is tolerated.

◆ Sulfite sensitivity can be tested by comparing the reaction after eating dried fruit without sulfite (available in many health food stores) to regular (sulfited) dried fruit available in supermarkets. When dried fruits or vegetables are treated with sulfites, they retain their natural color. Unsulfited fruits and vegetables are a uniform dull beige color, which makes it easy to identify those that are sulfite-free.

◆ To test for nitrates, test additive-free beef in comparison to a beef steak to which nitrates have been added to preserve the color. The butcher or supermarket manager will be able to supply that information.

◆ Monosodium glutamate (MSG) is available as a flavor enhancer in some specialty stores. Test food with and without MSG to determine sensitivity.

Instructions for the Sequential Incremental Dose Challenge of Individual Food Components

---

PULSE TEST

◆ Sometimes an adverse reaction to a food is accompanied by an increase in heart rate.

◆ Take your pulse before consuming the first test food. This is your baseline or resting pulse.

◆ Take it again 2 minutes, 5 minutes, 10 minutes, 20 minutes, and 30 minutes after eating the food. An increase of more than 10 beats above baseline (before eating the food) that may continue to increase over the test period (30 minutes) may indicate an adverse reaction.

Day 1

MORNING: BETWEEN BREAKFAST AND LUNCH

◆ Eat a small quantity of the test food.

◆ Monitor your response.

◆ Be aware of any adverse reactions.

◆ If a reaction occurs, you will have only the usual symptoms, but they may be more severe than usual.

Wait four hours before eating the test food again.

If you have had *no* adverse reactions, the reintroduction should proceed as follows:

AFTERNOON: BETWEEN LUNCH AND DINNER

◆ Consume *double* the quantity of the test food eaten in the morning.

◆ Monitor your response.

◆ Be aware of any adverse reactions.

◆ If a reaction occurs, you will have the usual symptoms, but they may be more severe than usual.

Wait four hours.

If you have had *no* adverse reactions, proceed as follows:

EVENING: AFTER DINNER

◆ Consume *double* the quantity of the test food eaten in the *afternoon*.

◆ Monitor your response.

◆ Be aware of any adverse reactions.

◆ If a reaction occurs, you will have only the usual symptoms, but they may be more severe than usual.

If an adverse reaction occurs at any time during the challenge, discontinue the test food.

Wait at least 48 hours after an adverse reaction has *subsided* before testing a new food.

Day 2

◆ Do not eat any of the test food challenged on Day 1.
◆ Eat only the foods allowed on the elimination diet.
◆ Monitor for any reactions throughout the day.
◆ Any adverse response may be due to a delayed reaction to the food tested yesterday; *discontinue testing that food component.*
◆ If there is no reaction, the food can be considered safe.

Day 3

If you have had no adverse reactions, test the next food on the list in the manner described for Day 1. *If results of the Day 1 test are unclear:* Test the same food as on Day 1 again on Day 3 as follows:

◆ At midmorning, eat a *greater* quantity of the test food than eaten at midmorning on Day 1.
◆ Continue to double the quantity every four hours and monitor all reactions as described for Day 1.

Day 4

This is another monitoring day, observing for delayed reactions as described for Day 2. If you do not have an *increased* adverse reaction by the end of Day 4, the food can be considered safe. Continue in a similar fashion until you have tested all suspect foods.

Record all your responses (positive or negative) to each test food on the chart provided in Appendix 2 (page 442).

RETESTING OF REACTIVE FOODS

The problem food can be tested again after eliminating it for a period of not less than two months for a child under the age of five years; a period of not less than six months for an adult.

Sequence of Testing Foods

◆ Individual components of each food are tested separately.

◆ The sequence of testing in each category is very important because each test adds an extra ingredient to the previously tested food.

◆ The "test component" is highlighted as each is added in sequence.

◆ After testing the first food in a category, (for example, milk and milk products, grain, vegetable), you should continue testing the foods in that category, in the sequence specified until each has been tested and the limit of tolerance has been established.

◆ Do *not* switch between food categories.

QUANTITY OF THE TEST FOOD

◆ Quantities given are for an adult.

◆ When testing foods for a child between two and ten years, use smaller quantities as indicated in the testing instructions given below.

◆ For an infant under two years old, a different reintroduction protocol is used.[2]

TESTING FOR SENSITIVITY TO MILK AND MILK PRODUCTS

TEST 1
Challenge for casein proteins

Test food: WHITE HARD CHEESE, without bleach (benzoyl peroxide)
Suggested types: mozzarella, Parmesan
Use a block of about 5 ounces; for a child under 5 years, use 2–3 ounces.
Cut into 7 equal cubes.
Quantities for test:

Morning:	1 cube
Afternoon:	2 cubes
Evening:	4 cubes

Interpretation of Results of Test 1

◆ If there is no reaction after Day 2 (monitoring day), CASEIN PROTEINS are tolerated.

◆ If there is a reaction, casein proteins are not tolerated and Tests 2, 3, 4, and 6 should not be attempted, since all of these foods contain casein.

---

[2] See J. M. V. Joneja, *Dietary Management of Food Allergies and Intolerances: A Comprehensive Guide*, 2nd ed. (Vancouver: J. A. Hall Publications, 1998), pp. 245–266.

◆ Test 5 (plain yogurt) can be tried, since some people who do not tolerate casein can tolerate yogurt.

◆ A separate test for whey proteins can be attempted (Test 7, see below).

TEST 2
Challenge for casein, annatto (natural beta-carotene yellow dye), and biogenic amines

Test food: ORANGE OR YELLOW AGED CHEESE
Suggested types: aged (old or vintage) cheddar
Test exactly as described for Test 1 (white cheese).
Use a block of about 5 ounces; for a child under 5 years, use 2–3 ounces.
Cut into 7 equal cubes.
Quantities for test:

Morning:	1 cube
Afternoon:	2 cubes
Evening:	4 cubes

Interpretation of Results of Test 2

◆ If there is no reaction after Day 2 (monitoring day), ANNATTO and BIO-GENIC AMINES are tolerated, in addition to casein proteins.

◆ If there is a reaction, biogenic amines and/or annatto are the culprits.

◆ If the reaction is to the biogenic amines, headache and hives are the most common symptoms.

◆ Annatto is more likely to induce a skin reaction such as hives (urticaria) and other signs of allergy, especially in asthmatics, but rarely headache.

◆ Biogenic amines and annatto can be tested separately.

TEST 3
Challenge for casein and whey proteins

Test food: LACTASE TREATED MILK
Suggested: Purchased Lactaid milk or Lacteeze milk (99% lactose-free)
OR milk treated with Lactaid drops as follows:

◆ Add 15 drops to 1 liter of milk (skim, 1%, 2%, or homogenized).

◆ Leave treated milk in the refrigerator for 24 hours before the test to allow the enzyme (lactase) to break down the lactose.

Quantities for test:

	Adult	Child
Morning:	¼ cup	⅛ cup
Afternoon:	½ cup	¼ cup
Evening:	1 cup	½ cup

Interpretation of Results of Test 3

◆ If there is *no* reaction after Day 2 (monitoring day), CASEIN and WHEY PROTEINS are tolerated.

◆ If there *is* a reaction to Test 3, but not to Test 1: Casein proteins are tolerated, but whey proteins are not.

TEST 4
Challenge for casein proteins, whey proteins, and lactose

Test food: REGULAR MILK
Suggested: Skim *or* partially skimmed, *or* 1%, *or* 2%, *or* homogenized milk
Quantities for test:

	Adult	Child
Morning:	¼ cup	⅛ cup
Afternoon:	½ cup	¼ cup
Evening:	1 cup	½ cup

Interpretation of Results of Test 4

◆ If there is *no* reaction after Day 2 (monitoring day), both milk protein allergy and lactose intolerance have been ruled out.

◆ When lactose-intolerant people exceed their limit of tolerance, they will have gastrointestinal symptoms of gas, bloating, sometimes abdominal pain, and diarrhea. If gastrointestinal symptoms occur after Test 4, but not after any of the previous tests for milk components, lactose intolerance is confirmed.

NOTE
1 cup of homogenized (3.3% milk fat) milk contains 12.0 grams of lactose
1 cup of 2% or 1% milk contains 11.2 grams of lactose
1 cup of skim (non-fat) milk contains 10.8 grams of lactose

- A person who tolerates ¼ cup of milk will be able to tolerate lactose in food and beverages to a total of about 3 grams.
- If ½ cup of milk is tolerated, lactose to a level of 6 grams in food and beverages will be safe.
- If 1 cup of milk is tolerated, lactose to a level of 12 grams in food and beverages will be tolerated.

TEST 5
Challenge for modified ("partially digested") milk components

Test food: PLAIN YOGURT
Suggested: Natural yogurt with live bacterial culture, free from additional ingredients such as fruit, color, flavor, and preservatives
If the taste of plain yogurt is unacceptable, you can add honey and a tolerated cooked fruit.
Quantities for test:

	Adult	Child
Morning:	¼ cup	⅛ cup
Afternoon:	½ cup	¼ cup
Evening:	1 cup	½ cup

Interpretation of Results of Test 5

- If plain yogurt is tolerated, yogurt can be considered safe, even if milk is not ("failure" of Tests 1, 2, 3 or 4).
- Manufactured yogurts with additional ingredients such as fruits, nuts, grains, color, and flavor must be challenged in separate tests to determine whether the added ingredients are tolerated.
- If yogurt causes symptoms, milk proteins or lactose intolerance is confirmed, depending on the results of the previous tests for milk components.

YOGURT AND LACTOSE INTOLERANCE
One cup of plain yogurt contains 8.4 grams of lactose. However, because the yogurt bacteria *Lactobacillus bulgaricus* and *Streptococcus thermophilus* can survive for a short time in the bowel and produce enough beta-galactosidase enzyme to break down most of the remaining lactose, some lactose-intolerant people can tolerate yogurt containing "live bacterial culture."

TEST 6
Challenge for curdled milk with lactose and minimal bacterial fermentation

Test food: COTTAGE CHEESE

Suggested: Any type of pure cottage cheese *without* additional ingredients, including soft curd, creamed, 2% milk fat

Quantities for test:

	Adult	Child
Morning:	¼ cup	⅛ cup
Afternoon:	½ cup	¼ cup
Evening:	1 cup	½ cup

Interpretation of Results of Test 6

◆ Test 6 is a confirmatory challenge of the milk components tested in Tests 1 to 5.

◆ Cottage cheese contains casein and whey proteins and lactose, as well as partially modified forms of these components.

◆ It is recommended that people who like to eat a lot of cottage cheese should carry out this challenge to ensure that the milk components in the product are tolerated in this form.

◆ If any of the components in Tests 1 to 5 is not tolerated, it is unlikely that cottage cheese will be tolerated.

ADDITIONAL INFORMATION

◆ One cup of cottage cheese contains 7.2 grams of lactose.

◆ In the manufacture of cottage cheese, milk is curdled and a bacterial culture is added.

◆ In cottage cheese, the degree of fermentation due to the bacterial culture is significantly less than it is in cheese or yogurt.

TEST 7
Challenge for complete milk proteins and lactose in a complex product

Test Food: ICE CREAM

SUGGESTED: Pure cream ice cream, plain vanilla flavor

NOTE ON THE MANUFACTURE OF ICE CREAM

In the manufacture of ice cream, vanilla is made first, then the lighter colored ice creams are made, usually ending with chocolate. If the vats are not cleaned adequately between different batches, residues from the previous batches may contaminate the later ones. Chocolate ice cream therefore is likely to contain the *greatest* number of potential allergens and should be *tested only after all other flavors have been shown to be tolerated*. This is an important consideration if a person is highly allergic to nuts: The nut-flavored ice creams are usually made before the chocolate-flavored ones. Cheaper brands of ice cream contain a number of additives such as artificial and natural flavors, colors, preservatives, emulsifiers, and texture modifiers. If these are suspected to be triggers of adverse reactions, ice creams containing these additional ingredients should be *tested only after ice cream made from pure cream has been tolerated.*

Each flavor of ice cream should be challenged *separately* if vanilla ice cream is tolerated.

Quantities for test:

	Adult	Child
Morning:	¼ cup	⅛ cup
Afternoon:	½ cup	¼ cup
Evening:	1 cup	½ cup

TEST 8
Challenge for whey proteins and lactose when casein (Test 1) is not tolerated

Test food: WHEY POWDER
SUGGESTED: Whey ("petit lait") free from other milk solids. The food powder is available in most health food stores.

NOTE ON WHEY POWDER

◆ Whey is the fraction of milk that contains lactose: Challenge tests for whey proteins and lactose can be carried out on complete whey powder in two stages (Tests 8a and 8b):

— Test 8a is a test for whey proteins without lactose; the complete whey powder is treated with lactase to digest the lactose and make the product lactose-free.

— Test 8b is a test for lactose intolerance when whey proteins are tolerated.

◆ Some whey powders have been treated with lactase and are sold as lactose-free: Lactose-free whey may be used in place of the lactase-treated whey powder described in Test 8a.

TEST 8A
Challenge for whey free from lactose

1. Dissolve 3 tablespoons of whey powder in 3 cups of water (*or* 2.4 ounces of powder in 24 ounces of water; *or* 45 milligrams of powder in 450 milliliters of water).
2. Add 7 drops of lactase (Lactaid) (refer to measurements of Lactaid in Test 3 on page 352).
3. Place in fridge for 24 hours.
4. Test quantities as follows:

	Adult	Child
Morning:	½ cup	¼ cup
Afternoon:	1 cup	½ cup
Evening:	1½ cups	1 cup

Interpretation of Results of Test 8a

◆ If no symptoms are recorded, whey proteins are tolerated; proceed to Test 8b to test for lactose intolerance.

◆ If symptoms occur, whey proteins are not tolerated; Test 8b for lactose in whey should *not* be carried out.

TEST 8B
Challenge for whey with lactose

1. Dissolve 3 tablespoons of complete whey powder (containing lactose) in 3 cups of water (*or* 2.4 ounces of powder in 24 ounces of water; *or* 45 milligrams of powder in 450 milliliters of water).
2. Test quantities as follows:

	Adult	Child
Morning:	½ cup	¼ cup
Afternoon:	1 cup	½ cup
Evening:	1½ cups	1 cup

Interpretation of Results of Test 8b

◆ If lactose-free whey powder is tolerated (Test 8a), but digestive-tract symptoms occur after Test 8b, whey proteins are tolerated and lactose intolerance is confirmed.

◆ For a complete explanation of lactose intolerance, see interpretation of Test 4 on page 332.

TESTING FOR SENSITIVITY TO EGG

Egg yolk and egg white are tested *separately* because each part contains different proteins. Eggs from different species of birds may be challenged in separate tests

◆ Hard-boil the egg.
◆ Separate the yolk from the white.

TEST 1
Challenge for egg yolk

Quantities for test:

	Adult	Child
Morning:	½ yolk	½ teaspoon
Afternoon:	1 yolk	1 teaspoon
Evening:	2 yolks	2 teaspoons

TEST 2
Challenge for egg white

Test exactly as described for egg yolk.
Quantities for test:

	Adult	Child
Morning:	½ white	½ teaspoon
Afternoon:	1 white	1 teaspoon
Evening:	2 whites	2 teaspoons

Interpretation of Results of Egg Challenge

◆ If egg yolk, but not egg white, is tolerated (no adverse reaction to egg yolk), egg yolks *separated from the white* can be used in baking, in making omelets, and in other egg-containing dishes, but they *cannot* be used in dishes that require egg white only.

◆ Egg Beaters or other similar products that are made from egg white only (often advised in cholesterol-lowering diets) *cannot* be used if egg white is not tolerated.

◆ If the egg white (albumin) is tolerated, but egg yolk is not, egg whites, separated from the yolk, *can* be used in recipes. Egg Beaters, and other products made from egg white only, *can* be used.

◆ Egg replacers made from vegetable oils and other non-egg ingredients *can* be used if egg yolk and egg white are not tolerated.

TESTING FOR SENSITIVITY TO YEAST

Test food: *Saccharomyces* species: brewer's and baker's yeast
Suggested: Debittered brewer's yeast (available from health food stores)

Morning: Mix ¼ teaspoon of yeast powder in warm water. Add to any tolerated beverage, such as fruit juice, or to cooked fruit such as applesauce.

Afternoon: Mix ½ teaspoon of yeast powder in water and add to chosen beverage or food.

Evening: Mix 1 teaspoon of yeast powder in water and add to chosen beverage or food.

INTERPRETATION OF RESULTS OF YEAST CHALLENGE

◆ Symptoms may develop at any time during the two-day testing period.

◆ A reaction to *Saccharomyces* species does **not** indicate sensitivity to other fungi such as the pseudo yeast genus *Candida*, mushrooms, molds, and the hundreds of genera within the fungal kingdom.

◆ Each of these must be challenged separately to determine a person's reactivity to them.

◆ If brewer's yeast is tolerated, it may be consumed regularly as a good source of natural B vitamins.

CEREAL GRAINS

◆ Each cereal grain is reintroduced as a single food before being challenged as an ingredient in baked goods such as breads and crackers.

◆ Most grains can be obtained as a "bulk food," so a small quantity suitable for the test can be purchased without incurring the expense of buying a large quantity of something that may not be eaten again.

Wheat

TEST 1
Challenge for wheat in its purest form

Test food: Pure wheat cereal, without additives
Suggested: Puffed Wheat
               Or Shredded Wheat (without sugar coating or additives)
               Or wheat flakes (cooked in water)
               Or Cream of Wheat (cooked in water)

Fruit juice, Rice Dream, or a soy beverage may be added *if allowed during the elimination phase of the program.*

Quantities for test:

	Adult	Child
Morning:	¼ cup	⅛ cup
Afternoon:	½ cup	¼ cup
Evening:	1 cup	½ cup

TEST 2
Challenge for wheat flour with ingredients commonly included in baked products, but without yeast

Test food: Yeast-free wheat cracker
Suggested: Triscuit crackers
Quantities for test:

	Adult	Child
Morning:	2 crackers	1 cracker
Afternoon:	4 crackers	2 crackers
Evening:	8 crackers	4 crackers

TEST 3A
Challenge for white (wheat) flour without benzoyl peroxide

Test food: Unbleached white flour
Suggested: Homemade bread made with unbleached white flour, or a purchased loaf of white bread made from unbleached white flour
Quantities for test:

	Adult	Child
Morning:	½ slice	¼ slice
Afternoon:	1 slice	½ slice
Evening:	2 slices	1 slice

TEST 3B
Challenge for white (wheat) flour when sensitivity to benzoates is suspected

Test food: "Bleached" (regular) white flour with yeast in a baked product
Suggested: Commercial white bread
Quantities for test:

	Adult	Child
Morning:	½ slice	¼ slice
Afternoon:	1 slice	½ slice
Evening:	2 slices	1 slice

TEST 4
Challenge for complete wheat product

Test food: Whole-wheat flour, with yeast and the usual bakery ingredients
Suggested: Commercial whole-wheat bread
Quantities for test:

	Adult	Child
Morning:	½ slice	¼ slice
Afternoon:	1 slice	½ slice
Evening:	2 slices	1 slice

Other Grains

◆ Test each grain in its purest form first.
◆ Follow with baked goods made from the flour (e.g., bread, crackers).
◆ Use the method and quantities described above for wheat.

Oats
(1) Test food: Oatmeal
    Suggested food: Cooked natural oatmeal, made into a breakfast porridge
(2) Test food: Oat cake
    Suggested food: Scottish oat cake (wheat-free, made with oat flour)

Rye
(1) Test food: Rye grain
    Suggested food: Rye flakes cooked in water, made into a breakfast porridge
(2) Test food: Rye cracker
    Suggested food: Ryvita rye cracker or Wasa Light rye crispbread without wheat
(3) Test food: 100% rye flour
    Suggested food: Commercial 100% rye bread (available in specialized bakeries)

Barley
(1) Test food: Barley grain
    Suggested food: Pearl barley or barley flakes cooked in water or tolerated broth
(2) Test food: Barley flour
    Suggested food: Barley bread, made with barley flour, wheat-free

Quinoa
(1) Test food: Quinoa grain
    Suggested food: Quinoa flakes cooked in water, made into a breakfast porridge
(2) Test food: Quinoa flour
    Suggested food: quinoa pasta or quinoa bread without wheat

Buckwheat
(1) Buckwheat grain
    Suggested food: Buckwheat groats
(2) Buckwheat flour
    Suggested food: Buckwheat pasta (soba); or buckwheat pancake without wheat

Corn

◆ Because corn is eaten in various ways such as the whole grain as a vegetable, and derivatives of corn are used as ingredients in the form of corn oil, corn syrup, cornstarch, corn flour, and cornmeal, it may be necessary to challenge each separately.

◆ Not all components of corn have the same potential for triggering adverse reactions.

◆ Thus it is important to assess a person's tolerance of each component.

◆ If whole corn is not tolerated, it is especially important to challenge corn derivatives because they are used in numerous manufactured foods.

◆ Eliminating corn from the diet is relatively simple and usually poses no nutritional risk; however, restricting all foods containing ingredients derived from corn can make life difficult, and it may lead to nutritional deficiency because so many convenience foods contain ingredients derived from corn.

◆ If corn derivatives are proven to be safe, it will make dietary choices much easier.

(1) Test food: Corn grain as a vegetable
Suggested: Corn on the cob (cooked)

	Adult	Child
Morning:	¼ cob	⅛ cob
Afternoon:	½ cob	¼ cob
Evening:	1 cob	½ cob

OR Frozen or canned corn niblets, cooked and served without additional ingredients such as butter:

	Adult	Child
Morning:	1 tablespoon	1 teaspoon
Afternoon:	2 tablespoons	2 teaspoons
Evening:	4 tablespoons	4 teaspoons

(2) Test food: Processed whole corn
Suggested food: Popcorn (use quantities as for corn niblets)

(3) Test food: Cornmeal
Suggested food: Cornmeal bread (use quantities as described for wheat bread, above)

(4) Test food: Cornstarch or corn flour
Suggested: Use as a thickener in gravy made from meat drippings, in which all the other ingredients are known and tolerated.

(5) Test food: Corn oil
Suggested: Add to pasta or a salad with known and tolerated ingredients.

6) Test food: Corn syrup
Suggested: Pour over pancakes made from known and tolerated ingredients.

Soy

◆ Soy is consumed in a number of different forms, for example:
   — Tofu (soy protein coagulated—not fermented—with calcium or magnesium sulfate)
   — Soy beverage ("soy milk") made from (usually) uncooked ground soybeans diluted with water
   — Soy sauce (fermented soy usually with wheat added)
   — Tamari sauce (fermented soy without wheat)
◆ It is important that each form of soy is challenged separately.
◆ The following schedule of challenge tests will evaluate a person's reactivity to each of these forms of soy.

TEST 1

Test food: Tofu, cooked
Suggested: Extra firm tofu cut into cubes, deep-fried in olive, safflower, or canola oil and drained
Use large cubes (2-inch cubes) for an adult; smaller (1-inch cubes) for a child.
Quantities for test:

Morning: 1 cube
Afternoon: 2 cubes
Evening: 4 cubes

TEST 2

Test food: Soy beverage
Suggested: Commercial soy "milk"

Quantities for test:

	Adult	Child
Morning:	¼ cup	⅛ cup
Afternoon:	½ cup	¼ cup
Evening:	1 cup	½ cup

TEST 3

Test food: Fermented soy derivative without wheat
Suggested: Tamari sauce; may be added to any known tolerated food
Quantities for test:

	Adult	Child
Morning:	1 teaspoon	½ teaspoon
Afternoon:	2 teaspoons	1 teaspoon
Evening:	4 teaspoons	2 teaspoons

TEST 4

Test food: Fermented soy sauce
Suggested: "Regular" soy sauce; may be added to any known tolerated food
Quantities for test:

	Adult	Child
Morning:	1 teaspoon	½ teaspoon
Afternoon:	2 teaspoons	1 teaspoon
Evening:	4 teaspoons	2 teaspoons

TESTING FOR SENSITIVITY TO FRUITS AND VEGETABLES

◆ Heat can change the allergenicity of vegetables and fruits.
◆ The cooked form is usually less allergenic, and thus better tolerated, than the raw form.
◆ When challenging vegetables and fruits, test the cooked form first, and follow with the food in its raw state.

Fruits

◆ The heat generated in the canning process is usually sufficient to change the allergenicity of the food, so fruit canned in its own juice can be challenged as "cooked."

◆ Alternatively, fruits can be "poached" by boiling in a little water, or cooked into a puree (for example, cooking apples into "applesauce") but without any added ingredient, such as sugar.

ORANGE

TEST 1

Test food: Cooked orange
Suggested: Canned mandarin orange
Quantities for test:

	Adult	Child
Morning:	2 sections	1 section
Afternoon:	4 sections	2 sections
Evening:	8 sections	4 sections

TEST 2

Test food: Raw orange
Suggested food: Fresh mandarin orange
Quantities for test:

	Adult	Child
Morning:	2 sections	1 section
Afternoon:	4 sections	2 sections
Evening:	8 sections	4 sections

TEST 3

Test food: Raw orange of a different variety than in Test 2 above
Suggested: Fresh navel orange
Quantities for test:

	Adult	Child
Morning:	2 sections	1 section
Afternoon:	4 sections	2 sections
Evening:	8 sections	4 sections

GRAPEFRUIT
Test food: (1) Cooked or canned grapefruit
          (2) Raw grapefruit
Challenge exactly as described for oranges in Tests 1, 2, and 3 above.

GRAPES
- Wash grapes well before testing, preferably with a detergent made for washing foods, to remove surface molds.
- Sulfites used as a preservative will not be removed entirely by washing.
- People sensitive to sulfites should *not* eat grapes.
- Because grapes are not usually eaten cooked, they may be challenged in the raw state only.

Quantities for test:

	Adult	Child
Morning:	2 grapes	1 grape
Afternoon:	4 grapes	2 grapes
Evening:	8 grapes	4 grapes

RAISINS
- Raisins (dried grapes) purchased in the grocery store or supermarket are raw.
- However, raisins are often eaten cooked in cakes, cookies, and other baked goods, whereas grapes are not.
- Occasionally a person will tolerate cooked raisins but will react adversely to raw raisins.
- It is wise to challenge cooked raisins before trying them raw.
- Most commercially produced raisins contain sulfite, which is added as a preservative.
- If sulfite sensitivity is suspected, nonsulfited raisins, available in health food stores, should be challenged before the sulfited kind.
- If non-sulfited raisins are tolerated, sulfited raisins should then be challenged.
- If sensitivity to raisins is suspected, raisins should be tested in the following sequence:
  1. nonsulfited cooked raisins
  2. nonsulfited raw raisins
  3. sulfited raw raisins

Raisins can be cooked by placing them in a little water to cover, then bringing them to a boil on the stove or in a microwave oven. Two minutes of boiling are usually sufficient to cook them.

◆ This sequence of testing will determine whether the person is
   1. sensitive to cooked raisins
   2. sensitive to raw raisins
   3. sensitive to sulfites
◆ For each challenge, the following quantities of raisins are suitable:

	Adult	Child
Morning:	¼ cup	⅛ cup
Afternoon:	½ cup	¼ cup
Evening:	1 cup	½ cup

APPLE
Test 1 Test food: Cooked apple

Boil
◆ Core and slice one large or two medium apples.
◆ Place in a saucepan with a little water and bring to a boil.
◆ Reduce heat and simmer until the apple is soft and mushy.

Microwave
◆ Alternatively, place cored, peeled, sliced apple into a covered dish.
◆ Microwave on high for five minutes.

Quantities for test:

	Adult	Child
Morning:	¼ cup	⅛ cup
Afternoon:	½ cup	¼ cup
Evening:	1 cup	½ cup

TEST 2

Test food: Raw apple

◆ Peel and core apple.
◆ For an adult, use a whole apple.
◆ For a child, use half an apple.
◆ Cut into seven equal slices.

Morning:	1 slice
Afternoon	2 slices
Evening:	4 slices

Vegetables

♦ Cook until the vegetable is soft and "limp"; for most vegetables, choose one of the following methods of cooking:
  — 5 to 7 minutes on high in a microwave oven
  — 15 to 20 minutes boiled in water
  — 20 to 30 minutes roasted in an oven at 400°F (200°C)
♦ This is usually enough to change the structure of the molecules sufficiently for the food to be tolerated.
♦ Make sure that the vegetable is cooked all the way through; if it isn't, the raw, uncooked center might cause an adverse reaction.
♦ Adjust the times given above to ensure thorough cooking.
♦ A few representative examples of challenge tests for vegetables are provided below.
♦ Test each type of vegetable separately.
♦ Adjust cooking times and quantities if necessary, depending on the characteristics of the vegetables being tested.

TOMATO
♦ Eat without dressing.

TEST 1
Challenge for cooked or canned tomato
without additional ingredients

Quantities for an adult:

Morning:	¼ tomato	or 2 slices cooked	¼ cup
Afternoon:	½ tomato	or 4 slices cooked	½ cup
Evening:	1 tomato	or 8 slices cooked	1 cup

Quantities for a child:

Morning:	⅛ tomato	or 1 slice cooked	⅛ cup
Afternoon:	¼ tomato	or 2 slices cooked	¼ cup
Evening:	½ tomato	or 4 slices cooked	½ cup

TEST 2
Challenge for raw tomato

Quantities for an adult:

Morning:	¼ tomato	or 2 slices	¼ cup
Afternoon:	½ tomato	or 4 slices	½ cup
Evening:	1 tomato	or 8 slices	1 cup

Quantities for a child:

Morning:	⅛ tomato	or 1 slice cooked	⅛ cup
Afternoon:	¼ tomato	or 2 slices cooked	¼ cup
Evening:	½ tomato	or 4 slices cooked	½ cup

TEST 3
Challenge for tomato ketchup

Test food: Commercial tomato ketchup
Carrier food: French fries (if tolerated)

◆ Ensure that the specified amount of ketchup is consumed.
◆ The number of french fries is unlimited.

Quantities for test:

	Adult	Child
Morning:	1 tablespoon	½ tablespoon
Afternoon:	2 tablespoons	1 tablespoon
Evening:	4 tablespoons	2 tablespoons

SPINACH

TEST 1
Challenge for cooked spinach

Test food: Raw or frozen spinach leaves

◆ Cook in a little water until leaves are limp and soft.

Quantities for test:

	Adult	Child
Morning:	¼ cup	⅛ cup
Afternoon:	½ cup	¼ cup
Evening:	1 cup	½ cup

TEST 2
Challenge for raw spinach

Eat as a salad vegetable with only tolerated ingredients if a dressing is used.

Quantities for test:

	Adult	Child
Morning:	¼ cup	⅛ cup
Afternoon:	½ cup	¼ cup
Evening:	1 cup	½ cup

OTHER FRUITS AND VEGETABLES

◆ Test each separately as described above.
◆ Adjust cooking times and quantities according to the characteristics of the food.

Juices

◆ Test cooked juice *before* testing the fresh, raw product.
◆ Fruit or vegetable juice can be heated in the microwave, or brought to boiling on the stove and cooled before drinking.
◆ Pasteurized juices will have been heated sufficiently to change the allergenicity of the fruit or vegetable antigens; pasteurized juices can be challenged in place of cooked juices.

LEMON OR LIME
◆ Squeeze juice from a fresh fruit into 2 glasses of water.
◆ Add honey or sugar to taste.

Quantities for test:

	Adult	Child
Morning:	Juice from ¼ fruit (½ glass)	Juice from ⅛ fruit (¼ glass)
Afternoon:	Juice from ½ fruit (1 glass)	Juice from ¼ fruit (½ glass)
Evening:	Juice from 1 fruit (2 glasses)	Juice from ½ fruit (1 glass)

OTHER FRUIT OR VEGETABLE JUICES (APPLE, ORANGE, CARROT, ETC.)

Quantities for test:

	Adult	Child
Morning:	¼ cup	⅛ cup
Afternoon:	½ cup	¼ cup
Evening:	1 cup	½ cup

VINEGAR

◆ Add to a tolerated carrier food such as french fries, salad vegetables, or the like.

◆ Any type of vinegar may be used.

◆ However, it is a good idea to start with distilled (white) vinegar and to test different types separately.

◆ Other types may include balsamic, rice, apple cider, and wine vinegars.

Vinegars containing herbs (e.g., tarragon, dill) should be challenged *only* when the herb or additional components (e.g., cranberry) are known to be tolerated.

Quantities for test:

	Adult	Child
Morning	1 tablespoon	½ tablespoon
Afternoon	2 tablespoons	1 tablespoon
Evening	4 tablespoons	2 tablespoons

Legumes

PEANUT

TEST 1
Challenge for cooked peanuts

◆ Roasted without added ingredients such as artificial barbecue flavor, etc

◆ Or: boiled peanuts

Quantities for test:

	Adult	Child
Morning:	4 peanuts	2 peanuts
Afternoon:	8 peanuts	4 peanuts
Evening:	16 peanuts	8 peanuts

TEST 2
Challenge for raw peanuts

◆   Eat after shelling.

Quantities for test:

	Adult	Child
Morning:	4 peanuts	2 peanuts
Afternoon:	8 peanuts	4 peanuts
Evening:	16 peanuts	8 peanuts

PEAS, DRIED PEAS, AND DRIED BEANS

TEST 1
Challenge for cooked peas and beans of any type with skins

These include peas and beans such as navy beans, green peas, pinto beans, dried peas, kidney beans, black-eyed peas, soybeans, and mung beans

Quantities for test:

	Adult	Child
Morning:	½ cup	¼ cup
Afternoon:	1 cup	½ cup
Evening:	1½–2 cups	up to 1 cup

TEST 2
Challenge for raw legumes

If legumes are sometimes eaten raw (e.g., green peas), challenge separately after testing them cooked.

BEAN SPROUTS

◆ Sprouting changes the composition of the bean.

◆ Bean sprouts are eaten cooked (as in stir-fries) or, more commonly, raw.

◆ Both cooked and raw sprouts from any beans should be challenged separately.

Quantities for testing cooked and raw sprouts:

	Adult	Child
Morning:	¼ cup	⅛ cup
Afternoon:	½ cup	¼ cup
Evening:	1 cup	½ cup

◆ Challenge sprouts from grains (such as wheat) and seeds (such as alfalfa) in the same way.

Nuts

◆ Nuts are the reproductive parts of trees of many unrelated species.

◆ Allergy to nuts from one species of tree does *not* indicate that nuts from botanically unrelated trees will cause allergy.

◆ Each type of nut should be challenged individually, for example, almond, cashew, chestnut, walnut, pistachio, hazelnut (filbert), pecan, macadamia, pine nut (pignoli), brazil nut, and coconut.

TEST 1
Challenge for cooked nuts

Suggested: Roasted nuts without additional ingredients such as artificial flavor, color, or preservatives

TEST 2
Challenge for raw nuts from the shell

Quantities for testing cooked and raw nuts:

	Adult	Child
Morning:	1 tablespoon	1 teaspoon
Afternoon:	2 tablespoons	2 teaspoons
Evening:	4 tablespoons	4 teaspoons

Seeds

Test food: Seeds, roasted, followed by raw if appropriate, without additional ingredients
Suggested seeds: sesame, sunflower, poppy, flax, pumpkin, or melon

Quantities for test:

	Adult	Child
Morning:	½ tablespoon	½ teaspoon
Afternoon:	1 tablespoon	1 teaspoon
Evening:	2 tablespoons	2 teaspoons

TESTING FOR SENSITIVITY TO MEAT AND POULTRY

◆ The easiest way to challenge meat of any animal and poultry is to start with pure ground meat, without additives such as preservatives, colors, or flavors. Ensure that no nitrates or nitrites have been added to preserve the color.
◆ Cook the meat well in a microwave, oven, or frying pan.
◆ Pour off excess fat and discard.
◆ The meat may then be consumed as a patty, or crumbled.

Quantities for test:

	Adult	Child
Morning	1 ounce (30 grams)	½ ounce (15 grams)
Afternoon	2 ounces (60 grams)	1 ounce (30 grams)
Evening	4 ounces (120 grams)	2 ounces (60 grams)

Processed Meats

TEST 1
Challenge for sliced meats

Suggested: Slices of any manufactured meats such as pepperoni, cured or smoked bacon, salami, cured or smoked ham, bologna, or summer sausage

Quantities for test:

	Adult	Child
Morning	2 slices	1 slice
Afternoon	4 slices	2 slices
Evening	8 slices	4 slices

TEST 2
Challenge for sausages

Suggested: Frankfurters, weiners, or other sausages

Quantities for test:

	Adult	Child
Morning	1 sausage	½ sausage
Afternoon	2 sausages	1 sausage
Evening	4 sausages	2 sausages

Note: "Sausage" refers to the small-size weiner. Cut "large" or "jumbo" size into the size of a small weiner.

Fish

TEST 1
Challenge for plain cooked fish without breading or batter

These include fish such as cod, perch, halibut, sole, salmon, mackerel, red snapper, tuna, or sea bass

TEST 2
Challenge for fish canned in water or oil, but without spices or sauce

These include fish such as tuna, sardines, salmon, or pilchards

Quantities for tests 1 and 2:

	Adult	Child
Morning	1 ounce (30 grams)	½ ounce (15 grams)
Afternoon	2 ounces (60 grams)	1 ounce (30 grams)
Evening	4 ounces (120 grams)	2 ounces (60 grams)

Shellfish

◆ Test cooked fish before testing it raw.
◆ Canned shellfish is cooked, so it can be eaten from the can.
◆ Amounts depend on the type of shellfish being tested.
◆ The following quantities are meant as guidelines.

TEST 1
Challenge for large shellfish such as crab, crayfish (crawfish), or lobster

Quantities for test:

	Adult	Child
	Adult	Child
Morning	1 ounce (30 grams)	½ ounce (15 grams)
Afternoon	2 ounces (60 grams)	1 ounce (30 grams)
Evening	4 ounces (120 grams)	2 ounces (60 grams)

TEST 2
Challenge for individual shellfish such as shrimp, mussel, prawn, clam, oyster, or scallop

Quantities for test:

	Adult	Child
	Adult	Child
Morning	4 fish	2 fish
Afternoon	8 fish	4 fish
Evening	16 fish	8 fish

TESTING FOR SENSITIVITY TO SUGARS

◆ Sensitivity to specific sugars can be due to several causes such as inborn errors of metabolism (e.g., abnormal galactose transport and metabolism, abnormal fructose metabolism); conditions involving abnormal regulation of serum levels of glucose such as hypoglycemia, hyperglycemia, and diabetes; and to allergy.
◆ If a person is *allergic* to sugar, it is the protein from the particular plant from which the sugar is derived that is the source of the allergen.
◆ In order to determine which sugar source causes the allergic symptoms, each is challenged separately.

◆ The instructions below are designed strictly and exclusively for determining whether a person is allergic to a specific sugar.

◆ The same quantity of sugar is consumed in each test. If desired, the sugar can be added to half a cup of warm water.

Quantities for test:

	Adult	Child
Morning:	1 teaspoon	½ teaspoon
Afternoon:	2 teaspoons	1 teaspoon
Evening:	4 teaspoons	2 teaspoons

Suggested sugars to be challenged individually:

◆ Maple sugar or maple syrup
◆ Cane sugar
◆ Beet sugar
◆ Corn sugar or corn syrup
◆ Date sugar
◆ Fructose (fruit sugar; sometimes called levulose)
◆ Honey (glucose and fructose)

Note on Allergy to Honey

◆ *Pollen Allergy*

If a person is allergic to the pollen of the plant from which the honey is derived, eating the honey may cause symptoms, whereas honey from a different plant may be tolerated. For example, alfalfa honey may cause an allergic reaction when clover honey is tolerated.

◆ *Bee Sting Allergy*

There is no evidence that allergy to bee sting is associated with allergy to honey. Bee venom is injected directly into the bloodstream during a bee sting, whereas the honey is eaten and undergoes digestion before entering the circulation. In any case, it is extremely unlikely that honey would contain any bee venom.

TESTING FOR SENSITIVITY TO ALCOHOLIC BEVERAGES

◆ Alcoholic beverages are usually consumed in the evening.
◆ The patient should consume the amount to which he or she is accustomed.
◆ Test each type of drink in this order:

1. Distilled alcohol (to test reactivity to alcohol alone): vodka, white rum, gin, or tequila. Mix with boiled and cooled fruit juice to taste, if desired.
2. White wine (to test sensitivity to biogenic amines, particularly histamine)
3. Red wine (to test sensitivity to biogenic amines, particularly histamine and tyramine)
4. Lager, beer, ale (to test sensitivity to fermented grains as well as histamine and tyramine)
5. Cider (to test sensitivity to fermented fruit, usually apple)

TESTING FOR SENSITIVITY TO TEA and COFFEE

◆ Tea and coffee contain caffeine.
◆ Both tea and coffee contain hundreds of potentially reactive chemicals in addition to caffeine.
◆ Challenge of decaffeinated tea and coffee will give some indication of a person's reactivity to the additional components of the beverages, but a complicating factor is introduced by the chemicals used in extracting caffeine.
◆ When the largest consumption of caffeine occurs in the evening, additional symptoms such as sleeplessness will appear.
◆ To minimize the effects of caffeine, challenge tea, coffee, and other beverages containing caffeine (e.g., colas) in a modified introduction schedule that does not entail increasing the dosage over a single day.
◆ During the modified reintroduction, increasing doses of the test beverage will be consumed in the morning on three successive days as follows:

	Adult	Child
Day 1	½ cup	¼ cup
Day 2	1 cup	½ cup
Day 3	2 cups or more	1 cup

Tea

Challenge each type of tea separately, for example, herbal tea, decaffeinated regular (black) tea, green tea, and regular (black) tea.

◆ Prepare tea as usual.
◆ Add ingredients such as milk and sugar only if they are tolerated.
◆ Do not add any spices unless they have been challenged and tolerated.

Coffee

TEST 1
Challenge for decaffeinated coffee

TEST 2
Challenge for regular coffee

◆ Prepare coffee as usual.
◆ Add ingredients such as milk and sugar only if they are tolerated.
◆ Do not use any flavored coffees until regular coffee has been challenged and tolerated.
◆ Coffee is not recommended for children under the age of five.

TESTING FOR SENSITIVITY TO CHOCOLATE

TEST 1
Challenge for pure chocolate

◆ Test food: Dark, bitter, baker's chocolate in blocks or chips.
◆ Melt in a pan over low heat.
◆ Add honey (if tolerated), sugar (if tolerated), or powdered fruit sugar (fructose) to taste.
◆ Pour onto a cookie sheet or baking tray.
◆ Place in the fridge to solidify.
◆ Break into pieces about one inch square.
◆ Eat one square in the morning, two in the afternoon, four in the evening.
◆ If any symptoms occur, stop eating chocolate and record reactions.

TEST 2
Challenge for milk chocolate (test only if milk is tolerated)

◆ Melt baker's chocolate as above.
◆ Add honey, fructose, or sugar as tolerated.
◆ Add powdered milk (1, 2, or 3 tablespoons depending on the amount of baker's chocolate in the pan) and stir until mixture is smooth and well mixed.
◆ Pour onto a cookie sheet or baking tray and proceed as for baker's chocolate test above.

TEST 3
Challenge for purchased chocolates

◆ Start with preservative-free pure chocolates, without fruit, nut, or other fillings.
◆ Test those with complex ingredients only when the additional ingredients have been shown to be tolerated by appropriate challenge tests.

TESTING FOR SENSITIVITY TO SPICES

◆ Spices are tested by adding appropriate quantities to a tolerated food.
◆ Some suggestions for "carrier foods" are provided.
◆ If the suggested carrier foods are not tolerated, substitute one that is.

TEST 1
Challenge for cinnamon (also a test for benzoates)

Carrier food: Homemade apple sauce sweetened with honey
Ingredients:
— One fresh apple that is peeled, cored, and sliced
— ½ cup water
— Honey or other sweetener as tolerated, to taste

◆ Place apples, water, and sweetener in a pan.
◆ Heat to boiling.
◆ Reduce heat and simmer for a few minutes until apple is soft.
◆ Add powdered (ground) spice to hot or cooled applesauce, as preferred.
◆ If apples are not tolerated, substitute pears or any tolerated fruit and cook as above.

Quantities for test:

Morning: 3 teaspoon cinnamon
Afternoon: 2 teaspoon cinnamon
Evening: 1 teaspoon cinnamon

TEST 2
Challenge for other spices that are frequently used in baked goods

Challenge in the same way as described for cinnamon (above).
Suggested: nutmeg, anise, allspice, carraway seed

TEST 3
Challenge for mixed spices

Curry spice (mixture)
Carrier food: Cooked tomatoes
Ingredients: Fresh tomato, peeled and diced

- Place tomato with any juice into a pan. Add a small amount of water to prevent burning.
- Bring to a boil, reduce heat, and simmer until tomato is soft.
- Add spice to hot cooked tomato.
- If tomato is not tolerated, substitute mango or any other tolerated fruit or vegetable.

Quantities for test:

Morning: ½ teaspoon spice
Afternoon: 1 teaspoon spice
Evening: 2 teaspoons spice

Individual spices
If curry powder is not tolerated, each spice in the mixture can be tested separately.

- Prepare carrier food as above (tomato, mango, or tolerated fruit or vegetable).
- Add each of the powdered (ground) spices to be tested *individually.*
- Use quantities as instructed for cinnamon (above).
- *Do not mix spices* until each has been tested and tolerated separately: turmeric, cumin, coriander, cayenne, ginger, clove, mace, cardamom.

Chili spice (mixture)
Test as described for curry spice mixture, Test 3 above. If chili spice is not tolerated, test each spice separately, as described above: cayenne, cumin, paprika, onion powder.

TESTING FOR SENSITIVITY TO ADDITIVES IN MANUFACTURED FOODS

Testing for food additive sensitivity is complicated by the fact that usually several different chemicals, such as flavor and texture modifiers, color, and preservatives, are added simultaneously to a manufactured food. It is not easy to obtain the additive in its pure form, or even to find it as a single additive in a manufactured food.

For home challenge tests, foods containing additives in the form and quantity in which they would normally be eaten are used as the test component. A food containing a high level of the suspect additive is compared to the results of challenge with the same food without the additive.

TARTRAZINE
◆ Kraft Macaroni and Cheese dinner contains tartrazine.
◆ Compare reactions to the manufactured product with a similar homemade meal *without* tartrazine, using cheddar cheese, which has a similar color, but contains the natural yellow color annatto instead.

BENZOATES
◆ Cinnamon contains a high level of naturally occurring benzoate; test applesauce with cinnamon, in the schedule outlined earlier for "spices."
◆ Compare to reactions after eating the same quantity of applesauce without the spice.

SULFITES
1. Test regular (sulfited) dried fruit (e.g., raisins, dried apricots, pears, peaches, apples) in comparison to nonsulfited dried fruit, which can be obtained in some specialty health food stores.
2. Wine and regular beer contain sulfites; test these in comparison to a wine or beer without the preservative.
   — Alcoholic beverages that have no added sulfites will usually be labeled "preservative-free."
   — In the United States, an alcoholic beverage that does contain added sulfites will have "sulfite" on the label. Choose a beverage that does *not* have a label reference to "sulfite" and compare it to the reaction after drinking the same type of beverage containing sulfite.
   —In Canada, government regulations do not require disclosure of any ingredients in alcoholic beverages, so "sulfite" will not appear on the label.

NITRATES AND NITRITES
◆ Test additive-free beef in comparison to a beef steak to which nitrates have been added to preserve color.
◆ Ask the butcher or supplier which meats have added nitrates or nitrites to preserve the red color while the meat is on display in the store under fluorescent lights.

Monosodium Glutamate (MSG)

◆   MSG can be obtained as a flavor enhancer in some specialty stores.
◆   Test food with and without MSG to determine sensitivity.
◆   Carrier food, as tolerated (minced chicken, turkey, beef; homemade sauces).
◆   Add MSG powder in increasing doses as follows:

Morning:	¼ teaspoon
Afternoon:	½ teaspoon
Evening:	1 teaspoon

— CHAPTER 29 —

THE FINAL DIET

When you identify all of the food components involved in your food-related reactions, it is time to formulate the diet that will allow you to remain symptom-free and, at the same time, to be well-nourished and nutritionally healthy. There are several essential goals that must be met in order for you to obtain the greatest benefit from your diet. This is an important step in the management program because if it becomes difficult to comply with the dietary strategies, you will lapse into eating the "reactive foods." Eventually, the diet will be virtually abandoned, and when your symptoms recur, you will be convinced that the whole exercise was a waste of time! Therefore, the diet should aim to meet several important goals:

- ◆ It must *exclude* all foods and additives to which a positive reaction has been recorded.
- ◆ It must be nutritionally *complete*, providing nutrients from non-reactive sources.
- ◆ It must be designed to take into account your lifestyle and finances.
- ◆ It should be flexible enough to accommodate "unusual" situations such as religious festivals, celebrations (e.g., as birthdays and weddings), vacations, travel, and eating in social settings where obtaining substitute foods might be a problem.

If dose-related intolerances are a problem, a rotation diet (described in this chapter) might be beneficial. However, at the present time there is no clear consensus on the benefits of rotation diets in the management of food allergies, although many practitioners seem to favor their use, and there are a number of popular books on the market that provide details about a variety of rotation diets and schedules.

Rotation Diets

The premise behind the use of the rotation diet holds that people who are mildly intolerant to certain foods may benefit from a diet that spaces those foods so that no one of them is eaten too frequently. Theoretically, if the foods that cause a reaction are not allowed to "build up" in the body, a person's "limit of tolerance" is not exceeded and symptoms do not occur or are kept to a minimum. In the "traditional" rotation diet, a food that is eaten on Day 1 is then avoided for from 3 to 30 days, depending on the type of rotation selected. The aim is to give the body a rest from each food family to prevent new or increased sensitivity to food developing. Four, five, seven, and thirty-one day rotations have been advised by various practitioners. Because two to four days is the approximate time for a food to pass through the gastrointestinal tract, a four-day rotation is considered to be the most effective schedule. After four days, the amount of a specific food in the body is considered to be sufficiently low that eating it again will not increase the level to a reactive threshold.

Rotation Diets and Food Allergy

There have been no well-designed controlled studies on whether rotation diets based on food families are of any real value in practice. In fact, most authorities consider rotation diets as a management strategy for food allergy to be controversial and of little or no benefit. Because cross-reactivity between foods within a food family is unusual, diets that are based on avoiding entire food families are illogical. Furthermore, following a strict rotation diet can be very tedious and time-consuming, and it can put a person at risk for nutritional deficiency.

Rotation Diets and Food Intolerance

In situations where the reason for an adverse response to foods is due to a non-immunologically mediated reaction, limiting the quantity of *all* foods containing the reactive component does make sense. In situations of enzyme deficiency, such as lack of lactase, consumption of a greater quantity of the enzyme substrate (in this case, lactose) than the enzyme is capable of processing will lead to the development of the symptoms of intolerance. A diet that *restricts* the intake of all lactose-containing foods will ensure that the limit of tolerance is not exceeded, and the patient can remain symptom-free. A similar situation probably exists for most food intolerances, so a type of "rotation diet" that restricts the number and quantity of foods known to contain the culprit component is necessary. Such diets need to be formulated on an individual basis to ensure that the "dose" of the reactive component is reduced to a minimum, while nutrients equivalent to those eliminated are supplied by alternative foods.[1]

THE FINAL DIET

While a person is focusing on the foods that are causing adverse reactions, and following often complex restrictive elimination diets, it is easy to lose sight of the most fundamental principle of dietary practice: Good health can be achieved and maintained only by providing the body with all of the macro- and micronutrients essential for its optimal functioning. At each stage of the process of determining the foods that are responsible for a person's adverse reactions, complete balanced nutrition must be provided, preferably from foods but, if this is not entirely possible, by adding appropriate supplements.

When the culprit food components and additives have been identified, a maintenance diet must be formulated that removes the reactive foods and supplies complete balanced nutrition from alternative sources. Because you will need to follow this diet for the long term, it is extremely important that it supply *every* essential nutrient, but at the same time be appropriate for your lifestyle and fit within your budget. If a diet is difficult to follow because of its emphasis on foods that are unacceptable to you; if it requires you to spend excessive time, money, and effort, or if it is inappropriate for your lifestyle, it will soon be abandoned. All of the effort and energy invested in identifying the culprit foods will have been wasted, and you will be left with the same degree of distress as before. Formulating the appropriate diet for your particular needs therefore requires a great deal of time and effort. This process is best achieved with the help of trained professionals, preferably your doctor and a registered dietician.

Ensuring That All the Essential Nutrients Are Present

The process of planning the ideal diet in each particular case starts with the identification of the nutrients that may be deficient when specific foods are removed,

---

[1] J. M. V. Joneja, *Dietary Management of Food Allergies and Intolerances: A Comprehensive Guide,* 2nd ed. (Vancouver, B. C.: J. A. Hall Publications, 1998).

and correcting the deficiency by substitution of different foods containing the same nutrients. The following guidelines will aid in this process. Tables 29-1 to 29-5 provide data that will help in formulating a nutritionally complete diet while eliminating the allergenic foods.

DIET FOR OPTIMAL NUTRITION

The most important directive is this: Consume a nutritionally balanced diet that supplies all required macronutrients (protein, fat, carbohydrate) and micronutrients (vitamins and trace minerals) *every day.*

To simplify the process, *each meal* should contain three components:

1. Protein (PRO)
2. Grain (GR) or Starch (ST)
3. Fruit and/or Vegetable (FR/VEG)

Supplements

When a food category supplying essential micronutrients (vitamins and minerals) needs to be restricted, supplemental sources of the nutrients should be provided. For example:

Multivitamin/mineral: You can take a multivitamin/mineral with iron once a day. The supplement should be free from artificial color, flavor, preservatives, and additional ingredients *if they are restricted in the diet* such as wheat, yeast, corn, lactose, sugar, salt. If histamine intolerance is a problem, the multivitamin should also be free from *niacin*. You will find multivitamins that replace niacin with *niacinamide*. This is acceptable. Recommended brands include (but are not restricted to) Quest, Jamieson, Nulife, Nutricology, Natural Factors, and Sisu. *Note:* These manufacturers also make supplements that do not conform to these recommendations, and other companies not listed here market suitable products. *Read all labels carefully* in order to find the right supplement for your needs.

Calcium: When all milk and milk products are restricted, you can take calcium gluconate, or calcium citrate, or calcium carbonate with Kreb's cycle derivatives according to recommended levels. See Table 29-2, which gives the Dietary Reference Intake (DRI) values for calcium and vitamin D. Dietary Reference Intake is the amount of a nutrient that has been deemed essential for good health, based on statistical analysis of all relevant research data.

Table 29-1
THE BALANCED DIET: EXAMPLES OF FOODS IN EACH IMPORTANT FOOD CATEGORY

Protein Foods

- Meat of all types
- Poultry
- Fish
- Shellfish
- Eggs
- Nuts
- Seeds
- Tofu
- Milk
- Milk products such as
  - Cheese of all types
  - Yogurt
  - Buttermilk

Grains (GR)

Grains should be whole grains as often as possible
- Wheat
- Rye
- Oats
- Barley
- Rice
- Corn
- Amaranth
- Quinoa
- Buckwheat
- Millet
- Varieties and derivatives of wheat such as
  - Spelt
  - Kamut
  - Bulgur
  - Triticale
  - Semolina

Starches (ST)

- Flours and starches derived from grains listed under "Grains"
- Starchy vegetables and fruits such as
  - Potato
  - Sweet Potato
  - Yam
  - High-starch root vegetables
  - Lentils
  - Dried beans
  - Dried peas
  - Garbanzo bean (chickpea)
  - Lima beans
  - Broad beans (fava)
  - Cassava
  - Plantain
  - Banana

Vegetables

- Green leafy vegetables such as
  - Lettuce
  - Chard
  - Spinach
  - Broccoli
- Beans
  - Green
  - String
  - French
  - Runner
  - Yellow wax
- Peas
  - Green peas
  - Sugar peas
- Green, red, yellow peppers
- Squashes of all types
- Onions
- Garlic
- Tomatoes
- Carrots
- Beets
- Radishes
- Cauliflower
- Asparagus
- Eggplant
- Others

Fruits

- Berries:
  - Strawberry
  - Raspberry
  - Blueberry
  - Cranberry
  - Others
- Stone fruits:
  - Peaches
  - Apricots
  - Nectarines
  - Cherries
  - Plums
  - Others
- Melons
  - Cantaloupe
  - Honeydew
  - Watermelon
  - Others
- Citrus
  - Orange
  - Grapefruit
  - Lemon
  - Lime
- Tropical fruits such as
  - Pineapple
  - Mango

Note: This list is not exhaustive.

Table 29-2
DIETARY REFERENCE INTAKE (DRI) VALUES FOR CALCIUM AND VITAMIN D

Life Stage Group Male and Female[a]	Calcium AI (mg/day)	Vitamin D [b,c] AI (mcg/day)
0–6 months	210	5
6–12 months	270	5
1–3 years	500	5
4–8 years	800	5
9–13 years	1,300	5
14–18 years	1,300	5
19–30 years	1,000	5
31–50 years	1,000	5
51–70 years	1,200	10
over 70 years	1,200	15
Pregnancy:		
Up to 18 years	1,300	5
19–50 years	1,000	5
Lactation:		
Up to 18 years	1,300	5
19–50 years	1,000	5

[a] Female only for pregnancy and lactation values
[b] As cholecalciferol (1 microgram [mcg] = 40 IU vitamin D)
[c] In the absence of adequate exposure to sunlight

AI = Adequate Intake (amount per day) required to maintain optimal health.

Source: Institute of Medicine, National Academy of Sciences, Office of News and Public Information, 2101 Constitution Avenue, NW, Washington, DC 20418. August 13, 1997.

Table 29-3
IMPORTANT NUTRIENTS IN COMMON ALLERGENS

Equivalent nutrients must be provided from alternative sources when the following foods are eliminated from the diet.

MILK AND MILK PRODUCTS

Calcium	*Smaller amounts:*
Phosphorus	*Vitamin A
*Vitamin D	Vitamin E
Vitamin B12	
Pantothenic acid	
Riboflavin	
Potassium	

Alternative sources of these nutrients:
Fortified rice beverages, soy beverages* and oat beverages* can be a good source of calcium, vitamin D, and vitamin A. Calcium-fortified juices and cereal products are also available. Riboflavin, pantothenic acid, phosphorus, and vitamin E can be found in meats and legumes (e.g., peanuts, peas, beans, soybeans), nuts, and whole grains.*

EGG

Vitamin B12	*Smaller amounts:*
Vitamin D	Vitamin A
Pantothenic acid	Vitamin E
Biotin	Vitamin B6
Folacin	Zinc
Riboflavin	
Selenium	
Iron	

Alternative sources of these nutrients:
Meat, fish and poultry products, legumes, whole grains, and vegetables can supply these nutrients.

SOYBEAN

Thiamin
Riboflavin
Vitamin B6
Folacin
Calcium
Phosphorus
Magnesium
Iron
Zinc

Alternative sources of these nutrients:
Soy is typically used in commercial products in amounts that are too small to be considered a significant source for these nutrients. Therefore, elimination of soy from the diet does not compromise the nutritional quality of most diets.

Table 29-3 (continued)
IMPORTANT NUTRIENTS IN COMMON ALLERGENS

PEANUTS

Niacin	*Smaller amounts:*
Vitamin E	Potassium
Manganese	Vitamin B6
Chromium	Folacin
Pantothenic acid	Phosphorus
Magnesium	Copper
	Biotin

Alternative sources of these nutrients:
These nutrients may be replaced by including meat, whole grains, legumes, and vegetable oils in the diet.

FISH AND SHELLFISH

Niacin	*Smaller amounts:*
Vitamin B6	Potassium
Vitamin B12	Magnesium
Vitamin E	Iron
Phosphorus	Zinc
Selenium	Vitamin A
Calcium (in shellfish and fish bones)	

Alternative sources of these nutrients:
These nutrients are also present in meats, grains, legumes, and oils.

WHEAT

*Thiamin	*Smaller amounts:*
*Riboflavin	Magnesium
*Niacin	Folacin
*Iron	Phosphorus
Selenium	Molybdenum
Chromium	

Alternative sources of these nutrients:
Alternative choices of foods include, oats, rice, rye, barley, corn, buckwheat, amaranth, and quinoa, which contain similar nutrients. Alternatives to wheat flour include flours and starches from rice, potato, rye, oats, barley, buckwheat, tapioca, millet, corn, quinoa, and amaranth.

RICE
*Thiamin
*Riboflavin
*Niacin
*Iron

CORN
*Thiamin
*Riboflavin
*Niacin
*Iron
Chromium

*Indicates nutrient added to the food product: May be labeled "fortified" or "enriched."

Table 29-4
SUMMARY: IMPORTANT NUTRIENTS IN COMMON ALLERGENS

Nutrient	Milk	Egg	Peanut	Soy	Fish	Wheat	Rice	Corn
Vitamins								
A	+	+			+			
Biotin	+	+				+		
Folacin (folate, folic acid)	+	+	+		+			
B1 (thiamin)			+		+	+	+	
B2 (riboflavin)	+	+		+		+	+	+
B3 (niacin)		+		+	+	+	+	
B5 (pantothenic acid)	+	+	+					
B6 (pyridoxine)		+	+	+	+			
B12 (cobalamine)	+	+			+			
C								
D	+	+			+			
E (alpha-tocopherol)	+	+	+		+			
K	+	+		+				
Minerals								
Calcium	+			+	+			
Chromium			+			+		+
Copper		+						
Iron		+		+	+	+	+	+
Magnesium				+	+	+		
Manganese			+					
Molybdenum						+		
Potassium	+		+		+			
Selenium		+			+	+		
Zinc		+		+	+			

Table 29-5
ALTERNATIVE SOURCES OF NUTRIENTS

Vitamins

Vitamin A	Liver, fish liver oils, dark green and yellow vegetables, tomato, apricots, cantaloupe, mango, papaya
Biotin	Organ meats, nutritional yeast, mushrooms, banana, grapefruit, watermelon, strawberries
Folacin	Organ meats, legumes, green leafy vegetables, asparagus, beets, broccoli, avocado, oranges, bananas, strawberries, whole grains, nutritional yeast
Vitamin B1 (thiamin)	Meats especially pork, dried and green peas, legumes, whole grains, nutritional yeast
Vitamin B2 (riboflavin)	Organ meats, legumes, green vegetables, whole grains, nutritional yeast
Vitamin B3 (niacin)	Organ meats, poultry, beef, legumes, whole grains, nutritional yeast
Vitamin B5 (pantothenic acid)	Organ meats, chicken, beef, fresh vegetables, whole grains, nutritional yeast
Vitamin B6 (pyridoxine)	Meats especially organ meats, legumes, whole grains, green vegetables, carrots, potato, cauliflower, banana, prunes, avocado, sunflower seeds, nutritional yeast
Vitamin B12 (cobalamin)	Meats especially organ meats, poultry
Vitamin D	Liver, fish liver oils, action of sunlight on skin
Vitamin E (alpha tocopherol)	Liver, legumes, green leafy vegetables, tomato whole grains, vegetable oils

Minerals

Calcium	Amaranth, baked beans, rhubarb, green leafy vegetables, broccoli, dates; molasses
Chromium	Vegetable oils, meats, liver, nutritional yeast, whole grains
Copper	Liver, meats, whole grains, green leafy vegetables, broccoli, potato, pears, banana, apple juice
Iron	Meats, liver, legumes, raisins, dried apricots, prunes, pumpkin, asparagus, broccoli, chard, green peas, spinach, molasses
Magnesium	Legumes, whole grains, meats, poultry, dark green vegetables
Manganese	Sunflower seeds, whole grains, legumes, nutritional yeast, green beans, broccoli, cranberry, grape, pineapple

Table 29-5 (continued) ALTERNATIVE SOURCES OF NUTRIENTS	
Minerals (continued)	
Molybdenum	Meats, legumes, whole grains, green vegetables especially spinach, lettuce, Brussels sprouts, carrots, squash, tomatoes, apple juice
Phosphorus	Meats, poultry, legumes, whole grains, seeds, green peas, artichokes, potato, Brussels sprouts
Potassium	Meats, oranges, banana, dried fruits, cantaloupe, honeydew melon, nectarines, papaya, tomato, avocado, dark green vegetables, sweet potato, winter squash, potato, molasses
Selenium	Whole grains, meats, broccoli, onions, tomato
Zinc	Meats, liver, green leafy vegetables, beets, green peas, oranges, strawberries, prunes, chocolate syrup

— APPENDIX 1 —

FEW-FOODS ELIMINATION DIET: RECIPES AND MEAL PLANS

When many foods and food additives are suspected to be a possible cause for your symptoms, but no specific foods are indicated as the culprits, a few-foods elimination diet is often the quickest and easiest way to determine whether foods are indeed causing your problems. The use and purpose of elimination diets is discussed in detail in Chapter 27. There are many few-foods elimination diets, and each one should be tailored for the needs of the person requiring it. Here we provide a diet that includes the foods that are the least likely to cause an adverse reaction in the majority of people. Inevitably, there will be some people who react to one or more of the foods allowed on this diet. In such a case, substitutions for the suspected "reactive foods" with ones of equal nutritional value, but without the risk of an adverse reaction, should be found.

The menus and meal plans that follow will allow you to prepare and consume attractive and tasty meals, in spite of the strict limitations on the range of foods you are allowed. But remember: A few-foods elimination diet should *never* be followed for more than 14 days; 10 days is preferable. Reintroduction of each food component should then be initiated, using one of the methods of food challenge described in Chapter 28, to precisely determine which foods and/or food additives are responsible for your symptoms.

Note on the Nutrition Information Tables

Each recipe in this section is followed by information on its nutritional content. The information includes the **energy** (in Kilocalories [Kcal] or Calories), **protein**, **carbohydrate**, and **fat** (all in grams) of a serving size of the recipe. Where the protein, carbohydrate, or fat content is less than half (0.5) of a gram, the value is recorded as 0 in the tables. The energy content of food is calculated in Kilocalories (commonly written as Calories). A (small) calorie is defined as the amount of heat required to raise the temperature of 1 kilogram of water 1 degree Celsius at a specified temperature. The large calorie (written as Kilocalorie, Kcal, or Calorie) is 1,000 (small) calories and is used almost exclusively in the field of nutrition, so when we talk about food calories we are actually referring to Kilocalories.

Table A-1		
FOODS ALLOWED		

All of the sources listed below should be free from all additives

Food Category	Food	Sources
Meat and Alternates*	Lamb Turkey Fish: – Red snapper – Perch	Fresh or frozen
Grains	Rice Tapioca Millet	Whole grains, flours, and cereals made from these grains
Fruits	Pears Cranberries	Pure bottled pear juice Pure infant pears in jars Homemade cranberry juice
Vegetables	Squash Parsnips Sweet potatoes Yams Lettuce	Acorn Butternut Chayote Hubbard Winter Summer Pattypan Spaghetti squash Crookneck Zucchini Pure infant squash in jars Pure infant sweet potatoes in jars Any tolerated varieties
Oils	Canola oil Safflower oil	
Condiments	Sea salt	
Beverages	Distilled water Juice	In glass bottles From the allowed fruits and vegetables only

* The choice of fish, poultry, or meat depends on the patient's sensitivity: Recipes are
  provided for all of these, but only those tolerated should be included.

FEW-FOODS ELIMINATION TEST DIET
INDEX TO RECIPES

MEAT, POULTRY, AND FISH

Lamb

BUYING

◆ Buy *only* plain, unprocessed lamb.
◆ Avoid prepared lamb sausage.

QUANTITY PER SERVING

◆ 4 oz (125 g) per serving of trimmed boneless lamb such as tenderloin
◆ 1–2 chops per serving depending on thickness

YIELD

◆ 1 leg of lamb with bone averages 8.5 lb (4 kg) = 16 servings
◆ 1 leg of lamb boned and rolled = 6 lb (2.7 kg) = 16 servings
◆ A boneless leg of lamb = 3 lb (1.4 kg) = 8 servings

THAWING

◆ Place frozen leg of lamb on a tray in the refrigerator.
◆ Allow 2 days to thaw.

ROAST LAMB

Half leg of lamb (bone in or boneless)
Sea salt

◆ Preheat oven to 325°F (160°C).
◆ Season lamb with sea salt.
◆ Place fat side up on a roasting pan.
◆ Calculate how long it will take to roast the meat at 30–35 minutes per pound (500 g). Add another 15 minutes for resting time on the counter before carving.
◆ *Or* use a meat thermometer. The lamb will be "medium" when the thermometer reaches 175°F (80°C) and "well done" when the thermometer reaches 182°F (83°C).
◆ Do not baste or turn the lamb while it is cooking.

Makes 6–8 servings

Nutrition Information for One Serving:

Size of Serving	Weight	Calories	Protein (g)	Carbohydrate (g)	Fat (g)
1½ slices	107 g	204	30	0	8

MARINADE FOR LAMB

Cranberry concentrate (see recipe on page 422)	¼ cup	(60 mL)
Canola oil	2 tbsp	(25 mL)
Distilled water	2 tbsp	(25 mL)
Sea salt	½ tsp	(2.5 mL)

◆ Combine all ingredients in a screw-top jar.
◆ Shake well before pouring over meat.
◆ Marinate meat a minimum of 1 hour.
◆ Marinade can be used for either lamb or turkey.

Makes ½ cup (125 mL) of marinade

Nutrition Information for One Recipe:

Size of Serving	Volume	Calories	Protein (g)	Carbohydrate (g)	Fat (g)
½ cup	125 mL	259	0	4	27

LAMB BROTH

Lamb bones and trimmings left over from roast, chops, or lamb shanks	1–3 lb (500 g–1.4 kg)
Distilled water	8 cups (2 L)
Sea salt	2 tsp (10 mL)
Outer lettuce leaves, shredded	8–10 leaves

For added flavor, roast the bones before simmering them in water: Spread bones in a roasting pan and bake at 400°F (200°C) for an hour or until browned. Transfer to a soup pot. *This step can be skipped but broth will have less flavor.*

◆ Add distilled water, sea salt, and lettuce leaves to the bones in a soup pot.
◆ Bring to a boil and skim off any scum.
◆ Reduce heat and simmer uncovered for 4 hours.
◆ Remove from heat and strain.
◆ Cover and refrigerate until chilled.
◆ Remove fat layer.
◆ Broth can be kept in the refrigerator for 2 days or frozen for longer storage.

Makes about 6 cups of broth

Nutrition Information for One Serving:

Size of Serving	Volume	Calories	Protein (g)	Carbohydrate (g)	Fat (g)
1 cup	250 mL	19	2	0	1

LAMB STEW

Lamb shoulder (bone in)	2 lb	(1 kg)
Or: Stewing lamb, boned	1¼ lb	(625 g)
Canola oil	¼ cup	(60 mL)
1 small yam peeled and cut in 1 in. (2.5 cm) cubes	1 cup	(250 mL)
1 small summer squash halved and cut into in. (2 cm) slices	1 cup	(250 mL)
Distilled water	2 cups	(500 mL)
Sea salt	½–1 tsp	(2.5–5 mL)
Plain rice noodles	4 oz	(125 g)
1 small zucchini halved and cut into ¾ in. (2 cm) slices	1 cup	(250 mL)

◆ Trim fat and bone from lamb and cut into 1 in (2.5 cm) cubes.
◆ Heat canola oil in a casserole or stew pot.
◆ Add the lamb and brown well on all sides.
◆ Drain off all excess oil. Leave brown lamb drippings in the pot.
◆ Add yam, summer squash, distilled water, and sea salt. Bring to a boil.
◆ Cover, and reduce heat to simmer for 1 hour.
◆ Add rice noodles and zucchini.
◆ Simmer another 10–15 minutes until the noodles are tender.

Makes 5 servings

Nutrition Information for One Serving:

Size of Serving	Weight	Calories	Protein (g)	Carbohydrate (g)	Fat (g)
⅕ recipe	approx. 250 g	347	22	33	14

MEAT SAUCE FOR PASTA OR SPAGHETTI SQUASH

Ground lamb (or turkey)	½ lb	(250 g)
1 medium pear, peeled and chopped	1¼ cup	(300 g)
Fresh or frozen cranberries	1 cup	(250 mL)
Pear juice	1 cup	(250 mL)
Sea salt to taste		

◆ Brown the lamb in a frying pan.
◆ If using turkey, add 1 tbsp (15 mL) canola oil to the pan.
◆ Add the pear, cranberries, and pear juice.
◆ Season to taste with sea salt.
◆ Bring to a boil; reduce heat and simmer until sauce thickens (20–30 minutes).
◆ Pour over cooked pasta, rice, or spaghetti squash.

Makes 3–4 servings

Nutrition Information for One Serving:

Size of Serving	Volume	Calories	Protein (g)	Carbohydrate (g)	Fat (g)
⅓ recipe	250 mL (1 cup)	336	14	25	20

LAMB SOUVLAKI

Lamb cut in 1 in. (2.5 cm) cubes	1½ lb	(750 g)
Small green zucchini	1–2	small
Small yellow zucchini or crookneck squash	1	small
Sea salt	to taste	
Canola oil	2 tbsp	(25 mL)

◆ If using wooden skewers, soak in water for 30 minutes before using them. Otherwise use flat bladed metal skewers.

◆ Slice zucchini and squash in half lengthwise, then slice ¾ in. (2 cm) slices.

◆ Thread the meat and the vegetables on skewers.

◆ Sprinkle prepared skewers with sea salt, and brush them with oil.

◆ Grill on a barbecue for approximately 10 minutes. They should be turned 2 or 3 times and brushed with oil while grilling.

◆ *Or* cook in the broiler. Preheat the broiler, and place the skewers on the unheated broiler rack 5 in. (12.5 cm) below the element. Brush with oil and turn every 3–4 minutes. They should be cooked in approximately 12 minutes.

Makes 4 servings

Nutrition Information for One Serving:

Size of Serving	Weight	Calories	Protein (g)	Carbohydrate (g)	Fat (g)
1 large or 2 medium skewers	Approx. 250 g (½ lb)	347	284	4	24

LAMB LETTUCE WRAPS

Canola oil	2 tbsp	(25 mL)
Lamb (or turkey), ground	½ lb	(250 g)
Zucchini, grated	½ cup	(125 mL)
Yellow squash such as acorn or butternut, grated	1 cup	(250 mL)
Sea salt	1 tsp	(5 mL)
Rice, cooked	1 cup	(250 mL)
Head (iceberg), Boston, or leaf lettuce	1	

◆ Heat canola oil in a saucepan.

◆ Add lamb or turkey, and fry until brown.

◆ Add the squash and salt, and cook for 5 minutes.

◆ Add the rice, and continue to cook until the rice is hot.

◆ Cut large lettuce leaves down the center vein. On the narrow end of each lettuce leaf, place 1 tbsp (15 mL) of the rice and lamb mixture. Roll into a cylindrical shape.

◆ Repeat with each lettuce leaf until all the filling is used up.

◆ Serve hot or chilled.

Makes 4 servings

Nutrition Information for One Serving:

Size of Serving	Weight	Calories	Protein (g)	Carbohydrate (g)	Fat (g)
¼ recipe	approx 250 g (½ lb)	283	11	14	20

Turkey

BUYING

◆ Buy only plain, unprocessed turkey. Check the label, as many brands have added butter, margarine, and so on.
◆ Plain ground turkey is excellent for meat sauces.
◆ Smoked turkey and turkey sausage are *not* suitable.

QUANTITY PER SERVING

◆ 8 oz (250 g) per serving of fresh young turkey or legs
◆ 6 oz (175 g) per serving of turkey breast
◆ 12 oz (350 g) per serving of turkey wings
◆ 4 oz (125 g) per serving of turkey cutlets or uncooked plain rolled turkey roast

YIELD

◆ 1 lb (500 g) raw boneless turkey = 2 cups (500 mL) cooked/diced.
◆ 1 lb (500 g) cooked boneless turkey = 3½ cups (875 mL) diced.

THAWING

◆ Refrigerator:
  – Place turkey on a tray in the refrigerator.
  – Allow 5 hours per pound (500 g) to thaw.
  – This is the safest method of thawing.
◆ Cold water:
  – Immerse turkey in cold water, changing water occasionally.
  – Allow 1 hour per pound (500 g).

ROASTING A TURKEY

◆ Remove the neck and giblets from the body cavity and save them for broth.
◆ Rinse turkey cavity with distilled water. Season the cavity with sea salt.
◆ Secure the legs by tucking them under the skin band or tying them with string.
◆ Fold the wings behind the back to secure the neck skin.
◆ Place the turkey on a rack in a shallow pan with the breast up.
◆ Brush with canola or safflower oil.
◆ Insert a thermometer into the inner thigh being careful not to touch the bone.
◆ Cover turkey with a loose tent of foil (dull side out). Tuck foil under the turkey at the ends, leaving open at the sides.
◆ To brown the turkey, remove the foil for the last 30 minutes of roasting time and baste with pan drippings.
◆ Refer to the following chart for roasting time.

ROASTING CHART (for unstuffed turkey only)

◆ Roast in 325°F (160°C) oven until the thigh records a temperature of 185°F (85°C) on a meat thermometer.
◆ If a thermometer is not available, the turkey is usually done when the leg moves easily and, when it is pierced with a knife, the juice is no longer pink.

	Weight	Cooking Time
Whole turkey	6–8 lb (2.7–3.6 kg)	1½–2¾ hours
	8–10 lb (3.6–4.5 kg)	2¾–3 hours
	10–12 lb (4.5–5.5 kg)	3–3¼ hours
	12–16 lb (5.5–7.3 kg)	3¼–3½ hours
	16–22 lb (7.3–10 kg)	3½–4 hours
Turkey leg	1 lb (500 g)	1–1¼ hours
Turkey wing	½ lb (250 g)	1–1¼ hours
Turkey breast	1 lb (500 g)	1¼ hours
Turkey roll	2½–3 lb (1.1–1.4 kg)	2–3 hours

Nutrition Information for One Serving:

Serving	Weight	Calories	Protein (g)	Carbohydrate (g)	Fat (g)
Light/dark meat, no skin	120 g (4.2 oz)	204	35	0	6

BASIC TURKEY BROTH

Turkey carcass, neck, giblets	4–5 lb	(1.8–2.3 kg)
Distilled water	16 cups	(4 L)
Sea salt	2 tsp	(10 mL)
Lettuce leaves, washed and shredded	2 cups	(500 mL)

◆ Place turkey pieces in a large pot.
◆ Add water and salt.
◆ Bring to a boil over low heat. Skim off the surface scum as necessary.
◆ Add lettuce. Bring to a boil, then lower the heat and simmer gently for 2 hours.
◆ Taste and add extra salt if desired.
◆ Reduce heat and simmer until tender (1½–2 hours).

Makes 4 servings

Nutrition Information for One Serving:

Size of Serving	Volume	Calories	Protein (g)	Carbohydrate (g)	Fat (g)
1 cup	250 mL	19	2	0	1

BRAISED TURKEY

◆ Place turkey parts (2 lbs or 1 kg) in a Dutch oven.
◆ Add two cups (500 mL) of distilled water.
◆ Season with sea salt.
◆ Cover and bring to a boil.
◆ Reduce heat and simmer until tender (1½–2 hours).

Nutrition Information for One Serving:

Size of Serving	Weight	Calories	Protein (g)	Carbohydrate (g)	Fat (g)
¼ recipe	250 g (½ lb)	347	22	33	14

TURKEY CUTLETS WITH CRANBERRY SAUCE

4 small turkey cutlets (meat only)	1 lb	(500 g)
Sea salt to taste	2 tsp	(10 mL)
Canola or safflower oil	2 tsp	(25 mL)
Distilled water	⅓ cup	(75 mL)
Fresh or frozen thawed cranberries	½ cup	(250 g)
Pear, peeled,cored, and finely chopped	1 cup	(250 g)

◆ Pound turkey cutlets to ¼ in. (.5 cm) thickness.
◆ Sprinkle lightly with sea salt.
◆ In a large frying pan, heat 2 tbsp (25 mL) oil over medium heat.
◆ Add turkey and sauté approximately 3–5 minutes per side, until turkey is no longer pink inside, but not overcooked
◆ Transfer turkey to a platter. Cover with foil to keep warm.
◆ Add distilled water, cranberries, and pear to frying pan.
◆ Bring to a boil, then reduce heat to simmer until cranberries have popped and pear is tender (approximately 5 minutes).
◆ Add sea salt to taste, and pour over turkey.

Makes 4 servings

Nutrition Information for One Serving:

Size of Serving	Weight	Calories	Protein (g)	Carbohydrate (g)	Fat (g)
1 cutlet with sauce	135 g (4.75 oz)	295	37	8	12

TURKEY KABOBS

Cranberry concentrate (see recipe on page 422)	1 tbsp	(15 mL)
Pear juice	1 tbsp	(15 mL)
Canola or safflower oil	2 tbsp	(25 mL)
Boneless turkey fillets	1 lb	(500 g)
Small zucchini		1 small
Small yellow zucchini or crookneck squash		1 small

- In a bowl, combine the cranberry concentrate, pear juice and oil.
- Cut turkey into ½ in. (1 cm) wide strips.
- Add to marinade, and marinate 30 minutes. Stir occasionally.
- Cut zucchini and squash in half lengthwise, then cut into ¾ in. (2 cm) slices.
- Preheat broiler without the broiler pan. The oven shelf should be placed far enough below the broiler elements that the kabobs will be 3–4 in. (7.5–10 cm) under the elements. In most ovens the rack will be 6–7 in. (15–17.5 cm) below the broiler element.
- Remove the turkey from the marinade. Keep the marinade.
- On 4 skewers, thread the turkey strips accordion style around the zucchini and squash.
- Place the kabobs on an unheated broiler pan, and brush kabobs with marinade.
- Broil kabobs for 5 minutes.
- Turn and brush with marinade.
- Broil another 3–5 minutes, until tender.
- Bring remaining marinade to a boil and serve as a sauce with the kabobs.

Makes 4 servings

Nutrition Information for One Serving:

Size of Serving	Weight	Calories	Protein (g)	Carbohydrate (g)	Fat (g)
1 skewer	135 g (4.75 oz)	239	38	5	5

Fish

TYPES

Perch   This fish is usually reasonably priced. It is sold as fillets with the skin on. The flesh is lean, white, and mild in flavor. Perch may be sautéed, baked, or broiled.

Snapper   This fish is a best buy year-around. It is sold in skinless fillets. It is lean and white-fleshed and may be fried, baked, broiled, or poached.

BUYING FISH

The best test of the freshness of fish is its smell. It should be very moderately fishy, nothing stronger. Don't be afraid to ask to smell the fish. The skin on perch should spring back when pressed lightly. If fresh fish is not available or very expensive, plain, frozen fish is acceptable.

THAWING FISH

It is very important to keep fish cold so that the outside of the fish doesn't deteriorate while the inside thaws. The best method is to thaw the fish in the refrigerator. If there is not enough time for that, the fish can be placed in cold water for 1½ hours.

QUANTITY PER SERVING

1 serving is usually 4 oz (125 g) of fish without bone.

Cooking

Measure the thickness of the fish at the thickest part. For each inch (2.5 cm) of thickness, allow 10 minutes of cooking time at 400–450°F (200–230°C). Add 5 minutes if the fish is wrapped in foil. Fish is cooked when it's slightly opaque and flakes easily.

BAKED FISH FILLETS

Fish fillets	1 lb	(500 g)
Canola or safflower oil	2 tsp	(10 mL)
Sea salt	to taste	

◆ Preheat oven to 425–450°F (220–230°C).
◆ Oil a baking dish just large enough to hold the fillets in a single layer, and arrange the fillets neatly in the dish.
◆ Drizzle or brush the oil on the fish and sprinkle with sea salt.
◆ Bake uncovered for 8–10 minutes or until the fish is opaque and flakes easily.
◆ Do not overcook.

Makes 3–4 servings

Nutrition Information for One Serving:

Size of Serving	Weight	Calories	Protein (g)	Carbohydrate (g)	Fat (g)
⅓ recipe	150 g (5.3 oz)	194	34	0	5

MICROWAVED FISH FILLETS

Fish fillets	1 lb	(500 g)
Canola or safflower oil	2 tsp	(10 mL)
Sea salt	to taste	

◆ Oil a microwave-safe baking dish just large enough to hold the fillets, and arrange them neatly in the dish.
◆ Drizzle or brush the oil on the fish.
◆ Cover with plastic wrap and turn back a corner to vent for steam.
◆ Microwave on high for 3–5 minutes.
◆ Let stand for 2–3 minutes before serving.
◆ Season to taste with sea salt after microwaving.
◆ Remove plastic-wrap cover before serving.

Makes 3–4 servings

Nutrition Information for One Serving:

Size of Serving	Weight	Calories	Protein (g)	Carbohydrate (g)	Fat (g)
¼ recipe sauce	150 g (5.3 oz)	194	34	0	5

FISH MIXED GRILL WITH SWEET POTATOES AND PEARS

4 red snapper fillets	about 1¼ lb	(625 g)
2–4 cooked and peeled sweet potatoes	1½–2 lb	(750g–1 kg)
2 poached pears, peeled, cored, and halved	4 halves	
Canola or safflower oil to drizzle	2–3 tbsp	(25–35 mL)
Sea salt to season	to taste	

◆ Preheat broiler with top rack of oven about 5 in. (12.5 cm) below the broiler element.
◆ Lightly oil the broiler pan.
◆ Arrange the fillets in a single layer in the pan.
◆ Slice cooked sweet potatoes in half lengthwise and place on broiler pan.
◆ Arrange poached pear halves on the same pan.
◆ Drizzle or brush food on broiler with oil and season with salt.
◆ Broil 6–8 minutes until fish is opaque and flakes easily and pears and sweet potatoes are hot and lightly browned.

Makes 4 servings

Nutrition Information for One Serving:

Size of Serving	Weight	Calories	Protein (g)	Carbohydrate (g)	Fat (g)
¼ recipe	500 g (approx. 16 oz))	321	28	40	5

STEAMED FISH FILLETS WITH SALSA

4 fish fillets	about 1¼ lb	(625 g)
Cranberries	½ cup	(125 mL)
½ pear, peeled and cored	½ cup	(125 mL)
1 small zucchini	½ cup	(125 mL)
sea salt	¼ tsp	(1 mL)

Steamed fish
◆ Add water to steamer and bring to a boil.
◆ If you don't have a steamer, put a rack in a wok or wide pan.
◆ Place fish on a heat-proof plate on the rack.
◆ Cover steamer tightly and steam for 5 minutes or until fish is opaque.
◆ Transfer fish to plates.

Salsa
◆ Chop cranberries, zucchini, and pear finely by hand or in a food processor.
◆ Add distilled water and sea salt.
◆ Transfer to a small saucepan.
◆ Bring to a boil, then lower heat and simmer for 10 minutes.
◆ If allowed, try the salsa raw, it has a sharper taste.

Makes 4 servings of fish and a cup of salsa

Nutrition Information for One Serving:

Size of Serving	Calories	Protein (g)	Carbohydrate (g)	Fat (g)
1 fillet with ¼ cup salsa (60 mL)	184	33	7	2

GRAINS

- Rice, tapioca, and millet can be eaten as the whole grain, refined grain, flour, and starch.
- Puffed rice and puffed millet are available in grocery stores and supermarkets.
- Rice cereals such as Cream of Rice and Ener-G Rice Flakes are fairly readily available.
- Rice polishings and rice bran are available in some specialty health food stores.
- White and whole-grain rice cakes are readily available in grocery stores. Choose rice cakes containing rice or rice and salt only.

Rice

- All forms of rice are allowed.
- Brown rice is the complete rice grain and as such is more nutritious than white.
- It retains more fiber, folacin, iron, riboflavin, potassium, phosphorus, zinc, and trace minerals such as copper and manganese than any other form of rice.
- Brown rice is the only rice that contains vitamin E.
- Brown rice takes longer to cook than white rice and has a richer flavor and chewier texture.
- In the production of white rice, milling removes the husk, bran, and most of the germ.
- Rice bran or rice polishings, removed in the production of white rice, contain not only bran but also rice germ, which is rich in oil and contains vitamin E.
- The inner white kernel is predominantly starch.
- Both brown and white rice can be used in desserts, stuffing, salads, soup, casseroles, or with a main course.

FORMS OF RICE

Rice is classified according to size: long-grain, medium-grain, and short-grain. All three sizes are available in both brown and white forms.

- *Long grain rice* grains are five times longer than they are wide. Properly cooked, the rice is fluffy and dry with separate grains.
- *Medium-grain rice* is twice as long as it is wide. Properly cooked, it is moister and more tender than long-grain rice. It is the type commonly used to make cold cereals.
- *Short-grain rice* is oval or round in appearance. Its high percentage of amylopectin (starch) causes the grains to clump or stick together when cooked. It is used in dishes such as sushi.
- *Wild rice* is not a grain, but a grass seed, and it belongs to a different botanic family (*Zizania aquatica*). Wild rice has about twice the protein of other rices and higher levels of B vitamins. It cooks up to a greater volume than regular rice grain (1 cup of dry wild rice makes 3–4 cups cooked), but is also more expensive than other types of rice. It is frequently served mixed with other types of rice in rice dishes.

In most cultures, white rice is eaten more frequently than brown. In North America it is available in a variety of forms:

- *Enriched white rice* has had thiamin, niacin, and iron added to it after milling to replace some of the nutrients lost in the bran layer.

◆ *Parboiled rice* (also called *converted rice*) has been soaked in water and steamed under pressure before milling. This process forces some of the nutrients into the grain so that they are not totally lost during milling. The rice is not precooked and is rather harder than regular white rice, so it takes a little longer to cook than white rice.

◆ *Enriched parboiled rice* has the same added thiamin, niacin, and iron as enriched white rice, but more potassium, folacin, riboflavin, and phosphorus (though less than brown rice).

◆ *Instant white rice* has been milled, polished, fully cooked, and then dehydrated. It takes only about 5 minutes to prepare, which is a process of rehydration rather than cooking. It is usually enriched and only slightly less nutritious than regular enriched white rice.

There are several *varieties* of rice, which are used in different types of cooking throughout the world. Examples of rice varieties include the following:

◆ *Arborio rice* is a short-grain (almost round) starchy white rice that is traditionally used for cooking Italian dishes such as risotto, paella, and rice pudding. It absorbs up to five times its weight in liquid during cooking.

◆ *Basmati rice* is traditionally grown in India and Pakistan, The grains elongate much more than they plump up as they cook. Basmati rice is lower in starch than other types, and cooked grains appear flaky and separate. It is most commonly used in Indian cooking, but can be successfully used in place of any long-grain rice in recipes. This rice is available as white and brown.

A variety of strains of rice have been developed in the United States, which approximate the flavor and texture of basmati rice. Most of them are basmati hybrids sold under trade names, such as Texmati, Wehani, and Wild pecan (also known as popcorn rice).

◆ *Jasmine rice*, a long-grain rice grown in Thailand, has a soft texture and is similar in flavor to basmati rice. It is available as white and brown.

◆ *Glutinous (sweet) rice* is a short-grain rice, not related to other short-grain rice varieties. It is very sticky and turns translucent when cooked. It is used to make rice dumplings and cakes, popular in China and Japan.

How to Cook Rice

PREPARATION

◆ *Domestic rice* (purchased in the United States, Canada, and most other Western countries) is almost always very clean. Do *not* rinse before cooking because the coating on the grains of enriched rice contains nutrients that will be lost during washing.

◆ *Imported rice*, or rice purchased in bulk, will need to be washed as it is likely to be dirty or dusty. There will be no nutrient loss in washing imported rice since it is not enriched. In Hispanic markets, rice may be coated in glucose, which is harmless.

COOKING

Rice is cooked in a number of ways, but the method most familiar to North Americans is simmering:

COOKING CHART FOR POPULAR RICE VARIETIES

Rice Type Quantity: ½ cup uncooked	Liquid (cups)	Cooking Time (minutes)	Yield (cups)
Brown, long-grain	1	25–30	1½
Brown, short-grain	1	40	1½
Brown, instant	½	5	¾
Brown, quick	¾	10	1
White, long-grain	1	20	¾
White, instant	½	5; plus 5 minutes standing time	1 1
Converted	1⅓	31	2
Arborio	¾	15	1½
Basmati, white	½	15	2
Jasmine	1	15–20	1¾
Texmati, long-grain, brown	1 plus 2 tbsp	40	2
Texmati, long-grain, white	1 plus 2 tbsp	15	1¼
Wehani	1	40	1¼
Wild	2	50	2
Wild pecan	1	20	1½

Source: S. Margen (ed.), *The Wellness Encyclopedia of Food and Nutrition* (University of California at Berkeley, Health Letter Associates, 1992), p. 307.

Nutrition Information for One Serving:

Type of Rice ½ cup cooked	Weight	Calories	Protein (g)	Carbohydrate (g)	Fat (g)
White, enriched long-grain	3½ oz cooked	129	3	28	<1
Brown, long-grain	3½ oz cooked	111	3	23	1

◆ In a saucepan with a well-fitting lid, add the required amount of rice to the quantity of distilled water specified in the chart below.
◆ Bring to a boil.
◆ Reduce heat, cover saucepan, and simmer for the length of time specified in the chart.
◆ Fluff rice with a fork before serving.
◆ For drier rice, fluff it, then cover the saucepan again and let it stand for 10–15 minutes.
◆ Converted, parboiled, "quick," and "Minute" rice should be cooked according to directions on the package.

◆ If different types of rice are cooked together, for example, white and brown rice, start the rice requiring longer cooking time first (the brown), then stir in the white rice about 20 minutes before the brown rice is done.

Reheating Rice

Leftover rice reheats well if you add a few tablespoons of extra liquid. Cooked rice will keep for about a week in the refrigerator

Method for Reheating Rice
Combine 1 cup (250 mL) of cooked rice with 2 tbsp (25 mL) of distilled water in a saucepan. Cover and cook 4 minutes or until heated through.

Rice Noodles, Rice Sticks, and Rice Vermicelli

Dried rice noodles are available in a variety of shapes and thicknesses. They may be labeled "rice noodles," "rice vermicelli," or "rice sticks." Follow the directions on the package for cooking each type. Rice noodles expand to 2–3 times their original size in cooking.

To use in soups or stir fries:
Soak the noodles in cold, distilled water for 20 minutes, then add to the other ingredients in the recipe.

To use in salads: Cover noodles with boiling distilled water and let stand for 5 minutes. Add to salad ingredients and toss.

Rice Wrappers

Thin flexible wrappers made from rice flour are available from Chinese and Vietnamese grocers. They can be wrapped around vegetables or fillings such as ground lamb, rice, and cranberries. To prepare, briefly dip the dry wrapper in cold water, and handle it carefully.

BAKED WHITE RICE (REGULAR AND PARBOILED)

White rice	1 cup	250 mL
Distilled water	2 cups	500 mL
Canola oil	1 tbsp	15 mL
Sea salt to taste	1 tsp	5 g

◆ Preheat oven to 35°F (180°C).
◆ In casserole greased with canola oil, combine white rice, boiling distilled water, and sea salt.
◆ Bake 60 minutes or until rice feels tender between fingers and all the liquid is absorbed.
◆ Uncover at once.
◆ Fluff up rice with a fork and serve.

Makes 3–4 servings

Nutrition Information for One Serving:

Size of Serving	Calories	Protein (g)	Carbohydrate (g)	Fat (g)
⅛ recipe	278	5	52	5

CREAM OF BROWN RICE

Canola oil	1 tsp	5 mL
Brown rice	1 cup	250 mL
Distilled water	2 cups	500 mL
Sea salt to taste	1 tsp	5 mL

- ◆ Heat canola oil in a frying pan.
- ◆ Add brown rice and sauté for a few minutes, stirring to ensure all grains are coated in oil.
- ◆ Put the rice into a blender and grind at high speed.
- ◆ Bring the water to a boil in a saucepan.
- ◆ Add the rice and sea salt. Bring to a boil.
- ◆ Cover, reduce heat, and simmer until the rice thickens, approximately 30 minutes.
- ◆ Stir frequently.

Makes 3–4 servings

Nutrition Information for One Serving:

Size of Serving	Calories	Protein (g)	Carbohydrate (g)	Fat (g)
⅛ recipe	265	5	50	4

BROWN RICE PUDDING

Canola oil	1 tsp	(5 mL)
Brown rice, cooked	1 cup	(250 mL)
Squash, cooked and mashed	¾ cup	(200 mL)
Pear, peeled and chopped	2 tbsp	(25 mL)

- ◆ Preheat oven to 325°F (160°C).
- ◆ Use canola oil to grease a small oven-proof casserole.
- ◆ Combine all ingredients in the casserole.
- ◆ Bake for 20 minutes.

Makes 3 servings

Nutrition Information for One Serving:

Size of Serving	Calories	Protein (g)	Carbohydrate (g)	Fat (g)
⅛ recipe	118	3	22	2

RICEOLA

White rice flour	1½ cups	(375 mL)
Brown rice flour	¼ cup	(60 mL)
Rice bran or polishings	¼ cup	(60 mL)
Canola oil	2 tsp	(10 mL)
Distilled water, hot	½ cups	(125 mL)
Sea salt to taste	½ tsp	(2.5 mL)

◆ Preheat oven to 250°F (130°C).
◆ Mix brown flour, white flour, rice polishings, salt, and water in a bowl.
◆ Spread on a cookie sheet oiled with canola oil.
◆ Bake for 1 hour or until lightly browned and dry.
◆ When cool, break into pieces and toss with 1½ tsp (7.5 mL) of canola oil to coat.
◆ Use as granola.
◆ Store leftovers in an airtight container.

Makes 4–6 servings

Nutrition Information for One Serving:

Size of Serving	Calories	Protein (g)	Carbohydrate (g)	Fat (g)
¼ recipe	279	4	57	3

RICE MILK

Cooked brown rice	1 cup	(250 mL)
Distilled water	4 cups	(1 L)
Sea salt to taste	¼ teaspoon	(1 mL)

◆ Combine all ingredients in a blender and blend until smooth.
◆ Let sit for 1 hour.
◆ Pour through a sieve.
◆ Refrigerate.
◆ Shake before serving.
◆ Use on cereals or in place of other liquids in recipes.

Makes 4 cups

Nutrition Information for One Serving:

Size of Serving	Calories	Protein (g)	Carbohydrate (g)	Fat (g)
1 cup (250 mL)	64	1	15	<1

Tapioca

Tapioca flour, starch, and granules are made from the root of cassava (manioc) plants. The flour forms a thick gel when heated with water. Tapioca is often used to thicken puddings, fruit pies, soups, and gravies.

For thickening: Use 1½ times as much tapioca flour as wheat flour.

TAPIOCA PUDDING

Distilled water, or pear and cranberry juice	1½ cups	(375 mL)
Tapioca granules	⅓ cup	(75 mL)
Sea salt	¼ tsp	(1 mL)

◆ Mix all ingredients in a double boiler over boiling water.
◆ Cook for 10 minutes.
◆ Turn off heat and let sit for 20 minutes, then stir well.
◆ The pudding may be eaten hot or cold.

Makes 4 servings

Nutrition Information for One Serving:

Size of Serving	Calories	Protein (g)	Carbohydrate (g)	Fat (g)
¼ recipe	52	0	13	0

Millet

Millet is nutritious and has a higher content of some B vitamins, copper, and iron than whole wheat or brown rice. Whole grains of millet are pale yellow to reddish orange in color. Millet flour and puffed millet are fairly easy to find in stores. Occasionally cracked millet may be sold as couscous, although most couscous is made from wheat. Millet is cooked like any other grain.

TO COOK MILLET

Simmering

Use 1½ (325 mL) cups of liquid to ½ cup (125 mL) grain.
Bring to a boil, cover, and reduce heat.
Simmer for 25 minutes.
Makes about 2½ cups (625 mL).

◆ If you keep the grain covered and undisturbed while cooking, it will be fluffy and separate, like rice.
◆ If you stir it frequently, and add a little liquid from time to time, the millet will acquire a creamy consistency like mashed potatoes.

◆ If you sauté the grain in a little canola oil before adding water, the cooking time will be cut in half.

Nutrition Information for One Serving:

Size of Serving	Calories	Protein (g)	Carbohydrate (g)	Fat (g)
½ cup (3½ oz)	121	4	24	<1

Millet Couscous

Cracked millet	1 cup	(250 mL)
Distilled water	2½ cups	(625 mL)

◆ Mix the grain with the water and let stand for 1 hour.
◆ Steam over boiling water (or simmering stew) for 30 minutes or until grain is cooked.

Makes 3–4 servings

Nutrition Information for One Serving:

Size of Serving	Calories	Protein (g)	Carbohydrate (g)	Fat (g)
½ cup (250 mL)	120	4	24	<1

MILLET RICE PITA BREAD (ROTI)

Brown rice flour	½ cup	(125 mL)
White rice flour	½ cup	(125 mL)
Millet flour	½ cup	(125 mL)
Sea salt	½ tsp	(2 mL)
Safflower oil	1 tbsp	(15 mL)
Distilled water	¼ cup	(60 mL)
		(or quantity needed to form firm dough)

◆ Stir flours and sea salt together in a mixing bowl.
◆ Add oil and mix well.
◆ Add water gradually and knead into a ball, using sufficient water to make a firm, but fairly soft, dough.
◆ Sprinkle rice flour on a flat counter or pastry board.
◆ Break off a piece of dough.
◆ Roll in the hands to make a round ball about 2 in. (5 cm) in diameter.
◆ Using hands, flatten the dough on the floured surface to make a pancake about 5 in. (13 cm) in diameter. The dough tends to break apart if a rolling pin is used.
◆ Heat a frying pan to medium-high heat on the stove.
◆ Cook flat bread on the dry pan, about 2 minutes. Press the surface of the bread gently with a cloth while cooking.

◆ Turn and cook the other side.
◆ Keep cooking each side alternately until small brown spots appear and bread is dry on the surface, but not burned.
◆ Serve hot, dry or spread with extra oil.

Makes about 8 breads

Nutrition Information per Bread:

Size of Serving	Calories	Protein (g)	Carbohydrate (g)	Fat (g)
1 bread	134	2.5	24.5	2.5

Millet Porridge

Whole-grain millet	½ cup	(125 mL)
Distilled water	1 cup	(250 mL)
Sea salt to taste	¼ tsp	(1 g)

◆ Soak millet overnight in distilled water.
◆ In the morning, add salt and cook covered for 20 minutes in the top of a double boiler. The mixture will be thick but can be thinned with more water.
◆ Serve with allowed fruit.

Makes 3–4 servings

Nutrition Information for One Serving:

Size of Serving	Calories	Protein (g)	Carbohydrate (g)	Fat (g)
⅓ cup (3½ oz) cooked	121	4	24	1

FRUIT

Suitable sources of fruits include

- Fresh or frozen pears
- Gerber First Food Pears
- Heinz Bartlett Pears (infant)
- Pears canned in pear juice (without preservatives or any other additives)
- Nonsulfited dried pears (available in health food stores)
- Fresh or frozen cranberries
- Cranberries canned without any additional ingredients

POACHED PEARS

Fresh pears, peeled, cored, and cut into halves	4 large (about 2–3 lb, or 1–1¼ kg)
Distilled water	1½ cups (375 mL)

- Place pears in a 3 quart (3 liter) saucepan.
- Add distilled water.
- Bring to a boil, reduce heat, cover, and simmer for 12–15 minutes until pears are tender but not mushy.
- Remove from stove and cool.

Makes 4 servings

Nutrition Information for One Serving:

Size of Serving	Calories	Protein (g)	Carbohydrate (g)	Fat (g)
2 pear halves	99	.5	23	.5

MIXED PEAR AND CRANBERRY COMPOTE

Fresh pears	4 large	(2–2½ lb, or 1–1¼ kg)
Fresh or frozen cranberries	2 cups	(500 mL)
Pear juice	1 cup	(250 mL)

- Peel and core the pears and cut into cubes.
- Place in a microwave-safe bowl.
- Add cranberries and pear juice.
- Mix, cover, and microwave for 4–5 minutes, or until pears are tender and cranberries have popped.
- OR cook in a saucepan on the stove for 12–15 minutes.

Makes 4 servings

Nutrition Information for One Serving:

Size of Serving	Calories	Protein (g)	Carbohydrate (g)	Fat (g)
1 cup (250 mL)	159	<1	37	<1

CRANBERRY SAUCE

| Pear juice | 1 cup | (250 mL) |
| Fresh or frozen cranberries | 2 cups | (500 mL) |

◆ Combine pear juice and cranberries in a small saucepan.
◆ Heat to boiling; reduce heat and simmer until cranberries are cooked and sauce has thickened.

Makes approximately 2 cups (500 mL) or eight ¼ cup (60 mL) servings

Nutrition Information for One Serving:

Size of Serving	Calories	Protein (g)	Carbohydrate (g)	Fat (g)
¼ cup (60 mL)	32	0	8	0

FRUIT BUTTER

| Dried pears, finely chopped | ½ cup | (125 mL) |
| Distilled water | ½ cup | (125 mL) |

◆ Combine dried pears with distilled water in a small covered saucepan.
◆ Bring to a boil, reduce heat, cover, and simmer for 15 minutes.
◆ Turn off heat and let stand for at least 30 minutes.
◆ The fruit will absorb more water as it cools. Add more distilled water if necessary to provide a good spreading consistency.
◆ Refrigerate.

Makes approximately ⅔ cup (175 mL) or twelve 1 tbsp (15 mL) servings

Nutrition Information for One Serving:

Size of Serving	Calories	Protein (g)	Carbohydrate (g)	Fat (g)
1 tbsp (15 mL)	16	0	4	0

Fruit Juice

Juice of pear or cranberries, including

◆ Pure pear juice can be extracted from the fruit using a juicer
◆ Gerber Pear Juice
◆ The water in which pears have been poached
◆ Gerber First Foods Pears or Heinz Bartlett Pears pureed and diluted with distilled water
◆ Pure cranberry juice without sweetener added (not available in all locations)

CRANBERRY CONCENTRATE

Fresh or frozen cranberries	2 cups	(500 mL)
Distilled water	2½ cups	(625 mL)

◆ Combine berries and distilled water in a stainless steel or enamel saucepan.
◆ Bring to a boil, reduce heat, cover, and simmer for 30 minutes.
◆ Strain, stirring and mashing berries until a fairly dry pulp remains in the sieve.
◆ Discard pulp.
◆ Store juice concentrate in the refrigerator.

Makes approximately 2 cups (500 mL) of concentrate

Nutrition Information for One Serving:

Size of Serving	Calories	Protein (g)	Carbohydrate (g)	Fat (g)
½ cup (125 mL)	32	0	8	0

CRANBERRY JUICE FROM CONCENTRATE

◆ Combine ¼ cup (60 mL) of cranberry concentrate with ¾ cup (200 mL) of distilled water.
◆ Serve chilled or add ice cubes made with distilled water if desired.

Nutrition Information for One Serving:

Size of Serving	Calories	Protein (g)	Carbohydrate (g)	Fat (g)
1 cup (250 mL)	16	0	4	0

FRUIT SLUSH

◆ Place in a blender or food processor:
   4–5 ice cubes made with distilled water
   ¾ cup (200 mL) of pear juice
   ¼ cup of cranberry concentrate
◆ Process on high speed until a "slushy" consistency is formed.
◆ Pour into glasses.

Nutrition Information for One Serving:

Size of Serving	Calories	Protein (g)	Carbohydrate (g)	Fat (g)
1¼ cups (310 mL)	107	0	26	0

FRUIT JUICE POPSICLES

◆ Combine ¼ cup (60 mL) of cranberry concentrate and ¾ cup (200 mL) of pear juice.
◆ Pour into an 8-portion, plastic popsicle maker.
◆ Add popsicle sticks.
◆ Freeze until firm.

Makes 8 popsicles

Nutrition Information for One Popsicle:

Size of Serving	Calories	Protein (g)	Carbohydrate (g)	Fat (g)
1 popsicle	16	0	4	0

FRUIT GLAZE

Cranberry juice	¼ cup	(50 mL)
Pear juice	¼ cup	(50 mL)
Safflower oil	1 tbsp	(15 mL)

◆ Combine cranberry juice, pear juice, and oil in a small saucepan.
◆ Bring to a boil.
◆ Reduce heat and simmer for 3 minutes.
◆ Remove from heat and, when cool, drizzle over turkey, fish, or lamb.

Nutrition Information for One Recipe:

Size of Serving	Calories	Protein (g)	Carbohydrate (g)	Fat (g)
5 tbsp (75 mL)	154	0	7	14

Vegetables

Vegetables Allowed

◆ Parsnips
◆ Squashes of all types
◆ Yams and Sweet potatoes
◆ Lettuce

Parsnips

◆ Parsnips are a good source of dietary starch and were very popular until the nineteenth century, when potatoes replaced them in popularity.
◆ Parsnips are a healthy stand-in for potatoes.
◆ Parsnips range in color from pale yellow to off-white.
◆ They can grow up to 20 inches long, but are most tender at about 8 inches.
◆ Very large parsnips tend to be overmature and have a tough, woody core.
◆ The vegetable should be firm and fairly smooth without many hairlike rootlets.
◆ Soft, withered parsnips are likely to be fibrous.
◆ Avoid parsnips with moist, dark spots.
◆ Parsnips should be stored like carrots, in a perforated plastic bag in the refrigerator crisper. They last 3–4 weeks when stored this way. Remove green leaves, if present, before storing.

Preparing and Cooking Parsnips
◆ Cut off the root and leaf ends. Trim off the large knobs.
◆ Scrub well or peel.
◆ Parsnips can be boiled, baked, steamed, or microwaved.
◆ The flavor of parsnips is sweetest when they are just cooked to the tender stage.
◆ Parsnips are too fibrous to be eaten raw.

Boiling
◆ Bring a saucepan of water to a boil.
◆ Drop in whole or cut-up parsnips.
◆ Reduce heat, cover, and simmer until tender.
◆ Cooking time: 5–15 minutes.

Baking
◆ Place whole or cut-up parsnips in a casserole dish with a cover.
◆ Pour about ½ cup (125 mL) distilled water or pear juice over the vegetables.
◆ Cover, and bake at 350°F (180°C) for 20–30 minutes.
◆ To reduce cooking time, parboil parsnips for 5 minutes before baking.

Microwaving
◆ Cut parsnips into large chunks.
◆ Place in a microwavable dish with 2 tablespoons (25 mL) of distilled water or pear juice.
◆ Cover with a lid or vented plastic wrap.
◆ Cooking time: 4–6 minutes per pound (500 g).

Steaming
◆ Place trimmed, well-scrubbed whole or cut-up parsnips in a steamer over boiling water.
◆ *Or*, place them in a saucepan with ½ in. (1½ cm) of boiling water.
◆ Cover and steam until tender.
◆ When cooked, allow to cool, or dip into cold water, and then peel.
◆ Cooking times: whole parsnips: 20–40 minutes; cut-up pieces: 5–15 minutes.

Nutrition Information for One Serving:

Size of Serving	Calories	Protein (g)	Carbohydrate (g)	Fat (g)
3½ oz raw (¾ cup sliced)	75	1	18	<1

BRAISED PARSNIPS

Parsnips	4 medium	(2 lb or 1 kg)
Safflower or canola oil		
Or lamb or turkey drippings	1 tbsp	(15 mL)
Sea salt	½ tsp	(3 mL) or to taste
Distilled water		
Or lamb or turkey broth	¾ cup	(175 mL)

◆ Preheat oven to 350°F (180°C).
◆ Peel and cut parsnips in half.
◆ Put parsnips in an oven-proof dish oiled with canola oil.
◆ Brush parsnips with oil or drippings.
◆ Sprinkle with sea salt and add water or broth.
◆ Cover and bake until tender (approximately 45 minutes).

Makes 4 servings

Nutrition Information for One Serving:

Size of Serving	Calories	Protein (g)	Carbohydrate (g)	Fat (g)
2 parsnip halves	126	1	16	6

PARSNIP AND YAM CASSEROLE

Fresh or frozen cranberries	½ cup	(125 mL)
Pear juice	½ cup	(125 mL)
Safflower or canola oil	2 tbsp	(25 mL)
Yams, peeled and sliced	1 cup	(250 mL)
Parsnips, peeled and sliced	1 cup	(250 mL)
Sea salt to taste		

- ◆ Preheat oven to 375°F (190°C).
- ◆ In a saucepan, combine cranberries and pear juice.
- ◆ Bring to a boil; reduce heat and simmer 15 minutes.
- ◆ Pour cranberry mix into an oven-proof dish.
- ◆ Wipe out saucepan and pour in oil.
- ◆ Heat oil and add yams and parsnips. Stir-fry for 5 minutes.
- ◆ Add yam mixture to cranberries. Stir and add salt to taste.
- ◆ Bake in oven for 30 minutes.

Makes 4 servings

Nutrition Information for One Serving:

Size of Serving	Calories	Protein (g)	Carbohydrate (g)	Fat (g)
¼ recipe	160	1	24	6

Squash

SUMMER SQUASH

Summer squash have edible skins and seeds. There are many varieties. All are mild and interchangeable in recipes. Their peak season is July through September, but in most places they are available year-round. Popular varieties include:

- ◆ Zucchini, both green and yellow
- ◆ Yellow straightneck or crookneck squash
- ◆ Chayote
- ◆ Pattypan squash (which is shaped like a top with a scalloped edge)

PREPARATION AND COOKING OF SUMMER SQUASH
- ◆ Trim off and discard ends.
- ◆ Wash the squash but do not peel unless the skin is thick. Beta-carotene is present in the skin, but there is none in the flesh.
- ◆ Chayote squash is the exception— it should be peeled because the skin is quite tough.
- ◆ Squash may be prepared and eaten whole, or diced, shredded, sliced, or cut into matchstick shapes.

Boiling
◆ Drop whole or halved squash into boiling water.
◆ Cook until tender.
◆ Cooking times: whole squash: 10–15 minutes; squash cut in halves: 5 minutes.

Microwaving
◆ Cut squash into slices.
◆ Arrange in layers in a microwavable dish.
◆ Add 3 tablespoons (35 mL) of distilled water.
◆ Cover.
◆ Cook until tender, stirring halfway through cooking time.
◆ Cooking time: 4–7 minutes.

Sautéing
◆ Cut squash into slices or chunks.
◆ Sauté in lamb or turkey broth with a little safflower oil added.
◆ Toss frequently to prevent the squash from browning.
◆ Blanch or salt the squash first if desired.
◆ Cooking times: summer squash: 3–6 minutes; chayote squash: 6–8 minutes.

Steaming
◆ Steam whole, sliced, diced, or cut into strips in a vegetable steamer.
◆ Cooking times:
   Whole summer squash: 10–12 minutes
   Halved or sliced summer squash: 3–5 minutes
   Chayote halves: 35– 40 minutes
   Chayote slices: 18–22 minutes

Stir-frying
◆ Cook sliced or diced squash in a wok or wide frying pan in a little safflower or canola oil.
◆ Keep stirring and tossing while cooking so that the slices cook quickly and do not turn watery.
◆ Cooking time: 4–5 minutes.

Nutrition Information for One Serving:

Size of Serving	Calories	Protein (g)	Carbohydrate (g)	Fat (g)
zucchini: 3½ oz raw (¾ cup sliced)	18	1	3	<1

Winter Squash

The skins and seeds of winter squash are inedible and need to be removed before eating. The yellow or orange flesh of the winter squashes is more nutritious than that of the summer varieties, being higher in carbohydrates and beta-carotene. There are dozens of varieties of winter squash, the most popular being

◆ Hubbard
◆ Acorn
◆ Butternut
◆ Spaghetti

Preparation and Cooking of Winter Squash *(excluding spaghetti squash; see separate instructions below)*
◆ Wash and cut acorn and butternut squash in half lengthwise.
◆ Cut Hubbard squash into serving-size pieces.
◆ Remove and discard seeds and fibers.
◆ Bake unpeeled, or peel with a sharp knife and cut into cubes or slices.

Boiling
◆ Place peeled squash pieces in a small amount of boiling water.
◆ Cook until tender.
◆ Drain well.
◆ Cooking time: 5–7 minutes.

Baking
◆ Cut small squash in half lengthwise and scoop out seeds and strings; cut large squash into serving-size pieces.
◆ Place the squash, cut side down, in a foil-lined baking pan.
◆ Pour about ¼ inch (1 cm) of water into the pan. Cover with foil.
◆ Bake at 350°F–400°F (180°–200°C) until squash is tender when pierced with a knife.
◆ Halfway through the baking time, turn the squash and brush the cut side with a little safflower or canola oil
◆ Cooking times: squash halves: 40–45 minutes; cut-up squash: 15–25 minutes.

Microwaving
◆ Arrange squash halves or large chunks in a shallow microwavable dish; cover with a lid or pierced plastic wrap.
◆ Cook until tender.
◆ Let stand for 5 minutes after cooking.
◆ Cooking times: squash halves: 7–10 minutes; chunks: 8 minutes

Sautéing
◆ Grated or peeled, diced squash can be sautéed in broth or a combination of broth and oil.
◆ Grated squash is best if it is cooked to the point where it is slightly crunchy.
◆ Cooking time: 8–15 minutes.

Steaming
◆ Place seeded squash halves cut side down, or peeled chunks or slices, in a vegetable steamer.
◆ Cook over boiling water until tender.
◆ Cooking time: 15–20 minutes.

Nutrition Information for One Serving:

Size of Serving	Calories	Protein (g)	Carbohydrate (g)	Fat (g)
Butternut: 3½ oz raw (1 cup cubed)	54	1	12	<1

Spaghetti Squash

The flesh of cooked spaghetti squash separates into slender strands that resemble spaghetti. This squash is a good substitute for pasta. Choose spaghetti squash as any other winter squash. It can be stored for up to 2 months. Spaghetti squash can be cooked whole or halved; do not peel.

PREPARATION AND COOKING OF SPAGHETTI SQUASH

Baking
◆ Pierce the shell several times with a fork.
◆ Place in a baking pan.
◆ Bake at 350°F (180°C) for 1 hour to 1 hour 45 minutes.
◆ Squash is cooked when the shell is no longer resistant to pressure.

Boiling
◆ Pierce the squash with a fork.
◆ Place in a large pot of boiling water.
◆ Reduce heat, cover, and simmer for 30–45 minutes or until tender when pricked.

Microwaving
◆ Pierce shell with a fork several times, or it may explode.
◆ Microwave 6–7 minutes, turn it over, and cook another 6–7 minutes.
◆ Let stand 5 minutes.

Steaming Squash Halves
◆ Cut the raw squash lengthwise (not cross-wise) through the middle.
◆ Place the halves, cut side up, in a pot and add 2 in. (5 cm) of boiling water.
◆ Cover and simmer until tender. Add more water if necessary, but ensure that the water remains below the cut edge of the squash so that the flesh cooks by steam.
◆ Or the halves may be cooked in the top of a vegetable steamer.

Preparation of the "Spaghetti"
◆ If squash was cooked whole, cut in half lengthwise. Scoop out the seeds and fibers.
◆ Take a fork and scrape the squash flesh along its length; the flesh will separate into pasta-like strands.
◆ Continue scraping down to the shell, transferring the forkfuls of strands as they are removed to a warm bowl or pot to keep warm.

Nutrition Information for One Serving:

Size of Serving	Calories	Protein (g)	Carbohydrate (g)	Fat (g)
1 cup (250 mL) cooked	71	3	15	1

BAKED SQUASH WITH PEARS

Acorn or other winter squash	1 small	
Safflower or canola oil	1 tbsp	(15 mL)
Sea salt	1 tsp	(5 mL)
Pears, peeled, cored and grated	2 medium	

◆ Preheat oven to 375°F (190°C).
◆ Rinse squash and pierce several times with a fork.
◆ Bake in a rimmed pan 30–40 minutes until almost soft.
◆ Remove from oven; cut in half, and scoop out seeds.
◆ Brush inside squash with canola oil and sprinkle with sea salt.
◆ Mound grated pear into squash halves and continue to bake 2–30 minutes or until tender.

Makes 2 servings

Nutrition Information for One Serving:

Size of Serving	Calories	Protein (g)	Carbohydrate (g)	Fat (g)
1 squash half	258	3	47	5

ZUCCHINI RICE

Safflower or canola oil	2 tbsp	(25 mL)
Zucchini, chopped	1 cup	(250 mL)
Long-grain brown rice	1 cup	(250 mL)
Sea salt to taste	¼ tsp	(1 mL)
Distilled water	2 cups	(500 mL)

◆ Heat oil in a saucepan.
◆ Add zucchini and stir-fry for 3 minutes.
◆ Wash rice well in a sieve.
◆ Add to saucepan and stir-fry for 3 minutes; ensure that all grains are coated with oil.
◆ Add distilled water and sea salt. Bring to a boil.
◆ Reduce heat and cover saucepan with a lid.
◆ Simmer for 1 hour.

Makes 4 servings

Nutrition Information for One Serving:

Size of Serving	Calories	Protein (g)	Carbohydrate (g)	Fat (g)
¼ recipe	255	4	40	7

ROASTED SQUASH SEEDS

Seeds from any type of squash
Safflower or canola oil

◆ Heat oven to 375°F (190°C).
◆ Remove fibrous strings and pulp from seeds and coat them lightly in oil.
◆ Place seeds in a single layer on a baking sheet.
◆ Bake in oven until seeds are lightly browned and slightly crisp, about 20 minutes.
◆ Stir seeds at about 10 minutes to ensure even browning.
◆ Be careful that seeds do not burn.
◆ Seeds can also be roasted in an open frying pan.
◆ Stir frequently while cooking.

Note: Roasted squash seeds can be ground in a food processor, blender, or coffee grinder to a fine flour. This may be added to rice, millet, or tapioca flour to provide extra nutrients and a "nuttier" flavor to the recipe. One tablespoon (15 mL) of squash seed flour to ½ cup (125 mL) grain flour works well, but quantities may be adjusted to individual taste.

Yams and Sweet Potatoes

Sweet potatoes are tuberous vegetables that resemble potatoes, but are not botanically related to them and belong to the morning glory family. True yams are large starchy roots (up to 10 lb) of plants of the *Dioscoreaceae* family. Both vegetables can be prepared in a similar manner.

SELECTION
◆ Choose potatoes that are heavy for their size.
◆ Choose those that are smooth, hard, and without bruises or decay, which appear as shriveled areas or black spots. Decay usually occurs first at the tips.
◆ The two varieties most readily obtainable are the moist orange-fleshed variety and the drier yellow-fleshed types. Both are acceptable.

PREPARATION AND COOKING
◆ Scrub vegetables well.
◆ They can be left whole or may be peeled, sliced, diced, or shredded.

Baking
◆ Preheat oven to 400°F (200°C).
◆ Pierce the skin in several places.
◆ Rub skin with safflower or canola oil.
◆ Arrange in a single layer in a rimmed baking pan.
◆ Bake uncovered for 45–50 minutes or until soft when squeezed.

Boiling
◆ Place 4 whole medium-size sweet potatoes or yams in a saucepan.
◆ Pour in distilled water to a depth of 2 in. (5 cm). Bring to a boil.
◆ Reduce heat; cover and boil for 20–30 minutes or until tender when pierced with a fork.
◆ Drain well.

Microwaving
◆ Pierce the skin of two medium-size sweet potatoes with a fork.
◆ Place on a double layer of paper towels in the microwave.
◆ Microwave on high for 5 minutes.
◆ Rotate the potatoes and cook for another 6–9 minutes.
◆ Let stand for 5 minutes. Potatoes should feel soft when squeezed.

Nutrition Information for One Serving:

Size of Serving	Calories	Protein (g)	Carbohydrate (g)	Fat (g)
1 cup cooked (250 mL)	158	2	37	<1

HASH BROWN SWEET POTATOES

Sweet potatoes	4 medium	(2 lb or 1 kg)
Canola oil	2 tsp	(10 mL)
Sea salt	Dash or to taste	

◆ Boil or steam potatoes in their jackets until they are crisp-tender when pierced with a fork (about 10–15 minutes).
◆ Chill.
◆ Peel, shred, or grate.
◆ Toss in oil and salt.
◆ Place in a frying pan and cook to desired brownness while stirring frequently (8–10 minutes or longer).

Makes 4 servings.

Nutrition Information for One Serving:

Size of Serving	Calories	Protein (g)	Carbohydrate (g)	Fat (g)
¼ recipe	136	1	28	2

SWEET POTATO PATTIES

Sweet potatoes, 2–4 depending on size	2 lbs	(1 kg)
Safflower or canola oil	2 tsp	(10 mL)
Sea salt to taste	½ tsp	(3 mL)

◆ Pierce potatoes several times with a fork.
◆ Boil or microwave sweet potatoes until they are tender-crisp when pierced with a knife.
◆ Chill and peel. Chop finely, grate, or mash.
◆ Mix in oil and sea salt.
◆ Pat into 4 thin patties.
◆ Brown in a nonstick skillet over medium heat for 10–12 minutes.
◆ Turn and brown another 8–10 minutes or to desired color.

Makes 4 servings

Nutrition Information for One Serving:

Size of Serving	Calories	Protein (g)	Carbohydrate (g)	Fat (g)
¼ recipe	235	3	46	3

MASHED SWEET POTATOES

Sweet potatoes	3 medium	
Safflower or canola oil	1 tbsp	(15 mL)
Sea salt to taste	¼ tsp	(1 mL)
Pear or cranberry juice	3 tbsp	(45 mL)

◆ Pierce potatoes several times with a fork.
◆ Boil or microwave potatoes until soft.
◆ Peel and mash, or process in a food processor.
◆ Add oil, sea salt, and juice. Add extra juice if potatoes are too dry.
◆ Process until well mixed and smooth.

Makes 4 servings

Nutrition Information for One Serving:

Size of Serving	Calories	Protein (g)	Carbohydrate (g)	Fat (g)
¼ recipe	248	3	47	4

SWEET POTATO PANCAKES

Sweet potatoes, peeled and grated	4 medium	(2 lb, or 1 kg)
Rice flour	2 tbsp	(25 mL)
Sea salt	½ tsp	(2.5 mL)
Safflower or canola oil	3 tbsp	(45 mL)

◆ Combine the grated potato, rice flour, and sea salt.
◆ Add more rice flour 1 tbsp (15 mL) at a time, if required to make the mixture stick together.
◆ Heat the oil medium-high in a frying pan or skillet.
◆ Drop the potato mixture in the oil by the spoonful. Flatten with the back of the spoon.
◆ Fry until brown and crisp on both sides.
◆ For variety, use a mixture of grated sweet potatoes, grated zucchini, and grated parsnips.

Makes 4 servings

Nutrition Information for One Serving:

Size of Serving	Calories	Protein (g)	Carbohydrate (g)	Fat (g)
¼ recipe	395	5	64	11

SWEET POTATO CHIPS

Sweet potatoes, sliced very thinly	2 medium potatoes
Safflower or canola oil	for frying
Sea salt	to taste

◆ Soak potato slices in ice-cold distilled water for 1 hour.
◆ Drain on paper toweling.
◆ Fry in 1 in. (2.5 cm) of oil heated to 400°F (200°C) until slightly brown. This will take only 1–2 minutes.
◆ Drain on paper towels and sprinkle with sea salt.
◆ The chips keep well in a tightly closed container.

Makes approximately 5 servings

Nutrition Information for One Serving:

Size of Serving	Calories	Protein (g)	Carbohydrate (g)	Fat (g)
⅕ recipe	230	2	24	14

Note: Zucchini chips can be made using the same method as sweet potato chips.

Lettuce

There are four basic types of lettuce available in most supermarkets and grocery stores:

◆ Butterhead, which includes the varieties Boston and Bibb lettuces.
◆ Iceberg (also known as head lettuce).
◆ Looseleaf, which consists of a number of varieties that don't form heads; instead, they consist of large, loosely packed leaves joined at a stem. The leaves are either green or shaded to deep red at the edges, and may be ruffled or smooth.
◆ Romaine (also known as cos lettuce).

All varieties are allowed in the Few-Foods Elimination Diet as long as they are tolerated. The variety that causes the largest number of reactions in sensitive people tends to be iceberg lettuce.

SELECTION AND STORAGE

◆ Lettuce should be fresh and crisp.
◆ Avoid wilted, limp, withered leaves that have brown or yellow edges or dark slimy spots.
◆ The darker outer leaves contain much more beta-carotene and vitamin C than the pale inner leaves, so you should select lettuce with healthy-looking intact outer leaves.
◆ Store in a plastic bag in the refrigerator crisper:
  – Iceberg lettuce will keep for up to 2 weeks.
  – Romaine lettuce will keep for about 10 days.
  – Butterhead and leaf lettuces will keep for about 4 days.

◆ Do not store greens near fruits such as apples and bananas, which give off ethylene gas as they ripen. The gas causes lettuce to decay rapidly and develop brown spots.

PREPARATION
◆ Wash lettuce, even if it is sold wrapped in cellophane.
◆ Remove the core of iceberg lettuce with a knife and wash under running water.
◆ Remove the stem and separate the leaves of looseleaf lettuce before washing.
◆ If the center ribs of the outer leaves of romaine lettuce are very thick, cut them away before using the leaves; the stems can be used in soup.
◆ Tear or cut lettuce into bite-size pieces.

Nutrition Information for One Serving:

Size of Serving	Calories	Protein (g)	Carbohydrate (g)	Fat (g)
3 oz raw (2 cups shredded)	16	2	2	<1

LETTUCE, ZUCCHINI, AND PEAR SALAD

Lettuce washed, dried, and torn into pieces	3 cups	(750 mL)
Zucchini, thinly sliced	1 cup	(250 mL)
Pear— peeled, cored, and sliced	1 large	
Oil-based salad dressing (recipe on page 437)	¼ cup	(60 mL)
Sea salt to taste	¼ tsp	(1 mL)

◆ In a salad bowl combine lettuce, zucchini and pears.
◆ Add salad dressing and toss
◆ Taste before adding more sea salt.

Makes 4 servings

Nutrition Information for One Serving:

Size of Serving	Calories	Protein (g)	Carbohydrate (g)	Fat (g)
¼ recipe	118	1	15	6

WILTED LETTUCE SALAD

Assorted varieties of lettuce	6 cups (approx. ¾ lb, or 375 g)
Oil-based salad dressing (recipe on this page)	½ cup (125 mL)

◆ Wash lettuce and cut or tear into bite-size pieces.
◆ Place lettuce in a large bowl.
◆ Bring salad dressing to a boil.
◆ Pour boiling dressing over lettuce and toss quickly.
◆ Serve immediately while salad is still warm.

Makes 4 servings

Nutrition Information for One Serving:

Size of Serving	Calories	Protein (g)	Carbohydrate (g)	Fat (g)
¼ recipe	118	1	15	6

OIL-BASED SALAD DRESSING

Safflower or canola oil	¼ cup	(60 mL)
Sea salt to taste	½ tsp	(2.5 mL)
Cranberry or pear juice	¼ cup	(60 mL)

◆ Place all ingredients in a small jar with a screw lid.
◆ Shake well before serving.

Makes 8 servings

Nutrition Information for One Serving:

Size of Serving	Calories	Protein (g)	Carbohydrate (g)	Fat (g)
1 tbsp (15 mL)	58	0	1	6

TRAIL MIX

Puffed rice
Puffed millet
Dried pear bits and cranberries with no preservatives or sweeteners
Roasted squash seeds

To puff rice or millet:
◆ Heat safflower or canola oil in a frying pan until a drop of water sizzles and jumps.
◆ Add millet or rice grains.
◆ Continue heating until most grains have popped.
◆ Remove from heat and transfer to a bowl.

MENU PLANNING

◆ There are many ways to combine the foods allowed, using the suggested recipes.

◆ It is fun to use one's creative talents in devising new and interesting meals in spite of what appears to be a very restricted ingredient list.

◆ A few ideas are suggested below.

◆ Make sure that a variety of *protein foods* (lamb, turkey or fish, and squash seeds), *grains* (rice, millet, tapioca, seed flours), *fruits* (pears, cranberries), *vegetables* (squashes, sweet potatoes, parsnips, lettuce), and *oil* (safflower, canola oil) are eaten every day to obtain the maximum nutritional benefit from the foods allowed.

Breakfast

◆ Cooked white or brown rice or millet with pureed pears or a jar of infant pears

◆ Hash brown sweet potatoes and a glass of pear juice

◆ Cream of brown rice with cranberries cooked in pear juice

◆ Riceola with poached pears

◆ Sweet potato pancakes with a glass of cranberry/pear juice

◆ On-the-run breakfast: a bottle of pure pear juice and trail mix

Soups

◆ Lamb or turkey broth

◆ To lamb or turkey broth add
  – rice noodles, rice, or millet
  – leftover chopped lamb or turkey
  – leftover cooked or chopped allowed vegetables
  – sea salt to taste

◆ Leftover vegetables such as yams and parsnips: Add distilled water, bring to a boil in a small saucepan, then puree in a blender or food processor. Add sea salt to taste.

Desserts

◆ Tapioca pudding with pears and cranberries

◆ Rice pudding with pears and cranberries

◆ Poached pears with cranberries and roasted squash seeds

Lunch or Dinner

1. Roast lamb
   Steamed rice
   Braised parsnips
   Mixed lettuce (romaine, red tip, iceberg) with oil-based dressing
   Fresh pear

2. Lamb meat sauce with spaghetti squash or pure rice noodles
   Tossed salad (romaine lettuce, yellow and green zucchini cubes) with oil-based dressing
   Tapioca pudding with cranberry sauce

3. Roast turkey breast half with fruit glaze
   Zucchini and yam casserole
   Head lettuce wedge with oil-based dressing
   Brown rice pudding

4. Turkey kabobs with zucchini
   Acorn squash slices (½ in./2.5 cm) slices brushed with oil and barbecued with kabobs
   Brown rice
   Fresh pear or poached pears

5. Baked fish fillets
   Baked winter squash
   Zucchini rice
   Mixed pear and cranberry compote

6. Fish mixed grill with sweet potatoes and pears
   Tossed salad (cooked rice, shredded zucchini, shredded lettuce) with oil-based dressing
   Fruit juice popsicle

7. Millet and rice pita bread
   Ground lamb
   Roast vegetables (parsnip, zucchini)
   Mixed lettuce leaves with oil-based dressing
   Poached pears

Snacks

◆ Ice-cold distilled water
◆ Chilled or hot pure pear juice or a mixture of pear and cranberry juice
◆ Cranberry or pear popsicles
◆ Raw pear
◆ Raw zucchini sticks with sea salt
◆ Lamb lettuce wraps
◆ Trail mix
◆ Toasted squash seeds with a sprinkling of salt
◆ Sweet potato or zucchini chips
◆ Leftover meat, vegetables, rice rolled in lettuce leaves
◆ Cooked rice or millet with fruit sauce or leftover meat and vegetables

— APPENDIX 2 —

SEQUENTIAL INCREMENTAL DOSE CHALLENGE

INSTRUCTIONS

- Carefully follow the detailed instructions for *sequential incremental dose challenge* provided in Chapter 28.
- Eat each test food in column two in the quantities and frequency described in the *challenge phase*, Chapter 28.
- Record any reactions you experience in column three.
- If you didn't have any reactions after the length of time specified on the Information Sheet, place a check mark by the "Pass" and follow the instructions in that column.
- If you recorded a reaction, place a check mark by the "Fail" and follow the instructions in that column.
- Proceed *exactly as instructed*, and in the *specified sequence*, for each selected food category.
- You can test the *food category* (dairy products, grains, fruits) in any order you wish.
- If the specific food you wish to challenge is not listed, test as described for the same type of food and enter results under "Other foods" at the end of the appropriate food category in the table

Do not test any food that is suspected to have caused a severe or anaphylactic reaction in the past by this method. Any foods that might cause a potentially severe reaction, especially in children, should be challenged only under medical supervision in a suitably equipped facility.

TEST COMPONENT	TEST FOOD	REACTION	PASS	FAIL
MILK AND MILK PRODUCTS				
TEST 1 **Casein**	White hard cheese; e.g., mozzarella, Parmesan		Pass___ Not sensitive to casein proteins **Proceed to Test 2**	Fail___ Sensitive to casein proteins **Proceed to Test 8**
TEST 2 Casein **Biogenic amines Annatto**	Orange/yellow aged cheese, e.g., aged (old) cheddar		Pass___ Not sensitive to annatto or biogenic **Proceed**	Fail___ Sensitive to biogenic amines or annatto[a] **Proceed**
TEST 3 Casein **whey**	Lactaid® milk or Lacteez® milk (99% lactose-free)		Pass___ Not sensitive to whey or casein proteins Not sensitive to cow's milk proteins **Proceed**	Fail___ Sensitive to whey proteins, but not to casein proteins **STOP HERE**
TEST 4 Casein Whey **lactose**	Milk: Homogenized, fat-reduced, 2%, 1%, or skim		Pass___ Not lactose-intolerant Not sensitive to cow's milk proteins **Proceed**	Fail___ Lactose-intolerant Not sensitive to cow's milk proteins **Proceed**
TEST 5 Modified milk proteins Partially digested lactose	Yogurt (plain only)		Pass___ Not sensitive to milk **Proceed**	Fail___ Lactose intolerance confirmed **STOP HERE**
TEST 6 Curdled milk with minimum fermentation	Cottage cheese		Pass___ Not sensitive to whole milk or lactose **Proceed**	Fail___ Sensitive to a component of cottage cheese Retest lactose Retest whole milk **STOP HERE**

a When you have a reaction, test each component (annatto [p. 461], biogenic amines [p. 454], histamine, and/or tyramine) separately.

TEST COMPONENT	TEST FOOD	REACTION	PASS	FAIL
MILK AND MILK PRODUCTS				
TEST 7 Complete milk in a complex manufactured product	Ice cream		Pass___ Not sensitive to milk Not lactose-intolerant Not sensitive to food additives Not sucrose intolerant	Fail___ *Suspect:* (1) Sucrose intolerance[b] (2) Sensitivity to food additives[c]
TEST 8a **Whey** (without casein) Lactose-free Test only if Test 1 for casein proteins is positive (failed Test 1)	Whey powder (contains whey but free from casein and milk solids) Lactose-free or treated with lactase enzyme (Lactaid™ drops)		Pass___ Not sensitive to whey proteins **Proceed**	Fail___ Sensitive to whey proteins **STOP HERE**
TEST 8b Whey with **lactose**	Complete whey powder		Pass___ Not lactose-intolerant	Fail___ Lactose-intolerant
YEAST				
Saccharomyces species	Debittered brewer's yeast		Pass___ Not sensitive to yeast	Fail___ Sensitive to yeast
GRAINS				
WHEAT				
TEST 1 Individual grain	Cream of wheat Puffed wheat Wheat flakes (cooked)		Pass___ Not sensitive to wheat **Proceed**	Fail___ Sensitive to wheat **STOP HERE**

b Challenge sucrose as described under "Sugars."
c Challenge food additives as described under "Food Additives."

TEST COMPONENT	TEST FOOD	REACTION	PASS	FAIL
GRAINS (continued)				
WHEAT (continued)				
TEST 2 Grain in a yeast-free baked product	Yeast-free soda bread Yeast-free flat bread Triscuit™ cracker		Pass___ Not sensitive to wheat Not sensitive to other ingredients in the product **Proceed**	Fail___ Sensitive to an ingredient in the product other than wheat Test other ingredients listed on the label of a manufactured food **STOP HERE**
TEST 3a White (wheat) flour without bleaching agent (contains yeast, but no benzoates)	White bread made with unbleached white (wheat) flour Use manufactured bread, or it can be made at home with unbleached white (wheat) flour		Pass___ Not sensitive to white (wheat) flour **Proceed to Test 3b**	Fail___ Sensitive to white (wheat) flour Sensitive to yeast if test for yeast (page 443) is positive **Proceed to Wheat Test 4**
TEST 3b White (wheat) flour with a bleaching agent (benzoate)	White bread or rolls made with "regular" bleached white wheat flour		Pass___ Not sensitive to to white flour, yeast, or benzoates	Fail___ Sensitive to benzoates Confirm by testing cinnamon, which contains a high level of benzoate (see page 4610)
TEST 4 Whole grain in a baked product with yeast	100% whole-wheat bread		Pass___ Not sensitive to wheat Not sensitive to yeast	Fail___ Possibly sensitive to proteins in wheat bran Sensitive to yeast if test for yeast (page 443) is positive

TEST COMPONENT	TEST FOOD	REACTION	PASS	FAIL
GRAINS (continued)				
RYE				
Single grain	Rye flakes (cooked)		Pass___ Not sensitive to rye **Proceed**	Fail___ Sensitive to rye **STOP HERE**
Whole grain in a yeast-free baked product	100% rye cracker: Ryvita™ (wheat-free) or Wasa Light™		Pass___ Not sensitive to rye Not sensitive to other ingredients in the product **Proceed**	Fail___ Possibly sensitive to an ingredient in the product Product label may identify possible reactive ingredients **STOP HERE**
OATS	*****	*****	*****	*****
Single grain	Oatmeal porridge made from natural oats (e.g., Traditional Quaker™ oatmeal)		Pass___	Fail___
Grain in a baked product	Traditional Scottish oat cake without wheat, made with oat flour		Pass___	Fail___
BARLEY				
Single grain	Barley flakes cooked as a porridge *Or* Pearl barley added to a meat-based stew		Pass___ Pass___	Fail___ Fail___
Grain in a baked product	Barley bread with only tolerated ingredients		Pass___	Fail___

***** From this point on, "Pass" means the food, or component part of food, being tested is tolerated; "Fail" means that it is NOT tolerated.

TEST COMPONENT	TEST FOOD	REACTION	PASS	FAIL
GRAINS (continued)				
CORN				
TEST 1 Single grain	Corn on the cob *Or* Corn niblets		Pass___ Pass___	Fail___ Fail___
TEST 2 Processed whole grain	Popcorn		Pass___	Fail___
TEST 3 Cornmeal	Cornmeal bread or muffins with tolerated ingredients		Pass___	Fail___
TEST 4 Cornstarch or corn flour	Used as a thickener in a product with tolerated ingredients		Pass___	Fail___
TEST 5 Corn oil	Added to a recipe with tolerated ingredients		Pass___	Fail___
TEST 6 Corn syrup	Add to recipe with tolerated ingredients		Pass___	Fail___
SOY				
TEST 1 Tofu	Extra-firm tofu, cooked		Pass___	Fail___
TEST 2 Soy beverage[d]	Boiled		Pass___	Fail___
	Uncooked		Pass___	Fail___
TEST 3 Fermented soy product without wheat	Tamari sauce		Pass___	Fail___

[d] Most commercial soy beverages are uncooked. Many people react to *raw* soy beverages, but tolerate them cooked.

TEST COMPONENT	TEST FOOD	REACTION	PASS	FAIL
FRUIT[e]				
ORANGE				
Orange juice, cooked	Pasteurized orange juice		Pass___	Fail___
	Or Diluted frozen orange juice, boiled and cooled		Pass___	Fail___
Orange juice	Fresh squeezed		Pass___	Fail
	Or Reconstituted from frozen concentrate		Pass___	Fail___
Orange, cooked	Canned mandarin orange		Pass___	Fail___
	Or Fresh orange, cooked in microwave or oven		Pass___	Fail___
Raw orange	Fresh mandarin		Pass___	Fail___
	Fresh navel		Pass___	Fail___
GRAPEFRUIT				
Grapefruit juice, cooked	Pasteurized grapefruit juice		Pass___	Fail___
	Or Fresh or frozen grapefruit juice, boiled and cooled		Pass___	Fail___
Grapefruit juice	Fresh squeezed		Pass___	Fail___
	Or Reconstituted from frozen concentrate		Pass___	Fail___

[e] Canned fruit is cooked. Dried fruit is sold in the raw state.

TEST COMPONENT	TEST FOOD	REACTION	PASS	FAIL
FRUIT[e]				
GRAPEFRUIT (continued)				
Grapefruit, cooked	Canned grapefruit segments *Or* Grapefruit cooked in microwave or oven		Pass___ Pass___	Fail___ Fail___
Raw grapefruit	Fresh white grapefruit		Pass___	Fail___
	Fresh pink grapefruit		Pass___	Fail___
GRAPES AND RAISINS[f]				
Fresh grapes	Grapes, washed		Pass___ Not sensitive to grapes Not sensitive to sulfite	Fail___ Sensitive to grapes and/or sulfite Test sulfite separately
Raisins without sulfite	Nonsulfited raisins		Pass___ Not sensitive to raisins	Fail___ Sensitive to raisins and probably grapes
Raisins with sulfite	Regular (sulfited) raisins		Pass___ Not sensitive to raisins Not sensitive to sulfite	Fail___ If nonsulfited raisins are tolerated, sensitive to sulfite
APPLE				
Apple juice, cooked	Pasteurized apple juice *Or* Fresh or frozen apple juice, boiled and cooled		Pass___ Pass___	Fail___ Fail___

[f] Do *not* challenge grapes if sulfite sensitivity is suspected, until sulfite is proven safe by challenge.

TEST COMPONENT	TEST FOOD	REACTION	PASS	FAIL
FRUIT[e] (continued)				
APPLE (continued)				
Apple juice	Unpasteurized pure juice *Or* Reconstituted from frozen concentrate		Pass___ Pass___	Fail___ Fail___
Apple, cooked	Fresh apple, peeled, cored, and cooked *Or* Applesauce without added sugar		Pass___ Pass___	Fail___ Fail___
Fresh apple	Golden Delicious		Pass___	Fail___
	MacIntosh		Pass___	Fail___
	Granny Smith		Pass___	Fail___
	Other varieties (specify type)		Pass___	Fail___
OTHER FRUITS				
Apricot	Cooked		Pass___	Fail___
	Raw		Pass___	Fail___
Banana	Cooked		Pass___	Fail___
	Raw		Pass___	Fail___
Kiwi	Cooked		Pass___	Fail___
	Raw		Pass___	Fail___
Peach	Cooked		Pass___	Fail___
	Raw		Pass___	Fail___

TEST COMPONENT	TEST FOOD	REACTION	PASS	FAIL
FRUIT[e] (continued)				
OTHER FRUITS (continued)				
Pear	Cooked		Pass___	Fail___
	Raw		Pass___	Fail___
Pineapple	Cooked		Pass___	Fail___
	Raw		Pass___	Fail___
Nectarine	Cooked		Pass___	Fail___
	Raw		Pass___	Fail___
Other fruits (specify type)				

TEST COMPONENT	TEST FOOD	REACTION	PASS	FAIL
VEGETABLES				
TOMATO				
Tomato juice, cooked	Canned or boiled		Pass___	Fail___
Tomato juice, raw	Commercial or freshly made in blender		Pass___	Fail___
Tomato, cooked	Canned or cooked slices		Pass___	Fail___
Tomato, raw	Various varieties (specify types)		Pass___	Fail___
Tomato ketchup (catsup)	Commercial brand		Pass___	Fail___ It tomato is tolerated, suspect vinegar. Confirm by testing vinegar separately (page 453)
SPINACH				
Cooked	Fresh or frozen spinach leaves, boiled		Pass___	Fail___
Raw	Fresh spinach leaves, eaten as a salad		Pass___	Fail___
CARROT				
Carrot juice, cooked	Juice extracted from raw carrots, boiled		Pass___	Fail___

TEST COMPONENT	TEST FOOD	REACTION	PASS	FAIL
VEGETABLES (continued)				
CARROT (continued)				
Carrot juice	Juice from raw carrots		Pass___	Fail___
Carrot, cooked	Carrots, sliced and boiled		Pass___	Fail___
Carrot, raw	Carrot sticks, fresh		Pass___	Fail___
OTHER VEGETABLES				
Celery	Cooked		Pass___	Fail___
	Raw		Pass___	Fail___
Cucumber	Cooked		Pass___	Fail___
	Raw		Pass___	Fail___
Lettuce	Cooked		Pass___	Fail___
	Raw		Pass___	Fail___
Radish	Cooked		Pass___	Fail___
	Raw		Pass___	Fail___
Other vegetables (specify types)			Pass___	Fail___

TEST COMPONENT	TEST FOOD	REACTION	PASS	FAIL
SPICES				
Cinnamon			Pass___	Fail___
Anise			Pass___	Fail___
Nutmeg			Pass___	Fail___
Cayenne			Pass___	Fail___
Curry spice mixture			Pass___	Fail___
Chili spice mixture			Pass___	Fail___
Other spices (specify types)			Pass___	Fail___
VINEGAR				
Distilled vinegar	White vinegar		Pass___	Fail___
Wine components	Wine vinegar		Pass___	Fail___
Fermented rice products	Rice vinegar		Pass___	Fail___
Additional ingredients	Balsamic vinegar		Pass___	Fail___
Raw vegetables in vinegar	Dill pickles		Pass___	Fail___
	Other pickles and relishes (specify types)		Pass___	Fail___

TEST COMPONENT	TEST FOOD	REACTION	PASS	FAIL
ALCOHOL				
Distilled alcohol	Vodka *Or* Gin *Or* Tequila *Or* White rum		Pass___ Pass___ Pass___ Pass___	Fail___ Fail___ Fail___ Fail___
Histamine in wine	White wine		Pass___	Fail___
Tyramine in wine	Red wine		Pass___	Fail___
Fermented grain products	Beer *Or* Ale *Or* Lager		Pass___ Pass___ Pass___	Fail___ Fail___ Fail___
Fermented fruit products	Apple cider		Pass___	Fail___
Fermented beverage without alcohol (histamine)	De-alcoholized wine		Pass___	Fail___
Fermented beverage without alcohol (grain products)	De-alcoholized beer or equivalent		Pass___	Fail___
TEA				
Herbal tea			Pass___	Fail___
Green tea			Pass___	Fail___
Decaffeinated regular tea			Pass___	Fail___
Regular tea			Pass___	Fail___

TEST COMPONENT	TEST FOOD	REACTION	PASS	FAIL
COFFEE				
Decaffeinated coffee			Pass___	Fail___
Regular coffee			Pass___	Fail___
Flavored coffees (specify types)			Pass___	Fail___
SUGARS				
Maple sugar or syrup			Pass___	Fail___
Cane sugar			Pass___	Fail___
Beet sugar			Pass___	Fail___
Corn syrup			Pass___	Fail___
Date sugar			Pass___	Fail___
Fructose			Pass___	Fail___
Honey			Pass___	Fail___
CHOCOLATE				
Cocoa butter	Dark, bitter, baker's chocolate sweetened as described in Chapter 28 (page 379)		Pass___	Fail___
Cocoa butter with milk	Dark baker's chocolate with milk and sweetener added		Pass___	Fail___
Complete chocolate confectionery	Purchased chocolate		Pass___	Fail___

TEST COMPONENT	TEST FOOD	REACTION	PASS	FAIL
LEGUMES				
Peanut	Peanut, roasted or boiled		Pass___	Fail___
	Peanut, raw		Pass___	Fail___
Whole beans, cooked (many *raw* beans are toxic)	Green (French, string, runner) bean		Pass___	Fail___
	Yellow wax bean		Pass___	Fail___
	Broad bean (fava)		Pass___	Fail___
	Lima bean		Pass___	Fail___
Dried beans	Navy		Pass___	Fail___
	Pinto		Pass___	Fail___
	Kidney		Pass___	Fail___
	Black-eyed peas		Pass___	Fail___
	Lentils		Pass___	Fail___
	Split peas		Pass___	Fail___
	Others (specify types)		Pass___	Fail___
Bean sprouts	Mung bean		Pass___	Fail___
	Alfalfa		Pass___	Fail___
	Others (specify types)		Pass___	Fail___
Green peas	Cooked		Pass___	Fail___
	Raw		Pass___	Fail___

TEST COMPONENT	TEST FOOD	REACTION	PASS	FAIL
NUTS				
Whole nuts	Almond		Pass___	Fail___
	Brazil		Pass___	Fail___
	Cashew		Pass___	Fail___
	Chestnut		Pass___	Fail___
	Hazelnut (filbert)		Pass___	Fail___
	Macadamia		Pass___	Fail___
	Pine nut		Pass___	Fail___
	Pistachio *Or* Pecan		Pass___ Pass	Fail___ Fail___
	Walnut		Pass___	Fail___
	Coconut		Pass___	Fail___
	Other nuts (specify types)		Pass___	Fail___
SEEDS				
Whole seeds, roasted	Sesame		Pass___	Fail___
	Sunflower		Pass___	Fail___
	Flax		Pass___	Fail___
	Melon		Pass___	Fail___
	Poppy		Pass___	Fail___
	Pumpkin		Pass___	Fail___
	Other seeds (specify types)		Pass___	Fail___

TEST COMPONENT	TEST FOOD	REACTION	PASS	FAIL
MEAT AND POULTRY				
Meat	Beef		Pass___	Fail___
	Pork		Pass___	Fail___
	Lamb		Pass___	Fail___
	Other meats (specify types)		Pass___	Fail___
Poultry	Chicken		Pass___	Fail___
	Turkey		Pass___	Fail___
	Duck		Pass___	Fail___
	Other poultry (specify types)		Pass___	Fail___
Processed meats ("deli meats")	Pepperoni		Pass___	Fail___
	Salami		Pass___	Fail___
	Bologna		Pass___	Fail___
	Cured bacon		Pass___	Fail___
	Smoked bacon		Pass___	Fail___
	Cured ham		Pass___	Fail___
	Frankfurter		Pass___	Fail___
	Wiener		Pass___	Fail___

TEST COMPONENT	TEST FOOD	REACTION	PASS	FAIL
FISH				
Fresh or frozen, cooked	Cod		Pass___	Fail___
	Sole		Pass___	Fail___
	Red snapper		Pass___	Fail___
	Salmon		Pass___	Fail___
	Halibut		Pass___	Fail___
	Perch		Pass___	Fail___
	Others (specify types)		Pass___	Fail___
Canned fish	Tuna		Pass___	Fail___
	Salmon		Pass___	Fail___
	Sardines		Pass___	Fail___
	Others (specify types)		Pass___	Fail___
SHELLFISH				
Cooked	Lobster		Pass___	Fail___
	Prawn		Pass___	Fail___
	Shrimp		Pass___	Fail___
	Crab		Pass___	Fail___
	Others (specify types)		Pass___	Fail___
Raw	For example, as eaten in sushi (specify types)		Pass___	Fail___

TEST COMPONENT	TEST FOOD	REACTION	PASS	FAIL
FOOD ADDITIVES				
Tartrazine	TEST 1 Cheese without tartrazine: natural orange/ yellow cheddar cheese		Pass___ Not sensitive to cow's milk cheese **Proceed to Test 2**	Fail___ Sensitive to cow's milk cheese Choose another similar food and retest
	TEST 2 Similar cheese containing tartrazine: processed cheese food or processed cheese slides (label will read "tartrazine" or "artificial food color)		Pass___ Not sensitive to tartrazine	Fail___ Sensitive to tartrazine
Sulfites	TEST 1 Dried fruit without natural color—all fruits appear the same beige/brown. Usually available in health food stores. Label will not have the word "sulfite" in the ingredient list. Example: dried apricots		Pass___ Not sensitive to test fruit (apricot) **Proceed to Test 2**	Fail___ Sensitive to test fruit (apricot) Choose another fruit and retest
	TEST 2 The same dried fruit treated with sulfites—the fruit will retain its natural color. "Sulfite" will appear on the label. Purchase from a regular grocery store or supermarket. Example: dried apricots		Pass___ Not sensitive to sulfites	Fail___ Sensitive to sulfites

TEST COMPONENT	TEST FOOD	REACTION	PASS	FAIL
FOOD ADDITIVES (continued)				
MSG	Available as a powder to be added to a carrier food that is known to be tolerated		Pass___ Not sensitive to MSG	Fail___ Sensitive to MSG
Benzoates	Cinnamon (see page 453)		Pass___ Not sensitive to benzoates	Fail___ Sensitive to benzoates
Annatto	TEST 1 Cheese without annatto: white or natural (cream-colored). Choose a cheese that is available in both an orange/yellow color and a natural/cream color, for example, cheddar.		Pass___ Not sensitive to cow's milk cheese **Proceed to Test 2**	Fail___ Sensitive to cow's milk cheese Choose another similar food and retest
	TEST 2 The same type of cheese with annatto added, such as orange/yellow cheddar		Pass___ Not sensitive to annatto	Fail___ Sensitive to annatto
OTHER FOODS				
	Specify types:		Pass___	Fail___

— GLOSSARY —

acetylcholine Chemical that relays nerve impulses released at the synapses (meeting points) of the parasympathetic nerves and at neuromuscular junctions.

adrenaline See *epinephrine*.

adrenergic agents Chemicals that stimulate the release of the neurotransmitter norepinephrine from nerve fibers of the sympathetic nervous system. There are two kinds, alpha and beta. Alpha-adrenergic agents constrict blood vessels, and alpha-adrenergic drugs (such as phenylephrine) are used as nasal decongestants; beta-adrenergic agents relax smooth muscle, and beta-adrenergic drugs (such as salbutamol) are used as bronchodilators (dilate or widen bronchi in the lungs) in the treatment of asthma.

aerosol Suspension of solid or liquid particles in a gas.

albumin A type of protein classified on the basis of its solubility. Albumins are soluble in water at pH 6.6. They occur in different forms according to their function, for example, serum albumin in animals and humans, ovalbumin in eggs, parvalbumin in fish, and α-lactalbumin in milk. See also *globulin, glutenin, and prolamin.*

allergen Antigen or hapten that causes a hypersensitivity reaction (allergy) in a sensitized individual. An *antigen* is a foreign protein that causes a response of the immune system. A *hapten* is a small molecule that causes immune system response when coupled with a protein.

amino acid Organic compound containing amino (nitrogen-hydrogen) and carboxyl (carbon-oxygen) groups. Amino acids are the building blocks of all proteins.

anabolism Synthesis by cells of complex compounds from simpler substances. The reverse of catabolism. See also *catabolism.*

anamnestic response Rapid production of antibody in response to an antigen subsequent to a first exposure, as in natural reinfection or a booster shot of vaccine. It requires the presence of memory B- and T-cells remaining from the first exposure.

anaphylactic reaction (anaphylaxis) Type 1 hypersensitivity reaction (allergy) due to the release of chemical mediators from cells caused to degranulate (release inflammatory chemicals) by complexing of antibody (usually IgE) with its homologous (matching) allergen.

463

anaphylactic shock Acute generalized reaction to an allergen in which edema (swelling), constriction of smooth muscles in the lungs, stomach, and blood vessels, a fall in blood pressure, circulatory collapse, and heart failure can lead to death.

anaphylactoid reaction Reaction with anaphylactic symptoms *not* directly induced by an antigen-antibody complex. Type III hypersensitivity reactions (IgG-mediated) are often referred to as anaphylactoid; they are induced by anaphylatoxins (see below).

anaphylatoxin Substance produced during a complement cascade (specifically by complement components C3a and C5a) that causes the release of histamine and other vasoactive chemicals from mast cells and basophils. See also *complement cascade*.

anaphylaxis See *anaphylactic reaction*.

antibiotic Substance produced by microorganisms that can kill or inhibit the growth of other microorganisms by interfering with their metabolism (growth and reproduction), for example, penicillin and sulfa drugs.

antibody A protein of the gamma-globulin type (immunoglobulin) produced by lymphocytes (white blood cells) in the blood in response to a foreign substance called an *antigen*.

antigen Foreign substance that induces the production of specific (homologous, or matching) antibody by the immune system of the host it enters.

antigen determinant site Part of an antigen's molecular structure that induces the production of antibody. Each cell has several different antigen determinant sites.

antigen processing Display of antigens on the surface of a macrophage (white blood cell) that has engulfed and partially destroyed them, a preconditioning for recognition and a protective response by T-cell lymphocytes. See also *T cells*.

antihistamine Drug–for example, chlorpheniramine, diphenhydramine, and mepyramine–that inhibits the action of histamine and is widely used to treat hypersensitivity reactions in which histamine is the main cause of symptoms such as hay fever, urticaria (hives), and pruritus (itching).

antioxidant A substance added to food to keep oxygen from changing the food's color or flavor.

antiserum Fluid portion (serum) of blood containing antibodies to specific known foreign substances called *antigens*. Used in diagnostic serology (analysis of blood serum) to identify unknown antigens and in passive immunization to transfer temporary immunity against a microorganism that causes disease.

antitoxin Antiserum containing antibodies against a toxin or toxoid (poisonous substances).

arachidonic acid Polyunsaturated fatty acid component of membrane phospholipids (fats attached to phosphorus molecules). Tissue disruption by any cause, especially immunological mechanisms, allows enzymes (a type of protein that breaks down and builds up all organic material) to separate arachidonic acid from the phospholipid, to be metabolized into a large number of chemicals (known as *eicosanoids*), such as prostaglandins and leukotrienes, that contribute to an inflammatory response.

atopy, atopic allergy A Type 1 IgE-dependent hypersensitivity reaction with rapid onset of symptoms.

autoallergy Hypersensitivity response to an allergen that is part of the body itself. Similar to *autoimmunity*.

autoantibody Antibody produced against antigens on a body's own cells, often leading to *autoimmune disease*.

autoantigen Antigen that is part of the body's own cells and induces the production of autoantibody, often leading to *autoimmune disease*.

autoimmune disease Immune response against its own body tissues leading to disease states, for example, Graves' disease, Hashimoto's thyroiditis, multiple sclerosis, lupus.

autoimmunity Production of antibodies against antigens of the body's own tissues. Often leads to *autoimmune disease* and tissue damage.

autonomic nervous system "Independent nervous system" not under our control that regulates cardiac muscle, smooth muscle, and glands. Also known as the sympathetic nervous system.

avirulent Describes a strain of microorganism that cannot cause disease.

azo- Prefix denoting a nitrogenous (containing nitrogen) compound, as in the azo dye tartrazine.

basophil White blood cell containing granules that stain with basic (alkaline) dyes. Degranulation (release of contents of the granules) in hypersensitivity (allergic) reactions releases mediators (chemicals that cause symptoms) of the allergic response.

B cell Lymphocyte (white blood cell) that produces antibodies in response to a specific antigen.

blocking antibody Antibody of one type that couples with a specific antigen, thus denying access to antibody of another type; for example, desensitization to a particular allergen, say ragweed pollen, produces IgG antibodies that block IgE from forming a complex with the allergen, thus preventing Type 1 hypersensitivity reactions (atopic allergy).

bradykinin Vasoactive peptide (peptide active on blood vessels), released during a hypersensitivity reaction, that causes pain, dilation (widening) of blood vessels, edema (swelling), and smooth muscle contraction.

bronchitis Inflammation of lung passages (bronchi) caused by infection with a microorganism or other agents that damage the bronchial lining.

bronchoconstriction Narrowing of the bronchi (lung passages) by contraction of the smooth muscle surrounding them.

bronchodilation Opening of the bronchi (lung passages) by relaxation of their smooth muscle coating.

bronchospasm Narrowing of the bronchi (lung passages) due to spasmodic contraction of their smooth muscle coating, caused by some stimulus. Usually allows air to be inhaled but requires great effort to expel it effectively. Occurs in such conditions as asthma and bronchitis.

bronchus (plural: **bronchi**) Air passages in the lungs that branch off from the trachea (windpipe), lined with mucus-secreting cells and surrounded by smooth muscle.

carbohydrates Compounds containing carbon, hydrogen, and oxygen with the general formula $C_x(H_2O)_y$. They are one of the three main constituents of food (protein and fat are the others) and include the sugars and starches. They are an important source of energy in cellular metabolism. Carbohydrates constitute three-quarters of the biological world and about 80% of the caloric intake of humans. The most abundant carbohydrate is cellulose, the principal constituent of trees and other plants; the major food carbohydrate is starch.

catabolism Breaking down of compounds into smaller, often simple, molecules by means of proteins called *enzymes*.

chemotaxin Chemical that promotes movement of a cell or microorganism toward a target in the process of *chemotaxis*.

chemotaxis Movement of a cell or microorganism toward a target in response to a concentration gradient (movement from high concentration to lower concentration, or vice versa) of a chemical known as a *chemotaxin*.

chitin A white, insoluble, tough polysaccharide (carbohydrate composed of sugar molecules). Next to cellulose, it is the most abundant natural polysaccharide.

chitinase An enzyme that hydrolyzes *chitin* to produce a linear homopolymer acetyl glucosamine.

cholinergic Describes nerve fibers that release the neurotransmitter acetylcholine.

colostrum First secretion from the breast after childbirth. Contains serum, protein nutrients, antibodies, lymphocytes, and macrophages.

complement Group of over twenty enzymatic proteins in the blood that act together, in response to antigen and antibody, to destroy foreign cells by a process known as *lysis*.

complement cascade *Sequential* activation of complement proteins resulting in lysis (destruction) of a target cell. The cascade releases various chemical by-products that act as opsonins, chemotaxins, and anaphylatoxins to help destroy a threat to the body.

complement fixation (1) Combining of complement proteins with antigen-antibody complexes that trigger the classical-pathway complement cascade. (2) Serological (blood) test to determine whether an antigen and an antibody are homologous (match) by the addition of *complement*. If homologous, they form a complex that attaches to (fixes) complement so that it cannot destroy (lyse) cells. For example, if sheep red blood cells (the antigen) are not lysed by complement in the presence of antigen-antibody complex, it is a positive indication that the cells and their antibody are homologous.

conjunctiva (plural: **conjunctivae**) Membrane covering the front of the eye and lining the eyelids.

conjunctivitis Inflammation of the *conjunctivae*, causing redness, swelling, and a watery discharge.

cross-reacting allergens A rather loose term that indicates that a person sensitized to one allergen will react to another allergen related to the first, because it either is from the same botanic family or is structurally very similar.

cyclo-oxygenase pathway Enzyme system that converts a achidonic acid (a fatty acid with a 20-carbon chain) to the important regulatory chemicals known as the prostaglandins: important as secondary inflammatory mediators (facilitators) of allergy.

cyto- Prefix denoting cell.

cytokines Collective name for lymphokines and monokines (the interleukins and interferons), peptides produced by immune system cells such as lymphocytes and macrophages (white blood cells). Involved in sending signals between cells.

cytolysis Destruction (lysis) of a cell, usually by disruption of its membrane and other outer structures.

dalton Atomic mass unit, equal to 1.6605×10^{-27} kg, $1/12$ the mass of an atom of carbon 12. The molecular weight of molecules is measured in daltons. A kilodalton (kd or kD) is 1,000 daltons.

DBPCFC See *double-blind placebo-controlled food challenge.*

degranulation Release of chemicals from the intracellular granules of leukocytes (white blood cells) in the process of inflammation.

desensitization Prevention or reduction in the allergic response to an allergen by use of allergen injections of gradually increasing strength (aka "allergy shots"). Often used in treatment of hay fever caused by pollens.

double-blind placebo-controlled food challenge Test in which the identity of the food to be challenged is unknown to both the patient and the supervisor of the test. A placebo (nonreactive material that will not cause a response in the body) is similarly concealed and the patient's response to the food is compared to his or her response to the placebo. A positive test is the appearance of symptoms after the patient consumes the food, with no symptoms in response to the placebo.

eicosanoids Collective name for reactive chemicals, such as leukotrienes, prostaglandins, and thromboxanes, derived from eicosanoic acid (a fatty acid with a 20-carbon chain); such as a achidonic acid. Eicosanoids are active chemicals in the allergic response.

ELISA See *enzyme-linked immunosorbent assay*. A blood test for measuring antibodies, especially IgE, against foods, when allergy is suspected.

emulsifier An agent that is added to food to stabilize a mixture and prevent it from separating into its different ingredients. For example, it allows oil and water to mix without separating into two distinct layers. Lecithin is one of the most common food emulsifiers.

endo- Prefix denoting inside. For example, *endogenous* means "originating from inside an organism or a body."

endocrine system System of ductless glands and other structures, including the pituitary, thyroid, parathyroid, and adrenal glands, the ovaries, testes, placenta, and part of the pancreas, and the hormones they secrete internally and release into the bloodstream.

endorphins Chemicals in the brain derived from beta-lipotropin, produced by the pituitary gland. Endorphins appear to influence the activities of the endocrine glands and have pain-relieving properties similar to those of the opiates.

endotoxin Lipopolysaccharide (fat-sugar complex) that is part of the cell wall of Gram-negative bacteria, released only when the bacteria disintegrate. Endotoxins are responsible for the fever, gastrointestinal disorder, and shock of infections caused by disease-causing enterobacteria such as salmonella and shigella.

enteritis Inflammation of the small intestine.

enzyme Protein produced by a living organism, that catalyzes a biological reaction without itself being affected. Enzymes are essential for the normal functioning of the body.

enzyme-linked immunosorbent assay (ELISA) Immunological (blood) test for identification of antigen-specific antibody in blood serum. Usually used to identify IgE or IgG antibodies to allergens. The "indicator system" for positive reactions is antibody to IgE or IgG linked to an enzyme. This acts on the enzyme substrate (substance that is changed by the enzyme) to form a product that is usually indicated by a change in color.

eosinophil Granulocytic white blood cell whose granules stain with acidic dyes such as eosin. Eosinophils help defend the body against parasites and contribute to allergic reactions by releasing the chemicals within their granules when they reach the reaction site.

epinephrine (adrenaline) Hormone secreted by the adrenal gland that prepares the body for "fight or flight." It has an important role in the control of blood circulation, muscle action, and sugar metabolism.

epitope A single antigenic determinant. Functionally it is the portion of an antigen that combines with the antibody, at a site called the paratope.

erythema Abnormal reddening of the skin caused by dilation of small blood vessels.

erythrocyte Red blood cell. Its color comes from hemoglobin, which transports oxygen around the body.

estrogens Steroid hormones, such as estrone and estradiol, that are produced mainly in the ovaries and control female sexual development.

etiology Study of the cause of disease. Hence, etiologic agent: the specific cause of a disease.

exo- Prefix denoting outside. For example, *exogenous* means "originating outside the organism or body."

exotoxins Soluble toxic proteins, secreted by bacteria, that cause a variety of life-threatening diseases including botulism, gas gangrene, tetanus, and diphtheria. Exotoxins are among the most poisonous substances known.

FAST Fluorescence allergosorbent test. An immunoassay (blood tests) that identifies allergens in which the indicator reagent is a derivative of fluorescein, which emits polarized light.

fat Chemical composed of one or more fatty acids and the principal form in which energy is stored in the body.

GALT Gut-associated lymphoid tissue. Includes the tonsils; areas of the digestive tract known as Peyer's patches; lamina propria of the intestine; and the appendix.

gamma globulin Blood proteins, rich in antibodies, that move in the "gamma" region in electrophoreses. Includes the five classes of *immunoglobulin* found in humans: IgA, IgG, IgM, IgD, and IgE.

globulin Type of protein classified according to its solubility. Globulins (e.g., β-lacto-globulin in milk) are soluble in dilute salt solutions at pH 7.

glucan Polymer (a compound formed by the joining of smaller compunds, usually molecules) of glucose, often formed by the breakdown of sucrose by streptococci, especially *Streptococcus mutans*, in the mouth.

glutenin A protein classified on the basis of its solubility in acids or alkalis, but insoluble in water or ethanol. Glutenins are major proteins in wheat and other cereal grains.

glyco- Prefix denoting the combination of a sugar molecule (often glucose or galactose) with another type of chemical. For example, glycoprotein is a sugar combined with a protein; glycolipid is a sugar combined with a lipid (fat) molecule.

granulocyte White blood cell with a lobed nucleus, characterized by numerous granules within its cytoplasm. See also *polymorphonuclear granulocyte*.

growth hormone (somatotropin) Hormone, secreted by the pituitary gland, that controls growth of the long bones and promotes protein synthesis.

hapten Molecule too small to be an antigen by itself that induces the production of antibody when combined with a protein; e.g., a body protein.

heparin Anticoagulant chemical that inhibits the enzyme thrombin in the final stage of blood coagulation. Various cells, including white blood cells, produce it predominantly in the liver and lungs.

hevamines Hydrolytic enzymes (hydrolases, which split a compound into fragments by the addition of water) with lysozyme activity. In latex, hydrolases tend to be located in lutoids, intracellular organelles thought to be polydispersed vacuoles (chambers distributed throughout plant tissues).

histamine Chemical derivative of the amino acid histidine. It is produced in all body tissues, especially by mast cells. An important mediator (facilitator) of inflammation, it causes contraction of smooth muscle and increases the permeability of small blood vessels. It is the principal mediator of the wheal-and-flare skin reaction of allergy skin tests. See also *wheal-and-flare reaction*.

homologous The same, or "matching." Describes the relationship between an antigen and the specific antibody whose production it induces.

hormone Chemical produced by the body—for example, by the endocrine glands—that circulates in the bloodstream and has a specific regulatory effect on certain cells or organs. Well-known hormones include estrogen, progesterone, testosterone, adrenaline, and growth hormones.

human leukocyte antigens (HLAs) Antigens on the surface of body cells, coded for the major histocompatibility complex (MHC), which is unique to each individual. They allow the immune system to recognize self and non-self.

hydrolase Class of enzymes that catalyze (causes an altering effect on a substance) the addition of the elements of water to a substance, thereby breaking it into two products.

hydrolysis The process by which a molecule is broken apart with the addition of water. The process occurs under the influence of a class of enzymes known as *hydrolases*.

hyper- Prefix indicating excessive, more, or above normal, for example, hyperactivity, hypersensitivity, hyper-responsive, and hypertension (high blood pressure).

hypo- Prefix indicating deficiency, less, or below normal, for example, hyposensitive, hyporeactive, and hypotension (low blood pressure).

IBS Irritable bowel syndrome. A chronic non-inflammatory disease characterized by abdominal pain, altered bowel habits consisting of diarrhea, constipation, or both, with no detectable pathology. Also called spastic bowel or spastic colon.

immunity Resistance to a disease.

immunoassay Blood tests in which the amount of specific parts of the immune system, such as antibodies, are measured.

immunoglobulin (Ig) Glycoprotein that functions as antibody. The five classes (IgA, IgD, IgE, IgG, and IgM) differ in their structures. Immunoglobulins make up gamma globulin; all antibodies are immunoglobulins.

inter- Prefix indicating between, for example, intercellular (between cells).

interferons Cytokines produced by cells infected with viruses. The known interferons (alpha, beta, and gamma) play a variety of roles in immunity, particularly stopping viruses from multiplying (increasing in number).

interleukins Cytokines, produced principally by macrophages and T cells, that act as signals in controlling various stages of the immune response.

intra- Prefix indicating inside, or within, for example, intracellular (inside a cell), intracytoplasmic (within the cytoplasm).

in vitro "In glass." Describes biological activity made to occur outside a living body, usually under experimental conditions in a laboratory.

in vivo "In life." Describes biological activity within a living body.

kd or **kD** Kilodalton: One thousand daltons.

lactoferrin Iron-containing compound, present in secretions such as milk, that has a slight antimicrobial action due to its ability to attach to and remove the iron required by the microorganism.

lactose (milk sugar) A carbohydrate (disaccharide), present in milk, that is broken down by the body into glucose and galactose.

lectins Proteins found primarily in plant seeds, which link to the branching sugar molecules of glycoproteins and glycolipids on the surface of cells. Certain lectins selectively cause clumping together of erythrocytes (red blood cells) of certain blood groups; others stimulate the multiplication of lymphocytes (specific white blood cells).

leukocytes White blood cells that defend the body against disease. Classified into three major types: *granulocytes*, *monocytes*, and *lymphocytes*.

leukotrienes Hormone-like chemicals derived from building blocks of fatty acids, such as arachidonic acid, via the lipoxygenase pathway of enzyme activity. They contribute to inflammatory and allergic reactions as powerful chemotaxins (chemicals that cause movement of cells from one place to another), and some cause constriction of smooth muscle.

lipids Organic substances, including fats, steroids, phospholipids, and glycolipids, that are important as cell constituents and as a source of energy.

lipo- Prefix denoting fat or lipid.

lipopolysaccharide Molecule composed of a fatty acid (lipo-) and a sugar (-polysaccharide), for example, the endotoxin in the cell walls of Gram-negative bacteria that causes the symptoms of many intestinal infections. Endotoxin is the poisonous substance (toxin) incorporated into cellular structures rather than released from a cell (exotoxin).

lymph Transparent fluid in the lymphatic system that bathes body tissues. Similar in composition to blood plasma, but with less protein and some lymphocytes.

lymphatic system Network of vessels that convey *lymph* from body tissues to the bloodstream. Pathway for exchange of electrolytes, water, proteins, and other chemicals between the bloodstream and body tissues.

lymphocytes White blood cells that mature within the lymphatic system. Classified as B and T cells, essential in immunity.

lymphokines Chemicals, produced by *lymphocytes*, that act as control signals between cells of the immune system. Often referred to collectively as *cytokines*.

lymph nodes (glands) Small swellings, distributed in groups over the lymphatic system, that filter lymph and prevent foreign particles from entering the bloodstream. Most noticeable in the groin, armpit, and behind the ear.

lymphoid tissue A latticework of reticular tissue which contains lymphocytes; lymphoid tissue may be diffuse or densely aggregated into lymph nodes and nodules.

lysis Destruction of a cell by disruption of its membrane and outer structures, allowing cell contents to escape.

lysozyme An enzyme that causes the destruction of linkages between molecules; occurs in tears, saliva, egg white, and other tissues and causes destruction of cell walls especially in bacteria.

macrophages Large phagocytes (engulfing cells), closely related to monocytes (special white blood cells), present in many organ systems such as connective tissue, bone marrow, spleen, lymph nodes, liver, and the central nervous system. Fixed macrophages (histiocytes) are stationary; wandering macrophages move freely and collect at the site of infection or trauma, where they remove foreign microorganisms and damaged tissue by a process known as *phagocytosis* (engulfing and breaking down of the foreign matter).

major histocompatibility complex (MHC) Genes located on chromosome 6 and encoded for the human leukocyte antigens (HLAs), present on all body cells, that distinguish self from non-self. Their products are primarily responsible for the rapid rejection of grafts between individuals. The function of the products of the MHC is signaling between lymphocytes and cells that display antigens on the surface.

MALT Mucosa-associated lymphoid tissue. Term for lymphoid tissue associated with any mucous-membrane-lined organs such as the intestinal tract, bronchial tree, and vagina and genital tract.

mast cell Large blood cell, fixed within body tissue and characterized by numerous granules within its cytoplasm. The granules contain chemicals such as histamine, heparin, and enzymes released during an inflammatory or allergic reaction.

metabolic pathway Series of reactions whereby enzymes transform organic molecules into something else along the pathway.

metabolism Sum of the chemical and physical processes by which nutrients are converted into body tissue and energy. Includes catabolism (destruction) and anabolism (construction).

monocytes Single-nucleus, granulocytic white blood cells that phagocytose (engulf and break down) foreign particles such as bacteria, viruses, and dead body cells.

MHC See *major histocompatibility complex.*

mucus Viscous fluid, composed largely of glycoproteins, secreted by mucous membranes lining many body organs, such as the respiratory, gastrointestinal, and urogenital tracts.

natural killer (NK) cell Lymphocyte (white blood cell) that destroys foreign cells, particularly cancer cells, apparently by releasing digestive enzymes that perforate the cells' membranes and cause cell contents to leak out.

neuropeptide Peptide (chain of amino acids) with significant effects on the nervous system, but not, strictly speaking, a neurotransmitter. Neuropeptides include the encephalins, endorphins, somatostatin, substance P, thyrotropin-releasing hormone (TRH), and luteinizing hormone-releasing hormone (LHRH).

neurotoxin Nerve poison, such as botulinum toxin and tetanus toxin, that causes paralysis.

neurotransmitter Complex chemical substance–for example, acetylcholine, norepinephrine, dopamine, serotonin–that transmits signals across the synapses (gaps) between nerve cells and across the minute gaps between nerves and the muscles or glands they control. See also *synapse*.

neutrophil White blood cell containing a lobed nucleus and numerous granules within its cytoplasm that stain with neutral dyes. A powerful phagocyte that removes microorganisms and other foreign particles by engulfing and digesting them.

norepinephrine Hormone produced by the adrenal gland and also released as a neurotransmitter from nerve fibers of the sympathetic nervous system. Its actions include constriction and relaxation of smooth muscles (especially in blood vessels and intestinal walls), regulation of heart rate, and an influence on rate and depth of breathing.

OAS See *oral allergy syndrome*.

opsonins Components of the immune system that aid in the attachment of antigen to the surface of phagocytes (engulfing cells). Opsonins are antibodies and the C3b component of complement. See also *complement*.

opsonization Process by which opsonins aid attachment of antigen to the surface of a phagocyte (engulfing cell).

oral allergy syndrome (OAS) A complex of clinical symptoms (e.g., itching, swelling of lips and tongue, blistering) in the mucous membrane of the mouth and throat that result from direct contact with food allergens in a sensitized person who also has respiratory symptoms in response to inhaled allergens, usually tree, grass, or weed pollens (pollinosis).

ovalbumin A major protein in eggs classified as an albumin (a type of protein) on the basis of its solubility in water at pH 6.6.

parasite Organism that lives in or on another living thing (the host), receiving food and shelter but contributing nothing to its host's welfare and may cause harm. Human parasites include bacteria, viruses, fungi, protozoa, and worms. However, the term is used more specifically in biology, and in this book, to mean organisms other than bacteria, viruses, and fungi. It is used to indicate amoebae, nematode, and helminth worms, and related organisms.

parasympathetic nervous system The part of the *autonomic* (sympathetic) *nervous system* that controls the systems associated with the eyes, the "bulb" that controls respiration and circulation, and functions in the sacral (pelvic) area of the body. See also *autonomic nervous system*.

pathogen Microorganism that causes disease.

pathogenesis-related proteins (PRs) Proteins that are induced by pathogens, wounding, or certain environmental stresses in plants. PRs are presently classified into 14 distinct families of proteins, including chitinases, antifungal proteins, lipid transfer proteins, inhibitors of alpha-amylases and trypsin, profilins, and proteases.

parvalbumin A major protein in fish classified as an albumin (a type of protein) on the basis of its solubility in water at pH 6.6.

peptide Chain of two or more amino acids linked by peptide bonds between the end amino group of one amino acid and the beginning carboxyl group of the next. Peptides joined together form a *protein.*

phagocyte White blood cell that is able to engulf and digest microorganisms, cells, cell debris, and other small particles.

phagocytosis Process of engulfment and digestion of microorganisms and other small foreign particles by white blood cells called *phagocytes.*

placebo A "dummy" medication or nonreactive material that will not cause a response in the body; sometimes called a "sugar pill."

plasma Fluid portion of blood in which blood cells are suspended.

plasma cell Cell, derived from a B-cell lymphocyte that produces antibody.

platelet (thrombocyte) Disc-shaped blood cell principally involved in coagulation.

platelet activating factor (PAF) Phospholipid produced by leukocytes (white blood cells) that causes aggregation of platelets and other effects such as an increase in permeability (ease of movement of contents in and out) of blood vessels and bronchoconstriction (constriction of airways in the lung causing wheezing, as in asthma).

polymorphonuclear granulocyte (polymorph, granulocyte) White blood cell distinguished by a lobed nucleus and fine granules within its cytoplasm. Classified according to the type of stain absorbed by granules.

polysaccharide Carbohydrate composed of monosaccharides (sugar molecules) joined together in chains.

preservative "Antispoilant" added to foods to retain or stop the food from going bad. About 100 preservatives are in common use in food manufacture. The most common food preservatives are benzoates, sulfites, nitrates, and nitrites.

profilins Regulatory proteins in plants, usually associated with reproductive processes; usually present in pollens and may act as allergens in respiratory allergy.

prolactin Hormone secreted by the pituitary gland that stimulates milk production after childbirth and production of progesterone (a hormone) in the ovaries.

prostacyclin Hormone-like chemical related to the *prostaglandins.*

prostaglandins Group of hormone-like chemicals derived from precursor (building blocks) fatty acids, such as arachidonic acid, by the cyclo-oxygenase pathway. They have many important controlling functions in the body, including smooth muscle contraction and relaxation.

prolamin A protein usually found in plants, classified on the basis of its solubility in 70% ethanol. Zein and gliadin are examples of major plant proteins of the prolamin class.

proteins Organic substances, composed of chains of amino acids linked by peptide bonds, that are essential as structural components of body cells and of regulators of function such as enzymes and hormones. Proteins are one of the three main constituents of food.

pruritus Itching.

pyogenic Pus-forming, for example, a pyogenic microorganism causes pus formation in the body at the site of its infection.

pyrogen Substance that produces fever. Examples include the endotoxins of bacteria such as salmonella (causes salmonellosis) and shigella (causes dysentery) in which fever is part of the disease process.

RAST Radio-allergosorbent test. Technique for measuring allergen-specific antibody in serum using reagents labeled with radioactive substances. Usually used to measure allergen-specific IgE or IgG.

receptor Molecule on the surface of a cell that provides a selective attachment site for a particular substance, usually a protein.

reticuloendothelial system (RES) Aggregates of phagocytes (white blood cells such as monocytes and macrophages) spread throughout body tissues.

rhinitis Inflammation of the mucous membrane lining the nose.

rhino- Prefix meaning nose.

rhinorrhea Runny nose with watery discharge characteristic of the common cold.

sensitization Alteration of a body's responsiveness to a foreign substance, usually an allergen. The immune system produces antibody to the allergen without symptoms on first exposure, which is the sensitization event. Subsequent exposure releases more of the antibody and induces an allergic reaction.

serum Fluid portion of blood remaining after separation from clotted blood or clotted blood plasma. Similar to plasma, but lacks fibrinogen and other coagulatory components.

serologic reactions The results from serological tests (e.g., "positive" serologic reaction).

serological tests Immunological techniques to identify antigen-specific antibodies in serum.

serologically related Applied to antigens, the term indicates that antigens have been demonstrated to be related because they react with the same antibody.

serology Study of serum, especially of constituents, such as antibodies and complement, involved in the body's defense against disease.

somatostatin Hormone that inhibits the secretion of growth hormone by the pituitary gland.

stabilizer A substance added to a food product to give it body and to maintain a desired texture or consistency. Chocolate milk requires a stabilizer to keep the particles of chocolate from settling to the bottom of a container.

sympathetic nervous system One of the two divisions of the autonomic nervous system (the other is called *parasympathetic*) that controls the functions of the blood vessels, sweat glands, salivary glands, heart, lungs, intestines, other abdominal organs, and genital organs. Nerve endings of the sympathetic nervous system release the neurotransmitter norepinephrine; the parasympathetic system releases acetylcholine.

sympathomimetic amines Chemicals, including alpha- and beta-adrenergic drugs, that stimulate the sympathetic nervous system.

synapse Conjunction without physical connection (gap) between nerve fibers across which neurotransmitters carry impulses from one nerve cell to the next.

synergism Cooperative interaction between two systems that produces a greater effect than the sum of two systems acting alone. One enhances the effect of the other.

T cells Specialized lymphocytes (white blood cells) that produce lymphokines and participate in all functions of the immune system.

texturizer A chemical used to improve the texture of various foods. Calcium chloride is often added to canned fruits and vegetables to keep them from falling apart in the can after cooking and processing.

thrombocyte See *platelet*.

thrombocytopenia Decrease in the number of thrombocytes (platelets) circulating in the blood.

thromboxane Hormone-like chemical, related to the prostaglandins, produced from fatty acid precursors, such as arachidonic acid, by the cyclo-oxygenase pathway.

thymus Organ at the base of the neck whose principal function appears to be the maturation of lymphocytes (a type of white blood cell) into T-cells.

titer Measure of the amount of antibodies in serum (fluid portion of blood).

urticaria Hives. Itchy rash with round red wheals ranging in size from small spots to large patches several inches in diameter.

vascular Relating to blood vessels.

vascular system Network of blood vessels that circulates blood throughout the body.

vaso- Prefix meaning vessel, especially relating to blood vessels.

vasoactive amine Chemical (amine) that acts on smooth muscle, especially surrounding blood vessels, increasing or decreasing their diameter.

vasoactive peptide Chain of amino acids that together cause a reaction in blood vessels, increasing or decreasing their diameter and affecting their permeability (ease of movement of fluid through the walls).

vasoconstriction Decrease in the diameter of blood vessels, causing an increase in blood pressure, due to contraction of the muscles in their walls.

vasopressin Hormone released by the pituitary gland whose chief function is to increase the reabsorption of water in the kidneys, preventing excessive water loss from the body. Can also cause constriction of blood vessels.

virulence Measure of the disease-producing ability of a microorganism. Includes factors such as the organism's ability to invade the host, to evade the host's immune defenses, and to cause damage to the host's tissues.

wheal-and-flare reaction Skin reaction resulting from introducing an allergen into the skin in an allergy test. The wheal is a raised area in the center of a surrounding red flattened area (the flare). The size of the combined wheal and flare is measured as an assessment of the degree of reactivity to the allergen. The reaction is caused by the release of inflammatory mediators from mast cells in the skin in response to the allergen.

— INDEX —